The LEARN® Program for Weight Control

7th Edition

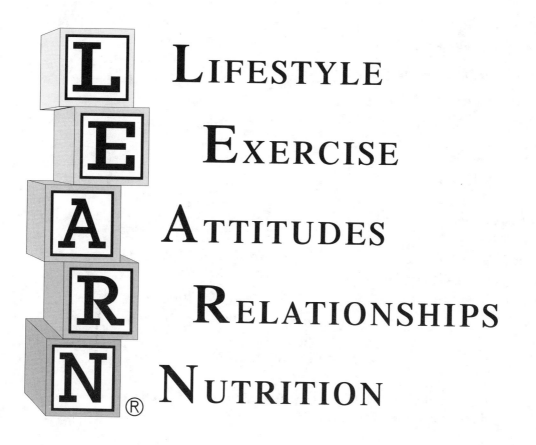

LIFESTYLE

EXERCISE

ATTITUDES

RELATIONSHIPS

NUTRITION

Kelly D. Brownell, Ph.D.
Yale University

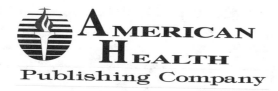

AMERICAN HEALTH Publishing Company

Library of Congress
ISBN   1–878513–13–3

Address orders to:

The LEARN® Education Center

P.O. Box 35328, Department 70

Dallas, Texas 75235–0328

World Wide Web address

E-mail address

In Dallas (817) 545–4500

Toll Free (800) 736–7323

Facsimile (817) 545–2211

www.LearnEducation.com

LearnCTR@aol.com

ACKNOWLEDGMENTS

I am grateful to several trusted colleagues and friends for providing comments and suggestions for this manual. Their help was invaluable. They are:

Dr. Steven N. Blair, Director of Epidemiology, The Cooper Institute for Aerobics Research, Dallas, Texas.

Dr. John P. Foreyt, Professor of Medicine and Director, Behavioral Medicine Research Center, Baylor College of Medicine, Houston, Texas.

Dr. G. Alan Marlatt, Professor of Psychology, University of Washington, Seattle, Washington.

Dr. Sachiko T. St. Jeor, Associate Professor and Director, Nutrition Education and Research Program, Department of Family and Community Medicine, University of Nevada School of Medicine, Reno, Nevada.

Dr. Thomas A. Wadden, Professor, Department of Psychiatry, University of Pennsylvania School of Medicine, Philadelphia, Pennsylvania.

Permission to reprint cartoons was granted by the Cowles Syndicate, Inc., the Universal Press Syndicate, Chronicle Features, King Features, North American Syndicate, Newspaper Enterprise Association, Tribune Media Services, *The Washington Post*, and the United Features Syndicate, Inc.

Finally, I thank my students, colleagues, and especially my clients for providing the challenges and stimulation that encouraged me to undertake this writing.

Table of Contents

When I travel in the U.S. and other countries to lecture, I am often greeted by professionals who use this manual in their work or by individuals who are using the manual to lose weight. Some even ask me to autograph their copy. Not only is this flattering, but it permits me to see how much the book has been used. Some of the manuals have hardly been opened, but in other cases the pages are ragged and bent at the corners, and sentences and paragraphs are underlined or highlighted with colored markers.

I am a great believer in feedback, and I'd very much like yours. If you can suggest changes to improve the program, please let me know. Additions, deletions, alterations—I am open to them all, and I can say with sincerity that this book, now in its seventh edition, has improved dramatically over the years with input from people using it. If you enjoy the book and it helps you, please let me know. It is always gratifying to hear good news. Also, your words may inspire other people, so if you contact me, let me know if I could use what you say (without citing names) in future versions of this book.

To send feedback to me, you may write a letter to my attention to:

American Health Publishing Company
P.O. Box 35328, Department 10
Dallas, Texas 75235–0328
Fax: 817–545–2211
E-mail: AMR Health@aol.com

I read every word.

I hope this manual and you make a nice pair. Bend the pages, underline liberally, and write notes in the margins. If you see yourself doing this, your motivation may be high enough to begin the program. If not, the following information may help you decide whether the time is right.

Is the time right for you?

I know you want to lose weight. You may marvel at my insight; after all, you *are* reading a weight-control guide! But before we begin, let us consider whether the time is right. With some simple guidelines, you can decide whether to move ahead now or to wait for a better time.

Losing weight is much easier than keeping it off. Some people have lost and regained as

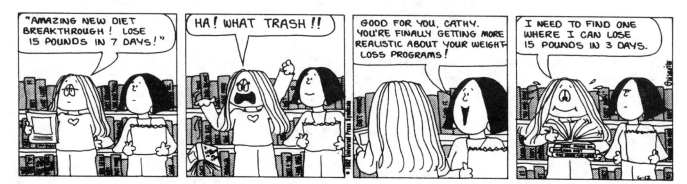

much as 1000 pounds in what nutrition expert Jean Mayer labeled the "rhythm method of girth control." Losing and regaining weight is discouraging, so it is best to begin a program when motivation is high.

The first step is to ask whether you are prepared for the rigors of a weight-loss program. Despite claims from diet books, most people cannot lose 15 pounds without trying, do not get addicted to exercise by buying designer shoes and jogging suits, and do not suddenly yearn for sprouts and tofu when they are used to bacon, pork chops, and hot fudge.

Right now you are probably saying, "Tell me something new!" You *know* that effort is required. Yet, many people start programs when they are only mildly motivated. They may be pressured by family, may be distressed by clothes that don't fit, or may be losing weight to look better for a special event, such as a wedding or reunion. Sometimes these provide sufficient motivation, but not always.

A key decision in any program is deciding whether to begin, but making the decision can be tricky. What follows are guidelines for deciding whether this program will meet your needs.

Weight-loss readiness

For most people who want to lose weight, the main question involves *which* program to follow. There is, however, a fundamental question that precedes this issue. The question is *whether* a person should begin a weight-loss program. With this is mind, I would like to introduce the issue of weight-loss readiness.

What is readiness?

People begin weight-loss programs for many reasons. Some have made an honest assessment of the effort necessary to stay with a program, while others enter expecting a rapid and simple solution. A health scare prompts some people to lose weight, while others may be motivated by family pressure, embarrassment, feeling uncomfortable, or just wanting to look better. These factors converge to form a person's readiness.

Readiness refers to whether you are truly prepared to begin a weight-loss program. It has several components. Among these are how motivated you are, whether the commitment exists to make a sustained effort, whether your life can tolerate the stresses of a program, and whether you can make significant changes in your dietary and activity patterns. It is important that you ask yourself the following question: "Is the time right for me?" You may be ready or you may not.

The consequences of not being ready

Far too often, individuals begin losing weight with a burst of energy that quickly fades. The result is initial weight loss followed by regain. Most overweight people have experienced this and know how unpleasant it can be. It is what some have referred to as "yo-yo dieting" or weight cycling.

The effects of regaining lost weight have not been studied in detail. Professionals must rely, therefore, on experiences with their clients to formulate a picture. It is a picture of discouragement and self-condemnation for failing at yet another attempt to lose weight. This adds to the legacy of failure that plagues so many people.

The feelings can be turned inside and affect mood (e.g., depression and anxiety) and wear away at self-esteem. They can be turned outside, into anger at the program and bitterness at having such a difficult problem. Recent research has also raised the possibility that increased weight variability is associated with negative health effects, such as elevated risk for coronary heart disease. Taken together, these consequences argue for being truly ready before beginning a program.

Assessing readiness

Weight loss can be a difficult and taxing process, and beginning when readiness is high can create an environment in which your success is more likely. It is important, therefore, to know about the concept of readiness and to think clearly about how the concept applies to you.

Assessing readiness can take place in two steps. The first is appreciating the importance

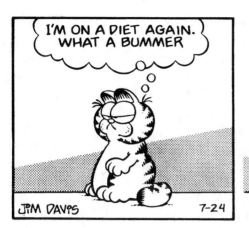
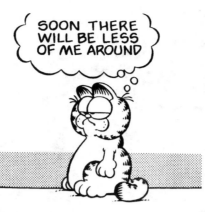
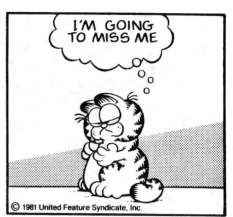

of the concept. You must recognize that beginning when the time is right is an important aspect of success. This is a novel concept to many people, so introducing yourself to the notion of readiness is necessary. It is also important to know that readiness is a fluid, changing condition, so that even if you are not ready at this specific point in time, the right time could arise as time changes. When the conditions are right, this manual can help you.

The second step is in assessing your readiness. For this purpose, I provide at the end of this section, *The Weight-Loss Readiness Test* (see page 9). It has 23 items divided into six sections with a scoring key at the end of each section. The sections deal with goals and attitudes, hunger and eating cues, control over eating, binge eating and purging, emotional eating, and exercise patterns and attitudes.

It is important that I convey to you what the test is and what it is not. I developed the test to pinpoint the areas you should consider when assessing your readiness. The questions were drawn from my experience with many people and from research on predictors of weight loss. The test is still in its early stages of development, so it must be considered an aid, not a fully-developed test.

The test should not be used, therefore, to make specific decisions on enrolling in a program. This is why I did not intend for the test to yield a single summary score for readiness. It can be used to help you think through the readiness concept and to decide how the concept applies to you. *You* are in the best position to make a judgment on readiness.

The weight-loss readiness test categories

The questions in The Weight-Loss Readiness Test are grouped into six categories. The discussion that follows covers the rationale for each section.

Section 1: Goals and Attitudes

The questions in this section are designed to help you evaluate how motivated you are, how long you anticipate the motivation will last (commitment), and whether you can envision a weight-loss program being woven into your lifestyle. In addition, it deals with setting realistic goals. This is relevant because many people have unrealistic expectations about how quickly they will lose weight and how easy the process will be. When the fantasies fail to become reality, you may feel discouraged and may be more likely to relapse.

Section 2: Hunger and Eating Cues

It is common lore that overweight people eat not in response to physical hunger, but rather eat out of habit, eat in response to some psychological need, or eat simply because food is available. This may or may not be true. It is also possible that overweight people experience physical hunger more often, perhaps because they are driven by internal pressures to have more energy.

Science *has* shown that many people, regardless of weight, are responsive to external cues to eat. Seeing a dessert cart after a meal, driving past a bakery, or realizing that it is a regular snack time can make many people

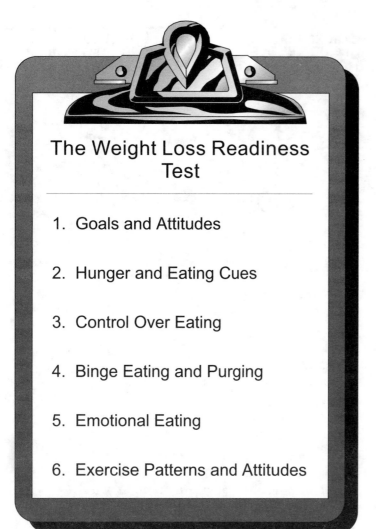

The Weight Loss Readiness Test

1. Goals and Attitudes

2. Hunger and Eating Cues

3. Control Over Eating

4. Binge Eating and Purging

5. Emotional Eating

6. Exercise Patterns and Attitudes

want to eat. This section of the test is designed to help you recognize how responsive you are to cues to eat.

Section 3: Control Over Eating

People vary in how much control they feel they have over eating. Some people exert strict control, while others can be thrown off course by seemingly trivial events. The questions in this section deal with whether external pressures to eat threaten your control.

Section 4: Binge Eating and Purging

Binge eating is a common problem in overweight persons. Research on this topic is relatively new, but what is known suggests that weight loss may be especially difficult when binge eating is hard to control. Purging, which involves the use of vomiting, laxatives, or diuretics to rid the body of weight, is less common, but is a serious matter. Individuals who indicate frequent binge eating and purg-

ing should be evaluated by an eating disorders specialist to determine whether additional help is necessary.

Section 5: Emotional Eating

Emotional upheaval can weaken dietary restraint which, in turn, sets the stage for overeating. This can occur when people are depressed, anxious, angry, or lonely. In some cases, even feeling good or relieved about some aspect of life can lead to overeating. This section of the test is designed to help you identify whether eating occurs in response to emotional changes.

Section 6: Exercise Patterns and Attitudes

As discussed elsewhere in this book, exercise is one of the key components to a comprehensive weight-loss program. People who exercise are most likely to keep off lost weight. This section contains questions about readiness to exercise. Your prediction on the likelihood of regular exercise should be discussed because of its central role in weight control.

A word of caution

I would like to underscore the readiness test should not be used as the only basis for deciding whether to begin a program. You should use it to ask yourself questions about readiness, not to make a final decision. As much information as possible should be gathered so that you can think through issues, such as motivation, commitment, and life circumstances. Then you decide on whether the time is right based on your feelings, attitudes, and behaviors.

Please note also that overall readiness may be a less helpful notion than thinking of readiness in different areas. For instance, most people enter a weight-loss program expecting to change their diet, so the majority would be in a high state of nutrition readiness. People vary more widely in their readiness to be physically active.

Low scores in one area may be a signal to take action to improve readiness in that specific area. A low physical-activity score might be a tip-off to think about obstacles to exercise, either physical or emotional, and then to devise ways to remove the obstacles. I will discuss such obstacles in an upcoming lesson.

Remember that readiness can change, if you take the right steps.

Having you assess your readiness is an important process. Even people who are not highly motivated may do an honest self-assessment and then find ways to motivate themselves. Low readiness is not necessarily permanent. It is a snapshot in time to show whether the conditions are right at this moment. Because you may not be ready at this point does not mean that you will not be ready later.

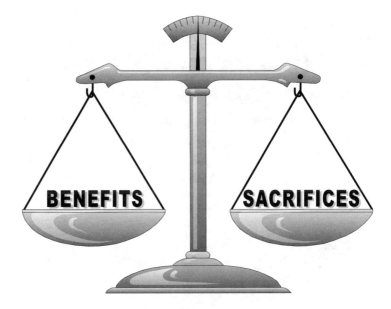

Weighing the benefits and sacrifices

Consider the benefits and sacrifices of starting a weight-loss program. Think of the benefits, such as improved health, better figure, self-confidence, better social life, more energy, attractive clothes, and whatever applies to you. The negative aspects should include *all* the factors like hunger, irritability, explaining your new lifestyle to others, problems eating out, and so forth.

The next page illustrates examples from two individuals contemplating a weight-loss program. Bob wants to lose 40 pounds and is being pressured from his wife to lose weight. Becky has 27 pounds to lose and is fed up with being heavy. She is applying for jobs after taking courses at night and wants to look as good as possible.

Bob and Becky weighed the positives and negatives and came to different conclusions. The positive side of the ledger was stronger for Becky, so she pressed ahead and achieved her goal. Bob was different. He decided against starting a program because it held so many disadvantages for him. He later found himself more motivated and lost his excess weight.

There are two morals from Bob's story. First, deciding not to go on a program is wise in some cases. A person who attempts to lose weight and fails can feel bitter and guilty. The decision to wait until later is not a failure—it may prevent a failure.

There is, however, a second side to Bob's story. People who decide the *time is not right* may be looking for a convenient excuse. They may deny or avoid the realities of their weight problem or may question their ability to succeed. I recommend that such people take a two-week trial of eating less and exercising more as a test of how they will do later. Difficulty may be a sign that starting a program should be set aside and undertaken later. If you do well, your attitude may continue to improve as you lose weight. Consider this two-week trial if you are uncertain about starting.

Fill out the blanks provided in the figure on page 7 to see if the balance of benefits and sacrifices leans in the direction of starting a program.

Your expected weight loss

This program produces average weight losses of 20–30 pounds. This has been documented in a number of studies from our research group and from scientists at other centers. This translates into a one to two pound loss per week for the 12–20 weeks the program is generally used. What does this mean for you?

Averages can be deceiving. If one person loses 50 pounds and another loses none, their average is 25 pounds. Whether the program is a success depends on which person you consider. Some people lose more than the average, and some lose less, but in general, the program aims for steady weight loss that will be maintained.

Bob's List

Benefits	Sacrifices
Stop wife's nagging	Give up favorite food
Look better	Must attend meetings
	Feel deprived
	Embarrassed about diet around my friends
	Fatigue
	Must exercise

Becky's List

Benefits	Sacrifices
More energy	Hard work & sacrifice
Better chance for job	Constant effort
Look better for dating	Must drink less
Wider choice of clothes	with friends
Improve health	

If you have 30 pounds or less to lose, this program provides a good opportunity for you to reach your goal weight. If you have more to lose, you can estimate the 20- to 30-pound loss for the initial program and then can continue to lose by applying the techniques you have learned. If you stop losing before reaching your goal, you may go through the program again or add another approach to take you further.

The best news is about the long-term results. Compared to the very high relapse rates from most programs, the maintenance of weight loss for this program is quite good. Again, some people lose even more after the program while some regain.

These numbers have more meaning when compared to the results of other approaches. Dr. Albert Stunkard, from the University of Pennsylvania, once estimated that fewer than 5 percent of people on weight-loss programs lose more than 40 pounds and keep it off. Many people (as many as 66 percent) who enter the popular commercial and self-help pro-

grams will drop out within six weeks, and techniques like hypnosis, herbal programs, and best-selling diet books are usually of little use. The key to successful weight control, of course, is maintenance. We will be working on maintenance from the first moment you dive into this program. I want to help you develop a mindset of *permanent lifestyle change*, of changing *fundamental behaviors and attitudes* that affect your eating and activity, and of *making changes that become part of the way you live*. Perhaps more than in any other program, methods to maintain weight loss are blended with ways to lose weight initially. Our vision is focused on both immediate and on long-term solutions.

Many programs and books promise quick and easy results, some as great as ten pounds in the first week. Such diets are drastic measures that may imperil your health. The weight losses are more water than fat, because the body rids itself of water when the intake of salt and carbohydrate decreases. This water returns when the rigid diets are abandoned in favor of more normal eating. Losing weight slowly allows your body to adjust to a new weight and will help you look and feel better as you reduce.

The slow and gradual weight loss is not as flashy as fad diets, but may ultimately be more effective. It is physically impossible to lose more than three to four pounds per week, even by fasting, so a one to two pound loss per week is pretty good. Slow and steady are the key words. This represents the most reasonable approach to weight control.

A description of The LEARN Program

I titled this program LEARN for two reasons. The first is that *learning* implies an educational process in which the learner must master crucial information and apply it in everyday life. The second reason is that the word LEARN is an acronym formed from the first letter of the five essential components of the program: **L**ifestyle, **E**xercise, **A**ttitudes, **R**elationships, and **N**utrition.

The program consists of 16 lessons. The five components of the program, Lifestyle, Exercise, Attitudes, Relationships, and Nutrition will be covered throughout the lessons. This is a departure from the usual approach in which each lesson covers only one topic. In the traditional approach, important information is delayed until late in the program. This new approach was born from experience with many clients and from the efforts of fellow scientists and clinicians.

There is a Self-Assessment Questionnaire and a Homework Assignment for each lesson. The Self-Assessment is for you to determine whether you have acquired the important information in each lesson. It will highlight the key points and will alert you to areas that need more detailed work. The homework lessons (the Monitoring Forms) are also serious business. They show you which techniques are working for you and will be a nice reminder of the progress you are making.

You will become a student of your habits. You will learn when, how, and why your habits occur and how to change them. You will

My List

Benefits	Sacrifices

practice your new techniques so they will become part of your lifestyle. We will also deal with the way you think about food, weight, and your body—all central features to long-term weight control. This is what separates the approach of The LEARN Program from most programs—the focus is on *permanent* results.

Two other aspects of the program should be mentioned. First, there are no legal or illegal foods. I resist the idea of dictating what you can and cannot eat. You will not be asked to rid your life of apple pie or faint with envy when your friends dip into the Haagen-Dazs. Likewise, you will not be running to the fruit stand for papaya and mangoes so you can abide by a senseless series of *magic* foods. The program is structured around your lifestyle, not vice-versa.

The second factor is that you can individualize the program to your unique circumstances. The focus is on learning new habits, whatever the necessary habits are for you.

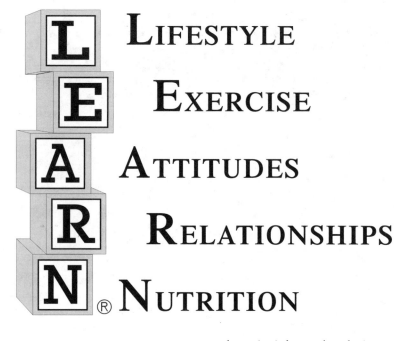

LIFESTYLE

EXERCISE

ATTITUDES

RELATIONSHIPS

NUTRITION

als and nonprofessionals to keep abreast of the latest developments in the field as well as keep up-to-date on the latest methods and techniques that help individuals maintain their weight. A complimentary copy of *The Weight Control Digest*, along with information on other materials, can be obtained by calling or writing to the address shown below.

The LEARN Education Center
P.O. Box 35328, Department 70
Dallas, Texas 75235–0328

Telephone	817–545–4500
Toll Free	800–736–7323
Fax	817–545–2211
E-mail	LearnCTR@aol.com
Web	www.LearnEducation.com

You can weave the principles and techniques of the program into the fabric of *your* life.

Additional materials have been developed which may be helpful to you while working through this program. *The LEARN Program Cassettes* contain four cassette tapes where I discuss the essential elements of The LEARN Program, lesson by lesson. These tapes were developed to help individuals acquire and apply the skills necessary for long-term weight control.

The LEARN Program Monitoring Forms were developed at the request of many people who had completed The LEARN Program. Although I provide you with daily monitoring forms throughout this manual that you may copy, some individuals find it more convenient to have a pocket-sized form that contains a week's supply of food monitoring.

Looking ahead, I want to alert you to *The Weight Maintenance and Stabilization Guide*, an in-depth companion and follow-up to The LEARN Program. After losing weight, a looming issue is how to make the changes permanent over time. There is a great deal of information on this in *The LEARN Program*, but more help is available for the long-term process of losing more weight, maintaining the loss, and stabilizing how you feel, how you think, and how you act in order to make your changes permanent.

And finally, *The Weight Control Digest* was developed as a newsletter for both profession-

So, without further delay, let's move on!

The Weight-Loss Readiness Test

Answer the questions below to see how well your attitudes equip you for a weight-loss program. For each question, circle the answer that best describes your attitude, then write the number of your answer on the line before each question number. As you complete each of the six sections, add the numbers of your answers and compare them with the scoring guide at the end of each section.

Section 1: Goals and Attitudes

____1.	Compared to previous attempts, how motivated are you to lose weight at this time?

   1   Not at all motivated

   2   Slightly motivated

   3   Somewhat motivated

   4   Quite motivated

   5   Extremely motivated

____2.	How certain are you that you will stay committed to a weight-loss program for the time it will take to reach your goal?

   1   Not at all certain

   2   Slightly certain

   3   Somewhat certain

   4   Quite certain

   5   Extremely certain

____3.	Consider all outside factors at this time in your life (the stress you're feeling at work, your family obligations, etc.). To what extent can you tolerate the effort required to stick to a program?

   1   Cannot tolerate

   2   Can tolerate

   3   Uncertain

   4   Can tolerate well

   5   Can tolerate easily

____4.	Think honestly about how much weight you hope to lose and how quickly you hope to lose it. Figuring a weight loss of one to two pounds per week, how realistic is your expectation?

   1   Very unrealistic

   2   Somewhat unrealistic

   3   Moderately unrealistic

   4   Somewhat realistic

   5   Very realistic

____5.	While losing weight, do you fantasize about eating a lot of your favorite foods?

   1   Always

   2   Frequently

   3   Occasionally

   4   Rarely

   5   Never

____6.	While losing weight, do you feel deprived, angry and/or upset?

   1   Always

   2   Frequently

   3   Occasionally

   4   Rarely

   5   Never

_____	**Section 1—TOTAL Score**

If you scored:

6 to 16:	This may not be a good time for you to start a weight-loss program. Inadequate motivation and commitment, together with unrealistic goals could block your progress. Think about those things that contribute to this, and consider changing them before undertaking a program.

17 to 23:	You may be close to being ready to begin a program but should think about ways to boost your readiness before you begin.

24 to 30:	The path is clear with respect to goals and attitudes.

Section 2: Hunger and Eating Cues

____7.	When food comes up in conversation or in something you read, do you want to eat even if you are not hungry?

   1   Never

   2   Rarely

   3   Occasionally

   4   Frequently

   5   Always

____8.	How often do you eat because of **physical hunger**?

   1   Always

   2   Frequently

   3   Occasionally

   4   Rarely

   5   Never

___9. Do you have trouble controlling your eating when your favorite foods are around the house?

1 Never
2 Rarely
3 Occasionally
4 Frequently
5 Always

_____ **Section 2—TOTAL Score**

If you scored:

3 to 6: You might occasionally eat more than you would like, but it does not appear to be a result of high responsiveness to external cues. Controlling the attitudes that make you eat may be especially helpful.

7 to 9: You may have a moderate tendency to eat just because food is available. Weight loss may be easier for you if you try to resist external cues, and eat only when you are physically hungry.

10 to 15: Some or most of your eating may be in response to thinking about food or exposing yourself to temptations to eat. Think of ways to minimize your exposure to temptations, so that you eat only in response to physical hunger.

Section 3: Control Over Eating

If the following situations occurred while you were on a weight-loss program, would you be likely to eat **more** or **less** immediately afterward and for the rest of the day?

___10. Although you planned on skipping lunch, a friend talks you into going out for a meal.

1 Would eat much less
2 Would eat somewhat less
3 Would make no difference
4 Would eat somewhat more
5 Would eat much more

___11. You "break" your diet by eating a fattening, "forbidden" food.

1 Would eat much less
2 Would eat somewhat less
3 Would make no difference
4 Would eat somewhat more
5 Would eat much more

___12. You have been following your diet faithfully and decide to test yourself by eating something you consider a treat.

1 Would eat much less
2 Would eat somewhat less
3 Would make no difference
4 Would eat somewhat more
5 Would eat much more

_____ **Section 3—TOTAL Score**

If you scored:

3 to 7: You recover rapidly from mistakes. However, if you frequently alternate between eating out of control and dieting very strictly, you may have a serious eating problem and should get professional help.

8 to 11: You do not seem to let unplanned eating disrupt your program. This is a flexible, balanced approach.

12 to 15: You may be prone to overeat after an event breaks your control or throws you off the track. Your reaction to these eating events can be improved.

Section 4: Binge Eating and Purging

___13. Aside from holiday feasts, have you ever eaten a large amount of food rapidly and felt afterward that this eating incident was excessive and out of control?

2 Yes
0 No

___14. If you answered yes to question 13 above, how often have you engaged in this behavior during the last year?

1 Less than once a month
2 About once a month
3 A few times a month
4 About once a week
5 About three times a week
6 Daily

___15. Have you ever purged (used laxatives, diuretics or induced vomiting) to control your weight?

5 Yes
0 No

___16. If you answered yes to question 15 above, how often have you engaged in this behavior during the last year?

1 Less than once a month
2 About once a month
3 A few times a month
4 About once a week
5 About three times a week
6 Daily

_____ **Section 4—TOTAL Score**

If you scored:

0 to 1: It appears that binge eating and purging is not a problem for you.

2 to 11: Pay attention to these eating patterns. Should they arise more frequently, get professional help.

12 to 19: You show signs of having a potentially serious eating problem. See a counselor experienced in evaluating eating disorders right away.

Section 5: Emotional Eating

___17. Do you eat more than you would like to when you have negative feelings, such as anxiety, depression, anger, or loneliness?

1 Never
2 Rarely
3 Occasionally
4 Frequently
5 Always

___18. Do you have trouble controlling your eating when you have positive feelings—do you celebrate feeling good by eating?

1 Never
2 Rarely
3 Occasionally
4 Frequently
5 Always

___19. When you have unpleasant interactions with others in your life, or after a difficult day at work, do you eat more than you would like?

1 Never
2 Rarely
3 Occasionally
4 Frequently
5 Always

_____ **Section 5—TOTAL Score**

If you scored:

3 to 8: You do not appear to let your emotions affect your eating.

9 to 11: You sometimes eat in response to emotional highs and lows. Monitor this behavior to learn when and why it occurs, and be prepared to find alternative activities.

12 to 15: Emotional ups and downs can stimulate your eating. Try to deal with the feelings that trigger the eating, and find other ways to express them.

Section 6: Exercise Patterns and Attitudes

___20. How often do you exercise?

1 Never
2 Rarely
3 Occasionally
4 Frequently
5 Always

___21. How confident are you that you can exercise regularly?

1 Not at all confident
2 Slightly confident
3 Somewhat confident
4 Quite confident
5 Extremely confident

___22. When you think about exercise, do you develop a positive or negative picture in your mind?

1 Completely negative
2 Somewhat negative
3 Neutral
4 Somewhat positive
5 Completely positive

___23. How certain are you that you can work regular exercise into your daily schedule?

1 Not at all certain
2 Slightly certain
3 Somewhat certain
4 Quite certain
5 Extremely certain

_____ **Section 6—TOTAL Score**

If you scored:

4 to 10: You are probably not exercising as regularly as you should. Determine whether your attitudes about exercise are blocking your way, then change what you must and put on those walking shoes.

11 to 16: You need to feel more positive about exercise so you can do it more often. Think of ways to be more active that are fun and fit into your lifestyle.

17 to 20: It looks like the path is clear for you to be active. Now think of ways to get motivated.

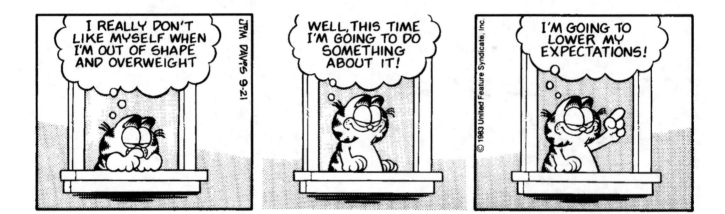

Today you begin The LEARN Program. It contains the best of what science and clinical practice have to offer. In writing this manual, my intention is for us to form a partnership. Together we can make it work.

When you lose weight on this program, only one person deserves credit. I would be happy to claim credit, but I deserve no more than Rand McNally does when you use their Atlas to drive from one city to the next. The Atlas supplies the possible routes, and may even suggest the best, but you choose the route and you determine whether you reach your destination. Most important, you do the driving. With that in mind, let's go!

The LEARN approach

The word "LEARN" represents the five components of this program: Lifestyle, Exercise, Attitudes, Relationships, and Nutrition. The lessons in this program contain information in each area. In some weeks the information in one area is particularly important, so it will receive the greatest emphasis.

Because we are partners in The LEARN Program, your role will be an active one. There will be forms and homework assignments. Upcoming weeks will be filled with experimentation because you will be trying many new approaches to eating and physical activity. It will be both exciting and challenging.

In some cases, this manual will be used in conjunction with classes or with some degree of professional contact. Be advised that such meetings do not replace the manual. Group sessions simply cannot cover the details of a program like a manual can. The manual permits you to examine the information at *your* pace and at a time when *you* can pay attention. Also, you can refer back to the manual at different points in the program. Remember to read the manual each week, and use it as a reference after the program ends.

Diet vs. lifestyle change

This program is not a diet. It is a system for lifestyle change. This is more than just a matter of words—it is a fundamental difference in philosophy that affects nearly every aspect of the LEARN approach.

The word *diet* conjures up a number of images. It implies deprivation and suffering, but most of all, it is something that you go on or off. Whether someone is "on a diet" or "off their diet" is part of modern language. This is a problem, of course, because changing habits is not

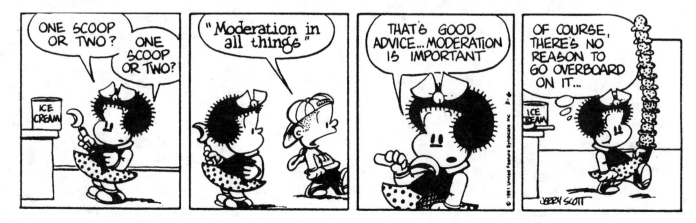

something that happens while a person is *on* a diet and then stops later when the diet ends. This implies a temporary solution, a quick-patch job that only requires minor effort over the short-term.

We are seeking a permanent solution. Instead of a quick but temporary solution, we want a reorientation of lifestyle. This involves establishing new habits and working hard to make these part of day-to-day life. Most people who struggle with weight have a chronic problem. Chronic problems require attention over the long-term.

Think for a moment of this difference between going on a diet and changing your lifestyle. The lifestyle approach, which emphasizes gradual, sustainable, and permanent changes in eating, exercise, thinking, and feeling, is the hallmark of this program.

Building skills and confidence

Albert Bandura, a highly respected psychologist at Stanford University, developed a concept known as self-efficacy. The concept states that an individual's chance of accomplishing some goal depends on having the skills to make the change and the confidence that the change can occur. The concept applies beautifully to weight control.

Skills are what this program is all about. You will be exposed to many approaches. You'll take each for a test drive and will find the ones that work best for you. The skills will deal with what you eat, whether you are active, and perhaps most importantly, the thoughts, feelings, and attitudes you have about many important factors. Thinking helpful thoughts, and looking at the world in a constructive way, involves skills that you can cultivate.

Confidence is the second part of the picture. If you are confident that you can handle high-risk situations, that you can bounce back when you falter, and that you can keep your motivation high, you'll have the strength to hang in there when things get tough. You'll approach situations with a new sense of control. We will be speaking many times about confidence.

Awareness is a key step to changing habits. Keeping records is a key to becoming aware of your habits.

Sometimes these discussions of confidence will sound like a pep talk, but pep talks can be pretty helpful. One of the most important things you can do is to hold your own internal pep talks. What you say when you do well, when you do not do well, or when you are pondering how best to proceed will be central to your success. You may be surprised by how often we will discuss the discussions you have with yourself.

Record keeping

Its purpose and importance

The first, and perhaps most important lifestyle behavior you will learn is to keep records. You will be keeping records of your eating, exercise, and weight. You will have more records than an accountant! Don't worry, there is a good reason for this.

This lesson introduces two records. The first is the Food Diary, which is a daily record of the food you eat. The second is the Weight Change Record, which is a weekly graph of your weight. Both will increase your awareness of eating and its effects on your weight.

Awareness is a key step in changing habits. You may already know a great deal about your habits and your weight patterns, particularly if you have kept records for an earlier program. You will be surprised by how much more there is to learn. The awareness you gain from record keeping has several benefits. These will become clear within a few weeks.

- **You learn about calories.** There are calories lurking where you least suspect. Do you think yogurt is a good diet food? One cup of fruit yogurt can have more calories than an ice cream cone. Ten innocent potato chips contain 110 calories, more than five cups of plain popcorn. Becoming a calorie expert insures you won't be derailed by calorie surprises.

- **You are aware of what you eat.** You might be thinking, "Of course I know what I eat." However, one does not always recall the exact number of Doritos consumed at happy hour or the ounces of milk poured into the bowl of Whea-

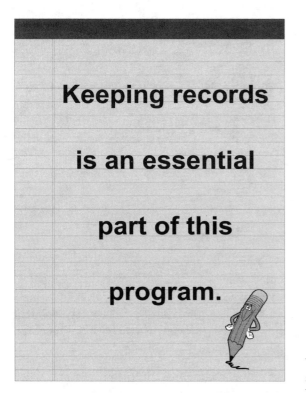

Keeping records is an essential part of this program.

ties. These are *forgotten* calories, sometimes because we like to forget them!

- **You increase control over eating.** Knowing exactly where you stand with the day's calorie count permits you to judge whether you can afford certain foods. You may have the calories *banked* to have that snack you are considering. Knowing where you stand makes the choice easier.

- **Eating patterns become clear.** You may discover that most of your eating is done between dinner and bedtime. Another person might eat throughout the day. Some people eat when they have certain feelings (anger, anxiety, etc.), and others find they eat when doing something else (watching TV). Knowing your patterns is a big help in changing habits.

- **The records help you *bank* calories.** Your body is like a bank account in which you make calorie deposits and withdrawals. If you eat less, you have some calories to bank for a special occasion. If you have a party to attend on the weekend, you can cut back during the week and can afford to indulge with some special dessert. Calorie records

give you the information to make such a decision.

- **The weight change record prevents despair.** There may be one or more weeks when you fail to lose weight, or even worse, gain weight! There are many reasons for this, as I will discuss later. Such a discouraging bout with the scale can make life difficult. This despair can be prevented by reviewing your change in weight over many weeks. A slight gain is easier to tolerate when you are reminded by your records that you have been losing weight in a steady manner.

The Food Diary

The Food Diary is your holy book during this program. You will use it to record amounts and calories of the foods you eat. You may resist this part of the program. It will be hard initially to record everything you eat and to estimate calories. When it becomes easy, you may find it repetitive. It is important to conquer this resistance and keep the records. Research has shown this to be one of the most, if not *the* most important part of habit change.

A blank Food Diary is provided on page 22, along with a sample that has a typical person's eating filled in (page 21). Make photocopies of the blank Food Diary and use it for your own. Here are the instructions for completing the Diary:

- **Record everything, forget nothing.** Every morsel of food goes in the Diary. If you eat pretzels, count how many. Every ounce of food or beverage must be entered. Don't forget when you taste foods you are preparing.

- **Record the food, the amount, the calories.** Record the type of food you eat, how it is prepared (baked, fried, etc.), how much, and the number of calories.

- **Record immediately after eating.** Do not wait until you are ready for bed, until the next morning, or worst of all, until right before your group session! It is hard to remember how many peanuts you ate at the cocktail party or how much juice you had for breakfast. As soon as you finish eating, whip out the Food Diary and make your entries. If you are with others and are embarrassed, excuse yourself and find a private place, like a phone booth. If Clark Kent can do it, so can you!

◆ **Carry the Food Diary always.** There is food everywhere waiting to leap into your mouth. Keep your Food Diary with you (except when swimming or in the shower) so you won't be caught unaware. Some people use a pocket notebook during the day and then transfer the information to their Food Diary later.

Using the calorie guide

You will need a calorie guide to estimate the calories in foods. The Calorie Guide for The LEARN Program appears at the end of this manual (Appendix F). In previous versions of this manual, I recommended that people purchase calorie guides at a bookstore, but I was convinced by my clients to develop an *official* guide. As you know, many calorie books are available, and they do not always agree. Feel free to use another guide if you wish, but first check it for accuracy against the guide given here.

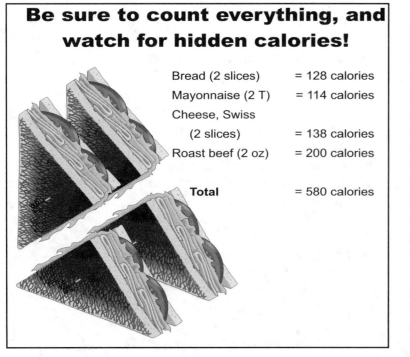

Be sure to count everything, and watch for hidden calories!

Bread (2 slices)	= 128 calories
Mayonnaise (2 T)	= 114 calories
Cheese, Swiss	
(2 slices)	= 138 calories
Roast beef (2 oz)	= 200 calories
Total	= 580 calories

Record EVERYTHING that you eat.

You will have to do some arithmetic to calculate calories. The guide may list one pat of margarine at 36 calories. If you have two pats on a roll, the contribution from margarine will be 72 (36 x 2) calories. If you have only half the pat, mark down 18 calories.

Your judgment is important when estimating calories because a calorie guide provides only estimates and may not apply to the food you are actually eating. For instance, a calorie guide may show that a roast beef sandwich has 347 calories. This refers to a regular sandwich with about two ounces of meat with no mustard, mayonnaise, or whatever else you use. If you get a deli sandwich with two inches (rather than two ounces) of roast beef, the calories could be three or four times what the guide lists.

The challenge is to estimate the *portion sizes* and *composition* of the foods you eat. This can be difficult, especially when you eat out. At home, the job can be simplified by using a food scale. Many people feel they do not need a scale, especially the veterans of weight-loss programs who have been keeping calorie records for years. My colleagues and I did a study on this by having individuals in our program estimate the quantities and calories in common foods and beverages, such as milk, green beans, meat, and soda. Some estimated high and some low, but the average error was 60 percent! Food scales are widely available and are not expensive.

It is also important to find the hidden calories in foods. Examples are butter on vegetables, whipped cream on desserts, dressings on salad, and sugar used as a sweetener. Be painfully honest since these are sources of extra pounds. Did you know that one extra pat of margarine per day, which has only 36 calories, can add up to four pounds of weight in one year?

As you progress through the program, you will be able to estimate food portions, the composition of foods, and calories more easily and accurately. The Food Diaries will be easier to keep and the exact calories will become less important.

The weight change record

The Weight Change Record is a weekly graph of changes in your weight. Once each week, record the date and your weight change from the previous week. A sample is given below.

Keeping the Weight Change Record has several advantages. First, it is a reminder of how you are faring with the program. Second, it shows the relationship between your eating and your weight. You can make a rough estimate of how many calories you need to lose weight by taking the average daily calorie values from several weeks of your Food Diary and checking weight changes from your Weight Change Record. Third, the graph puts your weight change in perspective. If you gain a pound during your eighth week, you can take heart from the steady loss in earlier weeks.

You will notice that the Weight Change Record is a graph of change, not of weight per se. This is done so people can place the graph in a public spot, like on the refrigerator door, if they wish. Your weight does not appear on the graph, just your progress. Many people like to have the graph posted in a place where they see it frequently, so it can act as a source of encouragement. The sample here shows how this could happen.

On the sample graph provided here, you will see a straight line. This represents what weight would look like if a person lost exactly the same amount of weight each week. Of course, life does not occur in a straight line. The *realistic* line on the graph shows some weeks where weight stays stable and even weeks when weight increases.

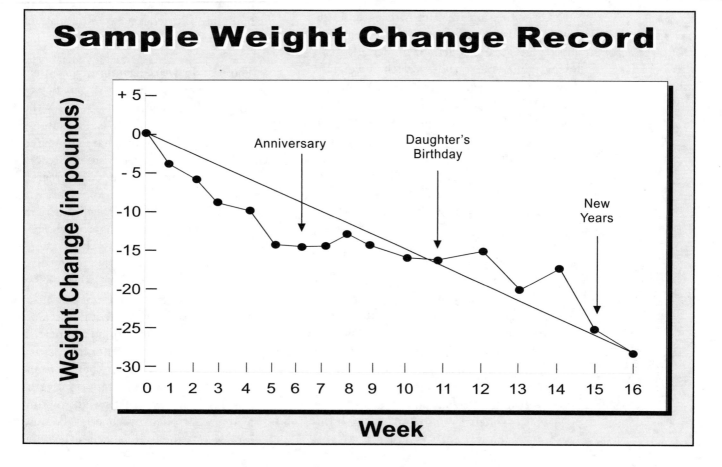

You should know right now that there may be weeks when your graph looks more like the realistic line than the straight line. What matters in a given week is where you are compared to where you started, not what you weighed the week before. Gaining a pound is a small setback in the scheme of your total program, but your *reaction* to the pound can be devastating. Therefore, think of this sample graph often, and remember that you are a real person and that the realistic line may best reflect your experience.

Reasons for overweight

Why people are overweight is still somewhat of a mystery, even though scientists from many countries have been working on the problem for years. Exciting discoveries occur frequently, yet there is still a long road to travel before we can unravel the complex causes and consequences of weight problems. In the meantime, it is helpful to examine the popular reasons people use to explain overweight.

I cover this information here because the reasons we use to explain weight problems create attitudes that can help or hinder efforts to lose weight. A person who feels their weight is determined by genetics may be discouraged from attempting to lose weight. The information that follows may counter some misconceptions.

- ◆ **Glands.** This is a popular reason given by heavy people. Many of my clients feel they have an underactive thyroid. The truth is, most overweight people have no gland problems, or if they do, the problems are not serious enough to account for much of their excess weight. If you suspect gland problems, do not hesitate to see your doctor, but remember that fewer than five percent of overweight persons have these difficulties.

- ◆ **Metabolism.** The issue of metabolism will be covered later in our discussion of exercise. Metabolic rate, which is the energy (calories) your body uses for living, varies widely among people. This influences the way they gain or lose weight.

Some women will lose weight rapidly on 1600 calories per day while there are rare individuals who lose very slowly on 800 per day. These people are cursed by a *thrifty* metabolism that conserves energy and promotes weight gain. Determining your exact metabolic needs is more costly than it is worth, because you approach weight loss in the same way regardless of metabolism. If you have a thrifty metabolism, exercise is especially important.

- ◆ **Genetics.** Overweight runs in families. A child with no overweight parents has less than a 20 percent chance of being overweight. If one parent is overweight, the chances increase to 40 percent. With two overweight parents, the odds are 80 percent. This could, of course, reflect the tendency of families to pass along their eating and exercise habits to children.

We have known for years that animals can be bred to be fat. The meat you buy at the supermarket comes from an animal bred to have a certain percentage of body fat. But what do we know about humans?

The past 15 years have brought an explosion of research on the genetics of body weight regulation. Among the ways to study genetics is to examine identical twins. Studies have compared body weights in twins who are reared together to weights in twins reared apart. If genetics is important, we would expect the weights within twin pairs to be similar regardless of whether they were reared together. If the twins reared apart are more dissimilar than twins reared together, the environment would seem to exert an important influence. The studies show that the similarity in body weights within twin pairs is nearly the same whether twins are reared apart or reared together. This indicates that genetics are important. Yet, this does not mean that weight is completely controlled by genetics, because how we eat and exercise will determine whether our genetic predisposition to be heavy or thin is expressed.

One virtue of this research is that it relieves some of the blame people place on themselves for being overweight. One danger is that people overstate the importance of genetics and come to feel they are destined to be heavy and there is nothing to be done.

- **Fat Cells.** The body accumulates and stores fat in fat cells, also called adipose tissue. Some people have too many fat cells (hyperplastic obesity) while others have the normal number but their fat cells are too large (hypertrophic obesity). Still others have both types. People who were overweight in childhood or are very heavy tend to have excessive numbers of fat cells as well as enlarged cells. Early researchers in this area speculated that people with too many fat cells would have difficulty losing weight. This has not been tested sufficiently to know whether it is true.

- **Family Upbringing.** Some families foster overeating for emotional or even cultural reasons. Some people may eat for psychological reasons related to family upbringing. A program aimed at behavior change is the right approach for these people because it helps to separate emotions from eating and helps to identify other sources of gratification.

- **Psychological Factors.** Many overweight people have trouble controlling their eating in response to stress, depression, loneliness, anger, and other emotions. Does this mean that being overweight is a symptom of deep psychological distress? If so, the remedy would be to root out the underlying psychological problems in hopes that the symptom (overeating) would disappear.

This theory rings true intuitively for many people, but does not have much support among experts. Many normal weight persons have psychological problems but cope without overeating. In people who undergo intensive psychotherapy, weight problems generally

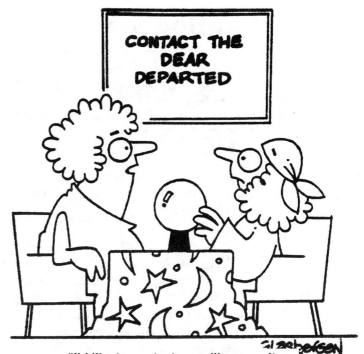

"I'd like to contact my willpower. It died last night at Angelo's Pizza Palace!"

remain after the psychological difficulties have been resolved. If you feel that psychological problems are at the root of your weight problem, deal with either the weight (through this program) or the psychological problems (with therapy). Do not labor under the notion that the psychological problems must be remedied before you can lose weight.

When all is said and done, and all the reasons for overweight are debated, the fact remains that people gain weight because they consume more calories than their bodies use. Becoming overweight is usually a gradual process and may result from small errors in what we eat. One business executive gained five pounds each year for 20 years. He did not notice the five pounds each year, but he was unhappy with the total of 100 pounds. This could have occurred from nothing more than two to three drinks per week. The solution to such a problem is gradual change in eating habits so that long-term weight loss can occur.

Rating your diet

Nutrition is one key to successful weight control. What you eat affects how you feel, whether you are healthy, and how you look. A great deal of information on nutrition awaits you in this program. To start the process, let's evaluate your diet.

I have provided on page 24 the "Rate Your Diet Quiz" developed by the Center for Science in the Public Interest and published in the *Nutrition Action Healthletter*. Take a few minutes to complete the quiz and to score your answers. You have probably changed your diet since beginning the program. Complete the quiz as you would have *before starting the program*, so you will see how you would score ordinarily. Then, toward the end of this program, you can take the quiz again to see how your eating habits have changed.

Better diets will receive higher scores on this quiz. You will see which choices for each question contribute to or subtract from the total score. Taking the quiz can be educational because it may help provide new ideas for healthy food choices.

A note about exercise and relationships

The emphasis this week is on lifestyle (record keeping), attitudes (causes for overweight), and nutrition. Exercise and relationships will be covered in detail later. They will receive much attention as we progress through The LEARN Program.

Your self-assessment

After each lesson there will be a Self-Assessment Questionnaire. This will be a simple true-false quiz to help you determine whether you have learned the important points of the lesson. If you answer all the questions correctly, you can boast about being a weight-loss whiz! When you answer a question incorrectly, check the material in the lesson.

Assignment for this lesson

The object this week is not to start a diet but to learn about your eating and weight habits from the Food Diary and the Weight Change Record. Specific calorie levels will be described in Lesson Two. Your assignment for this week is to make copies of the Food Diary provided here, fill one out for each day of the week, and to begin your Weight Change Record. Pocket-sized copies of the LEARN Food Diary Forms (enough for the entire program) can be ordered by calling 1-800-736-7323.

Completing these forms is *critical*, for three reasons. First, it is a good test of your motivation. Difficulty in keeping the records may reflect inadequate motivation. If this is the case, you might start the program later when motivation is higher. Second, the information will teach you about your habits. Third, the information will be valuable to a group leader or professional who may be working with you.

Self-assessment questionnaire

Lesson One
(Circle either T for true or F for false.)

T F 1. Discovering the psychological roots of your weight problem is the most important factor in weight reduction.

T F 2. All overweight people have an excessive number of fat cells.

T F 3. There is no such thing as a slow or underactive metabolism.

T F 4. Very few people can accurately estimate the quantity and calories of foods.

T F 5. Record keeping may be the most important aspect of a weight-loss program.

(Answers in Appendix C)

Food Diary—Lesson One *(sample)*

Today's Date_____

Description	Calories
Breakfast	
Orange juice, ½ cup	60
Cheerios, 1 cup	89
Skim milk, 1 cup	86
White toast, dry, 1 slice	64
Total calories from this meal	299
Lunch	
Apple, 1 medium	81
Vegetable soup, 2 cups	144
Chicken salad sandwich, 2 oz, with 2 T mayonnaise	332
Ritz crackers, 5	70
Diet Pepsi, 12 oz	1
Total calories from this meal	628
Dinner	
Sirloin steak, lean, 3.5 oz	208
Green beans, 1 cup	26
Cauliflower, 2 cups	60
Wheat bread, 1 slice	61
Apple pie, 1 slice (1/6 of pie)—water to drink	231
Total calories from this meal	586
Snacks	
Yogurt, low-fat, 8 oz	144
Total calories from snacks	144
Total calories for the day	1,657

Food Diary—Lesson One

Today's Date _____

Description	Calories
Breakfast	
Total calories from this meal	
Lunch	
Total calories from this meal	
Dinner	
Total calories from this meal	
Snacks	
Total calories from snacks	
Total calories for the day	

My Weight Change Record

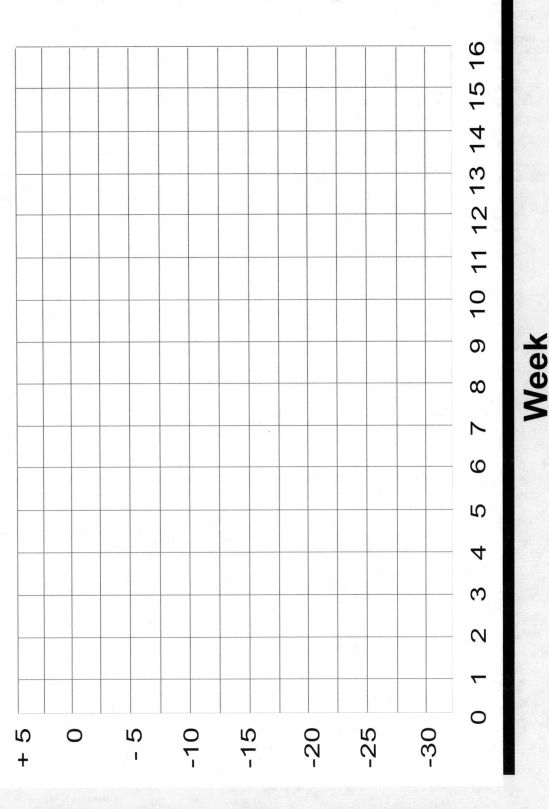

Weight Change (in pounds)

+5
0
-5
-10
-15
-20
-25
-30

0 1 2 3 4 5 6 7 8 9 10 11 12 13 14 15 16

Week

Rate Your Diet Quiz

The following questions will give you a rough sketch of your typical eating habits. The (+) or (-) number for each answer instantly pats you on the back for good eating habits or alerts you to problems you didn't even know you had. The quiz focuses on fat, saturated fat, cholesterol, sodium, sugar, fiber, and fruits and vegetables. It doesn't attempt to cover everything in your diet. Also, it doesn't try to measure precisely how much of the key nutrients you eat.

Next to each answer is a number with a + or - sign in front of it. Circle the number that corresponds to the answer you choose and write that score (e.g., +1) in the space provided in front of each question. That's your score for the question. If two or more answers apply, circle each one. Then average them to get your score for the question.

How to average. In answering question 19, for example, if your sandwich-eating is equally divided among tuna salad (-2), roast beef (+1), and turkey breast (+3), add the three scores (which gives you +2) and then divide by three. That gives you a score of +⅔ for the question. Round it to +1.

Pay attention to serving sizes, which are given when needed. For example, a serving of vegetables is ½ cup. If you usually eat one cup of vegetables at a time, count it as two servings. If you're ready, let's start.

Fruits, Vegetables, Grains, and Beans

____ 1. How many servings of fruit or 100% fruit juice do you eat per day? (*OMIT fruit snacks like Fruit Roll-Ups and fruit-on-the-bottom yogurt. One serving = one piece or ½ cup of fruit or 6 oz of fruit juice.*)
- -3 None
- -2 Less than 1 serving
- 0 1 serving
- +1 2 serving
- +2 3 serving
- +3 4 or more servings

____ 2. How many servings of non-fried vegetables do you eat per day? (*One serving = ½ cup. Include potatoes.*)
- -3 None
- -2 Less than 1 serving
- 0 1 serving
- +1 2 serving
- +2 3 serving
- +3 4 or more servings

____ 3. How many servings of vitamin-rich vegetables do you eat per week? (*One serving = ½ cup. Only count broccoli, Brussels sprouts, carrots, collards, kale, red pepper, spinach, sweet potatoes, or winter squash.*)
- -3 None
- +1 1 to 3 servings
- +2 4 to 6 servings
- +3 7 or more servings

____ 4. How many servings of leafy green vegetables do you eat per week? (*One serving = ½ cup cooked or 1 cup raw. Only count collards, kale, mustard greens, romaine lettuce, spinach, or Swiss chard.*)
- -3 None
- -2 Less than 1 serving
- +1 1 to 2 servings
- +2 3 to 4 servings
- +3 5 or more servings

____ 5. How many times per week does your lunch or dinner contain grains, vegetables, or beans, but little or no meat, poultry, fish, eggs, or cheese?
- -1 None
- +1 1 to 2 times
- +2 3 to 4 times
- +3 5 or more times

____ 6. How many times per week do you eat beans, split peas, or lentils? (*Omit green beans.*)
- -3 None
- -1 Less than 1 time
- 0 1 times
- +1 2 times
- +2 3 times
- +3 4 or more times

____ 7. How many servings of grains do you eat per day? (*One serving = 1 slice of bread, 1 oz of crackers, 1 large pancake, 1 cup pasta or cold cereal, or ½ cup granola, cooked cereal, rice, or bulgur. Omit heavily sweetened cold cereals.*)
- -3 None
- 0 1 to 2 servings
- +1 3 to 4 servings
- +2 5 to 7 servings
- +3 8 or more servings

____ 8. What type of bread, rolls, etc., do you eat?
- +3 100% whole wheat as the only flour
- +2 Whole-wheat flour as 1st or 2nd flour
- +1 Rye, pumpernickel, or oatmeal
- 0 White, French, or Italian

____ 9. What kind of breakfast do you eat?
- +3 Whole-grain (like oatmeal or Wheaties)
- 0 Low-fiber (like Cream of Wheat or Corn Flakes)
- -1 Sugary low-fibe (like Frosted Flakes or low-fat granola)
- -2 Regular granola

Meat, Poultry, and Seafood

___ 10. How many times per week do you eat high-fat red meats *(hamburgers, pork chops, ribs, hot dogs, pot roast, sausage, bologna, steaks other than round steak, etc.)*?

+3   None

+2   Less than 1 time

-1   1 time

-2   2 times

-3   3 times

-4   4 times

___ 11. How many times per week do you eat lean red meats *(hot dogs or luncheon meats with no more than 2 grams of fat per serving, round steak, or pork tenderloin)*?

+3   None

+1   Less than 1 time

0   1 time

-1   2 to 3 times

-2   4 to 5 times

-3   6 or more times

___ 12. After cooking, how large is the serving of red meat you eat? *(To convert from raw to cooked, reduce by 25 percent. For example, 4 oz of raw meat shrinks to 3 oz after cooking. There are 16 oz in a pound)*.

-3   6 oz or more

-2   4 to 5 oz

0   3 oz or less

+3   Don't eat red meat

___ 13. If you eat red meat, do you trim the visible fat when you cook or eat it?

+1   Yes

-3   No

___ 14. What kind of ground meat or poultry do you eat?

-4   Regular ground beef

-3   Ground beef that's 11 to 25% fat

-2   Ground chicken or 10% fat ground beef

-1   Ground turkey

+3   Ground turkey breast

+3   Don't eat ground meat or poultry

___ 15. What chicken parts do you eat?

+3   Breast

+1   Drumstick

-1   Thigh

-2   Wing

+3   Don't eat poultry

___ 16. If you eat poultry, do you remove the skin before eating?

+2   Yes

-3   No

___ 17. If you eat seafood, how many times per week? *(Omit deep-fried foods, tuna packed in oil, and mayonnaise-laden tuna salad—low-fat mayo is okay.)*

0   Less than 1 time

+1   1 time

+2   2 times

+3   3 or more times

Mixed Foods

___ 18. What is your most typical breakfast? *(Subtract an extra 3 points if you also eat sausage.)*

-4   Biscuit sandwich or croissant sandwich

-3   Croissant, Danish, or doughnut

-3   Eggs

-1   Pancakes, French toast, or waffles

+3   Cereal, toast, or bagel (no cream cheese)

+3   Low-fat yogurt or low-fat cottage cheese

0   Don't eat breakfast

___ 19. What sandwich fillings do you eat?

-3   Regular luncheon meat, cheese, or egg salad

-2   Tuna or chicken salad or ham

0   Peanut butter

+1   Roast beef

+1   Low-fat luncheon meat

+3   Tuna or chicken salad made with fat-free mayo

+3   Turkey breast or humus

___ 20. What do you order on your pizza? *(Subtract 1 point if you order extra cheese, cheese-filled crust, or more than one meat topping)*.

+3   No cheese with at least one vegetable topping

-1   Cheese with at least one vegetable topping

-2   Cheese

-3   Cheese with one meat topping

+3   Don't eat pizza

___ 21. What do you put on your pasta? *(Add one point if you also add sautéed vegetables.)*

+3   Tomato sauce or red clam sauce

-1   Meat sauce or meat balls

-3   Pesto or another oily sauce

-4   Alfredo or another creamy sauce

22. How many times per week do you eat deep-fried foods (*fish, chicken, French fries, potato chips, etc.)?*

- +3 None
- 0 1 time
- -1 2 times
- -2 3 times
- -3 4 or more times

23. At a salad bar, what do you choose?

- +3 Nothing, lemon, or vinegar
- +2 Fat-free dressing
- +1 Low- or reduced-calorie dressing
- -1 Oil and vinegar
- -2 Regular dressing
- -2 Cole slaw, pasta salad, or potato salad
- -3 Cheese or eggs

24. How many times per week do you eat canned or dried soups or frozen dinners? *(Omit lower-sodium, low-fat ones.)*

- +3 None
- 0 1 time
- -1 2 times
- -2 3 to 4 times
- -3 5 or more times

25. How many servings of low-fat calcium-rich foods do you eat per day? *(One serving = ⅔ cup low-fat or nonfat milk or yogurt, 1 oz low-fat cheese, 1½ oz sardines, 3½ oz canned salmon with bones, 1 oz tofu made with calcium sulfate, 1 cup collards or kale, or 200 mg of a calcium supplement.)*

- -3 None
- -1 Less than 1 serving
- +1 1 serving
- +2 2 servings
- +3 3 or more servings

26. How many times per week do you eat cheese? *(Include pizza, cheeseburgers, lasagna, tacos or nachos with cheese, etc. Omit foods made with low-fat cheese.)*

- +3 None
- +1 1 time
- -1 2 times
- -2 3 times
- -3 4 or more times

27. How many egg yolks do you eat per week? *(Add 1 yolk for every slice of quiche you eat.)*

- +3 None
- +1 1 yolk
- 0 2 yolks
- -1 3 yolks
- -2 4 yolks
- -3 5 or more yolks

Fats & Oils

28. What do you put on your bread, toast, bagel, or English muffin?

- -4 Stick butter or cream cheese
- -3 Stick margarine or whipped butter
- -2 Regular tub margarine
- -1 Light tub margarine or whipped light butter
- 0 Jam, fat-free margarine, or fat-free cream cheese
- +3 Nothing

29. What do you spread on your sandwiches?

- -2 Mayonnaise
- -1 Light mayonnaise
- +1 Catsup, mustard, or fat-free mayonnaise
- +2 Nothing

30. With what do you make tuna salad, pasta salad, chicken salad, etc.?

- -2 Mayonnaise
- -1 Light mayonnaise
- 0 Fat-free mayonnaise
- +2 Nothing

31. What do you use to sauté vegetables or other food? *(Vegetable oil includes safflower, corn, sunflower, and soybean.)*

- -3 Butter or lard
- -2 Margarine
- -1 Vegetable oil or light margarine
- +1 Olive or canola oil
- +2 Broth
- +3 Cooking spray

Beverages

32. What do you drink on a typical day?

- +3 Water or club soda
- 0 Caffeine-free coffee or tea
- -1 Diet soda
- -1 Coffee or tea (up to 4 a day)
- -2 Regular soda (up to 2 a day)
- -3 Regular soda (3 or more a day)
- -3 Coffee or tea (5 or more a day)

33. What kind of "fruit" beverage do you drink?
- +3 Orange, grapefruit, prune, or pineapple juice
- +1 Apple, grape, or pear juice
- 0 Cranberry juice blend or cocktail
- -3 Fruit "drink," "ade," or "punch"

34. What kind of milk do you drink?
- -3 Whole
- -1 2% fat
- +2 1% lowfat
- +3 skim

35. What do you eat as a snack?
- +3 Fruits of vegetables
- +2 Lowfat yogurt
- +1 Lowfat crackers
- -2 Cookies or fried chips
- -2 Nuts or granola bar
- -3 Candy bar or pastry

36. Which of the following "salty" snacks do you eat?
- -3 Potato chips, corn chips, or popcorn
- -2 Tortilla chips
- -1 Salted pretzels or light microwave popcorn
- +2 Unsalted pretzels
- +3 Baked tortilla or potato chips or homemade air-popped popcorn
- +3 Don't eat salty snacks

37. What kind of cookies do you eat?
- +2 Fat-free cookies
- +1 Graham crackers or reduced-fat cookies
- -1 Oatmeal cookies
- -2 Sandwich cookies (like Oreos)
- -3 Chocolate coated, chocolate chip, or peanut butter cookies
- +3 Don't eat cookies

38. What kind of cake or pastry do you eat?
- -4 Cheesecake
- -3 Pie or doughnuts
- -2 Cake with frosting
- -1 Cake without frosting
- 0 Muffins
- +1 Angle food, fat-free cake, or fat-free pastry
- +3 Don't eat cakes or pastries

39. What kind of frozen dessert do you eat? (Subtract 1 point for each of the following toppings: hot fudge, nuts, or chocolate candy bars or pieces.)
- -4 Gourmet ice cream
- -3 Regular ice cream
- -1 Frozen yogurt or light ice cream
- -1 Sorbet, sherbet, or ices
- +1 Nonfat frozen yogurt or fat-free ice cream
- +3 Don't eat frozen desserts

____ **Total Score**

Add up your score for each question and write it in the "total score" line above. **If your score is:**

1 to 29   Don't be discouraged. Eating healthy is tough, but you can learn to eat healthier.

30 to 59   Congratulations. Your are doing just fine. Pin your Quiz to the nearest wall.

60 or above   Excellent. You're a nutrition superstar. Give yourself a big pat on the back.

Source: Adapted with permission from *Nutrition Action Healthletter*, May 1996, V23/N4. (*Nutrition Action Healthletter*, 1875 Connecticut Ave., N.W., Suite 300, Washington DC 20009-5728. $24 for 10 issues.)

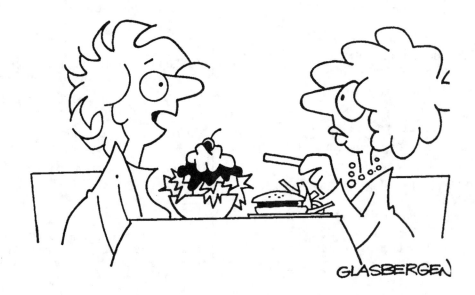

"I'm easing into my diet gradually. It's a hot-fudge salad!"

Welcome back after your first lesson! I hope you did well and are on your way to permanent weight-loss.

Reviewing your diary

One purpose of completing the Food Diary is to examine your eating patterns. Much of our eating is automatic and occurs with little thought or appreciation. We miss much of the pleasure in food and eat more than we need. Think of munching from a large bag of potato chips. Would you remember how many you ate? Would you taste each bite of each chip? Would you have just the right amount to satisfy yourself?

A nice example of automatic eating is from a client of mine named Ginny. She loved ice cream and would have a bowl every night. At my urging, she began counting her bites and noting the pleasure in each. She averaged 16 bites. She found that the first four bites were delicious, then there were about ten where she paid little attention (automatic eating). The final few bites were good again because she was nearly finished. With her increased awareness, Ginny decided that the middle ten bites were needless calories.

Searching for patterns

Examine your Food Diaries for the past week and look for patterns. The patterns you find will be the foundation for later parts of the program. This is where you and I work together. I will give you guidelines for tailoring techniques to your specific eating and exercise patterns. Here are some ideas for patterns.

- ◆ **Time.** Look for times of the day when you are likely to eat. A typical pattern shows little eating at breakfast and lunch, but much eating and snacking at dinner and after. Do you crave a snack just before bed? Do you always have something in mid-afternoon? Are your meals irregular? Do you skip meals?

- ◆ **Amount.** Look over the quantities and calories of the food you eat. One key is to enjoy the food you eat so there are no wasted calories. Are there foods you could eat less of or avoid completely? Do you eat specific amounts each time, without thinking about how much you need and want?

- ◆ **Foods.** Pay close attention to the foods you eat. Are there patterns to the foods you choose? Which foods contribute most to your calories? Can you think of substitutes for high-calorie foods?

- ◆ **Places.** Are there certain places where you eat? Do you frequently eat in places

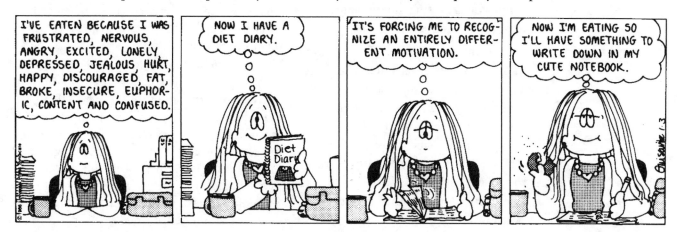

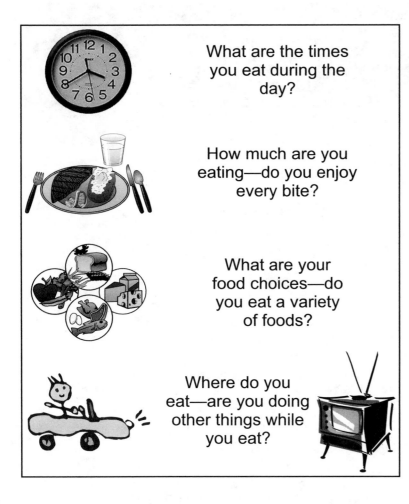

What are the times you eat during the day?

How much are you eating—do you enjoy every bite?

What are your food choices—do you eat a variety of foods?

Where do you eat—are you doing other things while you eat?

other than your kitchen or dining room? Some likely candidates are the den, the office, and the car.

An expanded food diary

This week you will find several categories added to your diary. These categories are Time, Feelings, and Activity. In addition to the food and calories, you will be able to record the time you are eating, how you feel, and whether you are doing something else.

These are important factors in the eating habits of many overweight people. Therefore, use the Expanded Food Diary as you did the Food Diary for Lesson One. In the next lesson, we will discuss the interpretations of the new diary. A blank diary is provided in this lesson, and a sample from one of my clients is given to show you how the diary might be completed. Make copies of the blank diary to use between now and the next lesson.

The role of exercise

It is hard to overstate the importance of increasing physical activity. Theoretically, you can eat less, exercise more, or do both to alter your energy balance and hence your weight. I feel strongly that doing both is the best approach. This comes from experience with hundreds of clients and from research showing that people who exercise are most likely to achieve long-term weight loss.

The importance of being active

Don't get nervous! Increasing your activity does not have to involve calisthenics, weight lifting, or marathon running. Many overweight people avoid exercise because it hurts, it takes time, they are embarrassed, and they are not skilled at athletic activities. There are solutions to these problems. I will discuss these in upcoming lessons. For now, I want you to be aware of the importance and benefits of being active.

A new view of exercise

Most of us labor under the old idea that exercise has to be taxing to be beneficial. In fact, this is what most experts preached for years and years. Much to the delight of people struggling with their weight, the view of exercise has changed entirely in the last several years. What we know now, and what has been emphasized by prestigious groups like the American College of Sports Medicine and the Centers for Disease Control and Prevention, is that low levels of activity can be beneficial for health. We also know that low levels can be helpful for weight loss.

This turns everything upside down. It means that making small increases in physical activity *counts* as exercise. It means that even with modest changes, you may improve your health. It also means that we can set aside the biggest barrier to exercise—the thought that high levels are the only acceptable amounts. I hope you don't tire of me saying that any amount of exercise is beneficial, because it will come up a number of times in the program.

The benefits of exercise

There are seven reasons why physical activity is central to weight loss. Most people know only the first—that it burns calories.

- **Burns calories.** Exercise does burn calories, but this may be its least important benefit. Be careful to avoid feeling that a modest amount of exercise entitles you to more calories at the table. You will probably eat more calories than the exercise expended.

- **Counteracts the ills of overweight.** Exercise can help change the physical and psychological problems associated with being overweight. It can lower blood pressure and cholesterol and improve carbohydrate metabolism.

- **Helps control appetite.** Studies with both animals and humans suggest that exercise can help control appetite. It certainly does not stimulate appetite when people exercise in moderate amounts. If you exercise and feel increased hunger, your mind is at work rather than your body.

- **Preserves the body's muscle.** Your body loses both muscle and fat when you lose weight. The aim is to maximize fat loss. Combining exercise with diet does this more effectively than using diet alone.

- **Increases metabolic rate.** Eating less and losing weight slow down your metabolism. This is bad news because your body then uses less energy (calories) for basic functioning at a time when you want to burn more calories. Exercise speeds up metabolism, although the degree and duration of this increase is subject to debate. Exercising while eating less may help offset this drop in metabolic rate.

- **Improves confidence and psychological factors.** Exercise makes people feel good. Each time you are active is a symbol that you are making positive changes. This improves confidence and gives you a boost that can carry over to your eating plan. In addition, many people exercise to relieve stress. If you are one of the people who eats to relieve stress, exercise may accomplish the same thing but will burn rather than add calories.

- **Correlates with long-term success.** Exercise is the factor which best predicts who will lose weight and keep it off. If people are followed a year or more after a weight-loss program, those who are exercising tend to be the ones who keep weight off. Furthermore, those individuals who are prescribed a structured exercise program during weight loss do better than those who just diet.

As you can see, the evidence in favor of exercise is clear and powerful. In the next lesson we will begin with specific suggestions for increasing activity. Walking will be the first step, so if you are walking now, keep up the good work! If not, don't hesitate to begin—but don't overdo it.

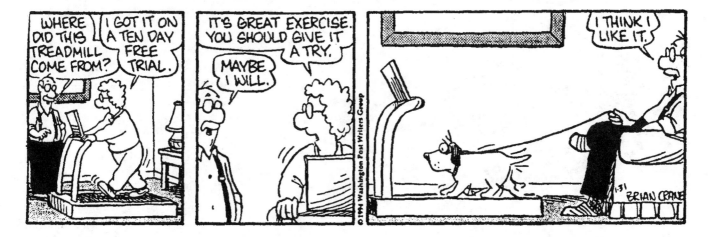

Dr. Steven Blair of The Cooper Institute for Aerobics Research in Dallas, has written an excellent book for those individuals who find it difficult to find time to exercise. *Living With Exercise* is a step-by-step guide designed to help people incorporate increased physical activity into their daily lifestyle. For more information on this guide, contact The LEARN Education Center (see Ordering Information in the back of this manual).

Why losing weight is difficult

Let's face it—losing weight is hard work. Most overweight people really want to lose weight, but find it difficult. There are many reasons. I will discuss several here. It is important for you to appreciate the complexities of weight loss so you don't get demoralized when you encounter tough times.

Eating is a complex activity. When you face temptation from food, say a piece of cake after dinner, many factors combine to determine whether you will eat it. There is physiology at work because hunger might be stimulated. Your family upbringing can enter the picture because you may have learned that foods (especially desserts) are associated with love. Culture plays a part, particularly if you are dining with someone else and you feel obliged to eat everything, including dessert. Psychology might take part if you are feeling depressed or lonely and want food for gratification.

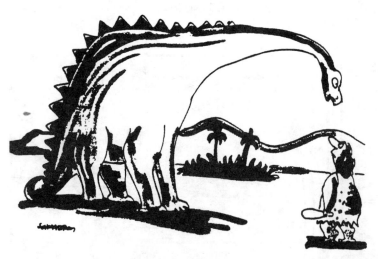

"How many calories are you?"

No one reason can be pinpointed. To keep your attitudes on the right track, remind yourself that getting the actual eating and exercise habits under control is the best course to weight loss. Instead of feeling guilty about what you eat or resentful about what you cannot eat, you can learn about food and calories and enjoy yourself!

The mysterious calorie

The word *calorie* is on the lips of millions of Americans. Food products boast about being *low calorie* and diet soft drinks sell because they have no calories. Just what is this thing we call a calorie?

A calorie is

The calorie is a measure of energy available to the body, much like a gallon is a measure of volume, the inch a measure of length, and the pound a measure of weight. When you eat something, the number of calories it contains is the number of energy units it provides to the body for its needs. The calorie is also a measure of energy your body uses, so it is a measure of both intake and expenditure. That is why we talk about the number of calories burned during exercise.

How do we measure the calories in foods? This is done by burning food in a special instrument called a bomb calorimeter. The food is first dried to remove water and then is placed in a special container which rests in water. When the food is burned, heat is transferred to the water. The amount the water is heated is the measure of calories. One calorie is the energy needed to raise the temperature of one gram of water one degree centigrade. Foods contain proteins, carbohydrates (sugars and starches), and fats, each of which provides calories. The water, vitamins, and minerals in food provide no calories.

Most foods are measured in kilocalories, which is 1,000 times the energy in a small calorie. In common usage, as in diet books and calorie guides, the word *calorie* actually refers to kilocalorie.

This may sound technical, but you need only know the calorie values of foods. A piece of apple pie has 400 calories, and a fresh apple has 100. The pie gives you four times the energy (calories) as the apple. This would be fine if you were starving, but when your basic energy requirements are met, the body stores the excess as fat. The pie contributes four times as many calories to your fat stockpile.

Not all people are created equal

People differ greatly in how their bodies use calories. We all know people who eat like crazy and gain very little. These fortunate folks are well served in a society where food is abundant and thin is in. In a famine, however, they would be the first to go because their bodies are not efficient at converting ingested calories to precious energy stores (fat).

The unfortunate ones among us are those who are *food efficient*. Their bodies make very good use of calories, so they are prone to gain weight. This is adaptive if food is scarce, but promotes weight gain when food supplies are adequate. To lose weight, such a person must cut intake to very low levels.

This is one reason why some heavy people have a more difficult time losing weight than others. Let's consider two individuals (Sheri and Bonnie) who fight different battles. Both weigh 180 pounds. Sheri eats 2500 calories each day to maintain that weight and will lose about one pound each week by cutting to 2000 calories. Bonnie, on the other hand, maintains the 180 pounds on only 1800 calories each day, and must reduce to 1000 calories to lose the one pound each week. Is it surprising, then, that Bonnie will have a more difficult time losing weight than will Sheri? Because of these individual differences, it would not be fruitful to prescribe the same calorie goal to these two different people.

In a related matter, we often hear that 3500 calories equals a pound (it takes 3500 extra calories to gain one pound). If we decrease intake by 3500, one less pound will adorn our bodies. The typical arithmetic is as follows. If you eat 500 fewer calories each day than your ordinary intake, you will create a 3500 calorie

deficit in a week and will lose one pound. These numbers are helpful to show how calories can be translated into pounds, but again, the numbers are rough averages. People are highly variable in the number of calories necessary to lose a pound, so these numbers may or may not apply to you. The key question is, therefore, "How do you choose a calorie goal for *you*?"

Determining your target calorie level

It is time to identify *your* target calorie level. As we explore your body's calorie requirements, you will soon learn (if you do not know already) whether you are more like Sheri or Bonnie, the two people mentioned above.

The guidelines are simple. We want to find the calorie level at which you can lose one to two pounds each week. Faster loss can be a clue that you are making drastic changes that can be difficult to maintain. You can probably make a good guess about what this level might be. Start there, and experiment to see whether you need to increase or decrease the calories.

If you are uncertain about the calorie level, consider using 1200 calories per day for women and 1500 for men. These are commonly used figures which represent calorie levels at which many people will lose weight. As you know, however, this is just an average, which means that some people will need fewer calories and some can afford more. In the space provided here, write in the calorie level you will use as the first step in identifying your long-term target.

Your Calorie Target

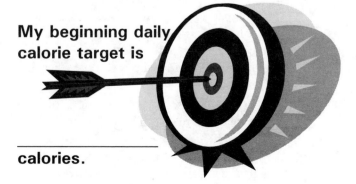

My beginning daily calorie target is

_____
calories.

Over the next few lessons, you will have time to experiment with this beginning calorie level and to arrive at your target number. This number is important and will be entered into the Monitoring Form for each week, beginning in Lesson Four. You will make note of your target number in each lesson and will have a record of whether you attained the goal each day of the program. The space for the precise calorie level in the Monitoring Form is left blank, so you can fill in your personal *number*.

It is not advisable to drop your calorie level below 1000 calories per day. It is extremely difficult to pack the necessary nutrients into fewer calories than this, so by eating fewer than 1000 calories, you may be losing weight at the expense of good nutrition. Diets of less than 1000 calories per day should be supervised by a physician.

Diets that fall below this level are labeled *very-low-calorie diets* (VLCDs). Again, these are to be used only under medical supervision, preferably in a program where a registered dietitian is available to provide expert nutritional input. The body goes through complicated changes when on such diets. There is the potential for danger if a person is not screened and monitored adequately and if the food or supplement to be eaten does not contain the right mix of nutrients.

Your vision of reasonable weight changes

People begin weight-loss programs with widely differing ideas about how much weight they will lose and how fast they will lose it. A common story might be of a person with 50 pounds to lose who begins a program in March in anticipation of swimsuit season. She may not consider how much weight might reasonably be lost in the few months ahead, and instead focuses on how she will look when she hits the beach.

Having unreasonable expectations of how fast weight will drop can be a problem. When this happens, people with perfectly respectable or even enviable weight losses can feel disappointed. Let's return to the beach example.

The woman we mentioned might lose 20 pounds in three months. This is terrific progress, but when she steps on the beach, she might feel like a failure knowing that she is still 30 pounds heavier than she wanted to be. This feeling could translate into self-doubt, anger, hurt, resignation, and the feeling that it was not worth trying in the first place.

To avoid this trap and allow yourself to have the good feelings you deserve when you do well, it is important to have a clear idea of how much weight you might lose. Here is how to proceed.

On page 37, I have provided another blank weight graph called "My Reasonable Weight Loss." Assume you will lose 20 pounds by Week 16. This is slightly less than 1.5 pounds per week. Draw a line from the zero mark (no pounds lost) at the beginning of the program to the 20 pounds at week 16. Next, at the bottom of the graph where the weeks are numbered, put in dates for each of the weeks so you have a specific date recorded for each week of the program. For instance, if you began the program on October 1, week 1 would be October 8, week 3 would be October 22, week 6 would be November 12, and so forth. Then, make a special mark on weeks in which some special date occurs (your birthday, your parent's or child's birthday, July 4th, Thanksgiving, Halloween, Valentine's Day, etc.).

When a specific week rolls around, like when your birthday arrives, you can look at your graph and evaluate your progress. This gives you a reasonable standard against which to do so. A person beginning a program on October 1 could pull out this graph on Halloween, see that a reasonable loss is about five to six pounds, and then feel great about a nine pound loss.

Completing this exercise is important. Referring to it could make the difference between feeling good (as you should) or bad (as is possible) later in the program. Feeling bad is a good state to avoid.

On being a good group member

Many people who use this program do so on their own. Others are part of a group program. If you are part of a group and are with others who struggle with problems like yours, there are several important matters to consider.

Being in a group can be a wonderful experience, with support, encouragement, and good ideas flowing from one member of the group to another. This is why groups can be so beneficial. To make a group a positive experience, each member must realize that working in a cooperative way, with a team spirit, will allow the group to reach its potential. Each member has the opportunity, the **responsibility**, to follow certain guidelines. Some effort will be required, but the payoff will make it worthwhile.

Detailed guidelines for being a good group member are presented in Appendix D. If you are participating in a group program, I urge you to read these over, and to take the advice seriously. Being a contributing and constructive member of the group will support the other group members, who in turn will support you. This can go a long way toward motivating you when times are tough and providing you with fresh ideas for specific problems.

Counting grams of fat

As I discuss later in this program, there are many reasons why dietary fat is a central issue in a weight management program. Among the reasons are that fat has many calories and that fat intake is related to risk of heart disease and some cancers. For these reasons, some nutrition experts recommend that individuals keep a record of their grams of fat intake, in addition to or in lieu of counting calories.

Whether one counts fat or calories depends on the aim of dietary change. If the purpose of the diet is to reduce the risk for chronic disease, counting fat grams would be sensible. If weight control is the issue, counting calories is the reasonable choice. A diet high in fat is typically high in calories, and vice-versa, but there are exceptions. For instance, one could drink 25 cans of Coca Cola each day, take in little fat, and still gain weight because of the high sugar content.

Some individuals who use this program choose to record grams of fat as well as calories. Because fat intake is so important, I have provided the grams of fat as well as calorie values in The Calorie Guide (Appendix F) and in many tables throughout this book. Feel free to record fat grams if you wish, but remember that it is essential to keep an accurate record of your calorie intake.

Reduced fat foods

The food companies have been working hard to develop products with less fat. The enormous popularity of reduced sugar items such as diet soft drinks has led to a frantic search for ways to preserve the taste of foods while lowering the amount of nutrients that may contribute to health problems.

More and more we will see food items that are reduced in fat. Some will have other nutrients replace the fat, and fat substitutes will be more common. For the most part, I believe these are positive developments as they will allow people to enjoy some of the foods they like but with fewer calories and grams of fat. One risk lies in the way people interpret and then make use of terms like "low fat."

Low fat does not mean low calorie. In fact, many of the low-fat cookies now on the market have nearly as many calories as the cookies they hope to replace. True, if one is destined to eat a certain number of cookies, then it would be better to have the reduced-fat versions, but we cannot assume this will cut calories. Some people feel that because a food seems healthy that more can be eaten. So, if you encounter cookies, crackers, and other foods that are reduced in fat, be certain to check the calories. For some people, the marketing of these products has had a paradoxical effect—people feel they can eat more and thus increase their calorie intake.

Assignment for this lesson

Your assignment is to copy the Expanded Food Diary from the one provided here and to fill one in each day. Remember that you can order blank week-at-a-time food diaries by calling the LEARNEducation Center at 1-800-736-7323 or checking the web site www.LearnEducation.com. Also, your prescribed calorie level is 1200 (for women) or 1500 (for men), so stick to this tenaciously. Set another level only if you have a good reason. Be sure to check with your physician if you have any medical problems which require special attention.

Self-assessment questionnaire

Lesson Two

T F 6. Automatic eating is common in overweight people and distracts them from the taste of food.

T F 7. The Food Diary helps uncover patterns in your eating habits.

T F 8. Exercise isn't of much use for weight loss because it burns relatively few calories.

T F 9. Exercise can help prevent the loss of muscle tissue during weight loss.

T F 10. The calorie is the measure of the amount of fat in food.

T F 11. The calorie level necessary to lose weight is the same for all people.

(Answers in Appendix C)

My Reasonable Weight Loss

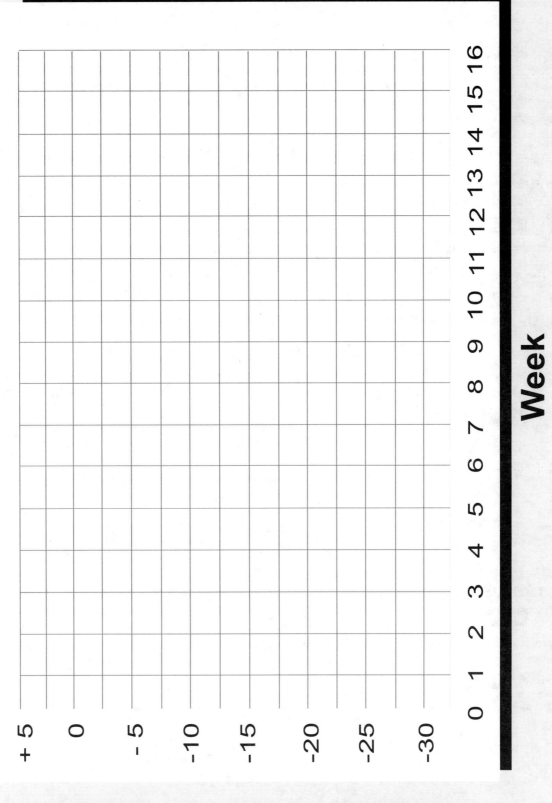

Weight Change (in pounds)

Week

Expanded Food Diary—Lesson Two *(sample)*   Today's Date_____

Description	Time	Feelings	Activity	Calories
Breakfast				
Coffee, 6 oz	7:30	Tired	Reading paper	0
Poached egg, 1 med				79
Bagel, ½ med				92
Orange juice, 1 cup				111
Total calories from this meal				282
Lunch				
Roast beef sandwich, 2 oz, with 2 T mayonnaise	12:30	Hurried	Working at desk	442
Water, 1 glass				0
Raspberry yogurt, 8 oz				90
Total calories from this meal				532
Dinner				
Chicken breast-grilled, 3.5 oz	7:30	Relaxed	Watching TV	193
Green beans, 1 cup				44
Carrots, 1 cup, cooked				70
Wheat bread, 1 slice, dry				61
Skim milk, 1 cup				86
Total calories from this meal				454
Snacks				
Celery, 4 stalks	10:00	Tense	Working at desk	24
Apple, 1 med	3:00	Frustrated	On break	81
Total calories from snacks				105
Total calories for the day				1,373

Expanded Food Diary—Lesson Two

Today's Date_____

Description	Time	Feelings	Activity	Calories
Breakfast				
Total calories from this meal				
Lunch				
Total calories from this meal				
Dinner				
Total calories from this meal				
Snacks				
Total calories from snacks				
Total calories for the day				

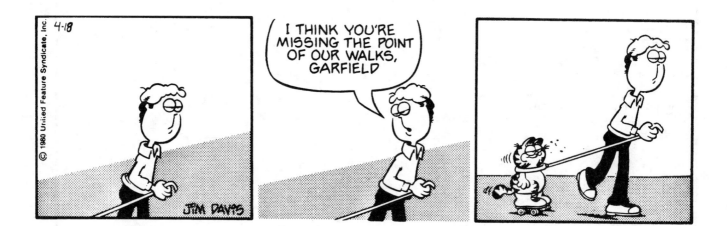

Wе are ready to move on to new and exciting things. Our emphasis in this lesson will be on Lifestyle and Exercise, with information also on the other parts of The LEARN Program. You will begin to see how the areas of the LEARN model complement each other. For example, we will begin a structured walking program (Exercise) and will discuss the virtues of walking with a partner (Relationships). Our interpretation of the Expanded Food Diary (Lifestyle) will teach you to be aware of when you are eating from hunger or habit, and the section on Attitudes will help you distinguish actual hunger from psychological cravings. You can see how the different aspects of the program are woven together.

Analyzing your expanded food diary

Now that you have experience with the Expanded Food Diary, let's discuss what the information means. We are looking for several things. The first are eating *patterns* that tell us whether your eating follows a reliable course from day-to-day. The second are *triggers*—the circumstances which provoke overeating.

The search for patterns

The Expanded Food Diary included spaces for the time of eating, feelings, and other activities. Did you find any patterns?

- **Time.** Did your eating cluster in certain parts of the day? Your eating times may vary depending on the day of the week. Some people keep a strict schedule on weekdays and then have less control on weekends. If you find times when control is difficult, think about scheduling alternative activities (like exercise).

- **Feelings.** Did you eat when you were bored, depressed, anxious, angry, or lonely? Other feelings may also be involved, like resentment, hostility, jealousy, or even joy. Seeing a pattern is a sure sign that you can learn more adaptive ways to cope with difficult feelings.

- **Activity.** What do you do while eating? Watching television is the main culprit, but reading a newspaper, listening to a radio, or browsing through magazines can also be a problem. Doing two things at once insures that neither gets full attention. Eating already gets less attention than it deserves. Later we will discuss how eating can be separated from other activities.

Searching for Patterns

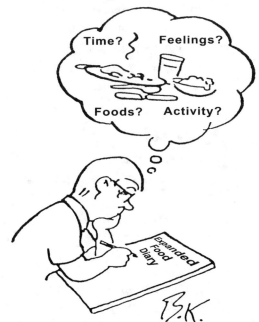

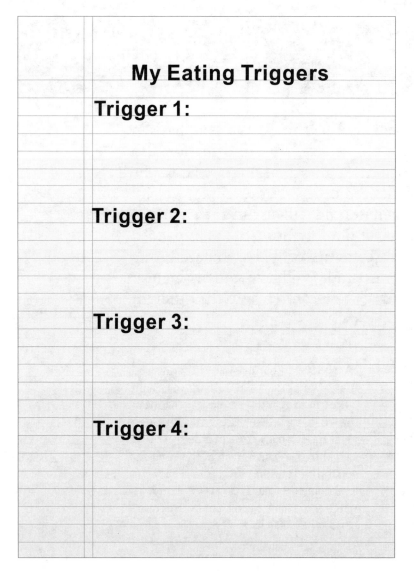

My Eating Triggers

Trigger 1:

Trigger 2:

Trigger 3:

Trigger 4:

- ◆ **Foods.** What types of foods do you eat? Do you crave carbohydrates at certain times? Do you eat foods because they are available or do you seek out the foods you love? Are some foods very difficult to eat in moderation?

High-risk situations—triggers for eating

What are your triggers for eating? Talking to your mother-in-law may do it, being bored at home, or having your spouse eat ice cream in front of you. It could be a trying day at work, a fight with someone, or fear about money matters. Most people have well-defined triggers. What are yours?

This is where the concept of *high-risk situations* becomes so important. Throughout the program, you will learn methods for avoiding or coping with situations that spell trouble. Identifying these situations, or triggers, is the first step. What you learn from the Food Diary and from your own study of yourself will provide valuable information for later stages of the program. You can learn to predict the situations which increase your risk and to plot your course accordingly.

Triggers are typically a mix of the factors included in your Expanded Food Diary. Given the right time, feelings, and other circumstances, eating is hard to resist. There may be positive pressure, like offers of food from friends, or negative pressure, like feeling upset. Once the trigger loosens a person's control, it is difficult to stop.

Make a list of your four main triggers in the spaces provided here. Remember these, as there will be many suggestions later about how to counter them.

How often should you weigh yourself?

One popular self-help group, Overeaters Anonymous, does not weigh its members at all. The theory is that more frequent weighing gives "too much power to the scale." Other programs recommend that members weigh regularly to get feedback on their progress. Some people weigh themselves many times each day. The average for people who enter weight-loss programs is about once per day.

Feedback from the scale can be a nice incentive for some individuals. It reminds them of the progress they have made and spurs their efforts. Others despair when the scale shows no change, and they look with horror at how much weight they have to lose to reach their goal. Since the scale represents various things to different people, it can be either friend or foe. Please remember that it can be a *powerful* friend or foe, so think seriously about how often you and the scale should communicate.

This is where *your* judgment must prevail. Weigh yourself as often as you see fit. I recommend no less than once each week and no more than once each day. If you are a frequent weigher you may get discouraged by weight gains beyond your control. Fluid shifts alone can lead to gains or losses of several pounds. However, if you feel the scale can be a motivating factor, try weighing more often.

One problem with paying too much attention to the scale is that it can lead to undeserved euphoria or despair. An example would be a person who does not do well on their eating plan, but shows a weight loss anyway, perhaps due to water loss from a menstrual cycle. This may lead a person to think they can stray from the plan and still lose weight. The opposite side of the coin is the person who does well on the program and gains weight anyway. Again, this can happen for several reasons, including fluid shifts. The danger lies in the person assuming that their efforts are going for nothing.

The scale should be a general guide about progress, not a day-to-day index of whether your program is working. This is why the Food Diaries (Monitoring Forms) at the end of each lesson ask you to record your calorie intake, your behavior changes, and your exercise. If these change, you will lose weight. Paying attention to these will make you less vulnerable to the vagaries of the scale.

Being on the move

Much has been said about the glories of exercise. Some joggers boast of a *runner's high*, and others feel that sweating and panting are the path to heaven. Some overweight people react to this hysteria by giving up on exercise. However, the LEARN concept of physical activity is not your usual exercise program. The object is to make it fun and to increase the number of activities you consider *exercise*. The first example is walking. Other activities will follow later in the program.

Is exercise safe for you?

Today we begin a walking program. If you are doing more vigorous activity, keep it up if you feel comfortable and have medical clearance. If you are not exercising regularly, the

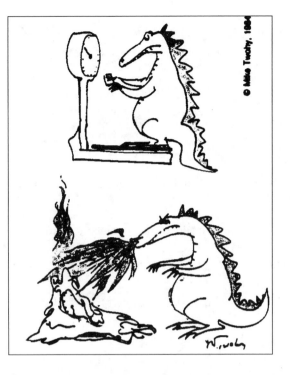

walking program may be for you. Walking has many virtues. It is healthy and helps you lose weight. It is easy and poses little physical risk (depending on where you walk!). But before we begin, we must ask if it is safe for you to exercise.

Moderate activity, including the walking discussed here, is safe for most people. There are, however, some people with physical problems who should not begin an exercise program without being checked carefully by a physician. This should extend beyond a simple checkup, and the physician should be alerted that the person is being checked to determine whether regular exercise is advisable.

The Physical Activity Readiness Questionnaire (PAR-Q) on page 44 provides a simple questionnaire you can complete to see if it is safe for you to increase your physical activity. Read and answer each question carefully. If any factor applies to you, see your physician before doing any exercise. This is serious and goes beyond the usual warning to *see your doctor* which is found in every diet book. If you are uncertain about what the terms mean or about whether you qualify, play it safe, and consult a physician. The list is adapted from the Canadian questionnaire by Dr. Steven Blair of The Cooper Institute for Aerobics Research.

The Physical Activity Readiness Questionnaire (PAR-Q)

The PAR-Q is designed to help you help yourself. Many health benefits are associated with regular exercise, and the completion of the PAR-Q is a sensible first-step to take if you are planning to increase the amount of physical activity in your life.

For most people, physical activity should not pose any problem or hazard. The PAR-Q has been designed to identify the small number of adults for whom physical activity might be inappropriate or those who should have medical advice concerning the type of activity most suitable for them.

Common sense is your best guide in answering these few questions. Please read them carefully, and circle the YES or NO for each question as it applies to you.

1. YES NO Has your doctor ever said you have heart trouble?

2. YES NO Do you frequently have pains in your heart and chest?

3. YES NO Do you often feel faint or have spells of severe dizziness?

4. YES NO Has a doctor ever said your blood pressure was too high?

5. YES NO Has your doctor ever told you that you have a bone or joint problem, such as arthritis, that has been aggravated by exercise, or might be made worse with exercise?

6. YES NO Is there a good physical reason, not mentioned here, why you should not follow any activity program, even if you wanted to?

7. YES NO Are you over age 65 and not accustomed to vigorous exercise?

If you answered YES to one or more questions:

If you have not recently done so, consult with your personal physician by telephone or in person BEFORE increasing your physical activity and/or taking a fitness test. Tell him or her what questions you answered YES.

After a medical evaluation, seek advice from your physician as to your suitability for:

Unrestricted physical activity, probably on a gradually increasing basis, or

Restricted and supervised activity to meet your specific needs, at least on an initial basis. Check in your community for special programs or services.

If you answered NO to all questions:

If you answered the questions on the PAR-Q accurately, you have reasonable assurance to your present suitability for:

A graduated exercise program. A gradual increase in proper exercise promotes good fitness development while minimizing or eliminating discomfort.

An exercise test. Simple tests of fitness may be undertaken if you so desire.

Postpone exercise or exercise testing:

If you have a temporary minor illness, such as a common cold.

Adapted with permission from Blair SN. *Living With Exercise* 1991. American Health Publishing Company: Dallas.

Starting your walking program

Walking has many advantages. Here are a few:

- **Almost anybody can do it.** Compared to many activities like swimming, basketball, or horseback riding, walking is an activity available to most people.
- **Do it at your pace.** You can walk fast or walk slow, and you can do it whenever *you* want, not just when the health club is open.
- **Walking is easy.** You need not strain with exertion when you walk. Even low levels are helpful.
- **Walking is enjoyable.** Think of all you can see while walking. You can enjoy the sights, listen to a portable tape player, or walk with friends.
- **It is cheap.** You do not need a health club membership or expensive equipment.
- **It can be a social event.** You may like company while you walk. It is a nice time to be with someone you enjoy.

This may surprise you, but walking burns almost the same number of calories as running the same distance. How *far* you go is more important than how *fast* you go. It needn't knock you out for it to help.

Clothes, shoes, and weather

Before you begin, consider clothes, shoes, and weather. Wear clothes that make you feel comfortable. There is nothing special about expensive jogging suits. Walking will help just as much if you are adorned with an old sweatshirt and jeans.

Shoes are important and may be worth the money for a good pair. Go to a sporting goods store and try on several brands. Pick one that feels good. Good shoes can help your feet, keep you from tiring, and reduce the chance of orthopedic injury.

Weather can be tricky. It is wise to avoid exercise when it is too hot or too cold. If the temperature is above 90 degrees or is below zero, it is best to get your exercise inside. This still leaves most days of the year available. Most people manage to do their walking in nearly any weather.

Wear layers of clothing in cold weather. When it gets quite cold you might wear a cotton T-shirt, several sweatshirts, and a windbreaker. The cotton will absorb the perspiration. You may feel cold for the first few minutes, but you will warm up rapidly. If you get too hot you can remove one of the layers. Wear a hat because much of the body's heat loss occurs through the head (especially if you are a hot head!). Mittens will keep hands warmer than gloves.

It is also important to be careful in hot weather. Walking in the morning or evening may help avoid the hottest parts of the day. Wear as few clothes as possible, and *never* wear rubber suits or other clothes designed to make you sweat. Whatever weight you lose in sweating will be regained, and trapping the body's heat in hot weather can be dangerous. Drink plenty of water. It is safe to drink water before, during, and after exercise.

Mall walking

Shopping malls are a good place to walk in inclement weather, or even when the weather is nice. In many parts of the country, *mall walkers* go to malls early in the morning and walk alone or in groups. This is a terrific idea.

The walkers who go with friends or who make new friends find the social contacts helpful in adhering to a regular schedule. Also, walking by the stores each morning leaves you poised for action the minute new "SALE" signs are posted!

Barriers to exercise

Many overweight people are reluctant to exercise because they are embarrassed. This occurs for several reasons. The extra weight can make exercise physically difficult. People who have been overweight all their lives may have little experience with vigorous exercise, and the experiences they do have may be unpleasant (being picked last for teams, teasing, etc.). Most important, however, is the fear of what others will think when a heavy person jogs by or cruises past on a bike.

Put aside these feelings right now! You have nothing to be ashamed of. Your weight-loss program is more important than being shy or embarrassed. Losing weight is a long process as it is and will be even longer if you wait to trim down before starting to exercise. Don't worry about what others think. In fact, most normal-weight people give heavy people much credit for making positive changes.

The 15-minute prescription

After all this information on walking, it is time to begin. Begin gradually and work your way up. There is no danger in starting with less than you can tolerate, but starting with more can be painful and discouraging.

Begin walking for 15 minutes each day. If you have difficulty doing this all in one bout, try three five—minute walks. When you can do this with ease, increase by five minutes each day to the point you feel some exertion. If the 15—minute walk is too difficult, subtract time until you feel comfortable. *The goal is to walk 30 minutes to one hour each day.* Try to gradually increase your walking to this level, so as not to make it difficult or unpleasant.

You know best when your schedule can accommodate your walking. Here are six suggestions:

❶ Get up 30 minutes early to walk

❷ Walk at lunch

❸ Walk during work breaks

❹ Walk after work

❺ Walk after dinner

❻ Walk before bedtime

Do your level best to walk every day. It is important to make it part of your routine, like brushing your teeth, making your bed, or taking a shower. This is the only way it will be integrated into your lifestyle. However, do not despair if you miss a day now and then. The long-term picture is more important than if you miss a day occasionally. Your attitudes about exercise will be discussed later in the program.

Your weight-loss program is more important than being shy about physical activity.

Experiment with walking different places, at different times, and with different people (or try it alone). Find the way you like it best. In Lesson Four, I will present specific ideas about making walking fun.

You can win a presidential sports award

A program sponsored by the President's Council on Physical Fitness and Sports now makes awards available to adults for participation in a number of activities. The award, called the *Presidential Sports Award*, can be earned by participation in one or more of 43 qualifying sports. Examples of these sports are backpacking, bicycling, bowling, fitness walking, golf, jogging, racquetball, rowing, running, sailing, swimming, tennis, and general types of exercise that you might do at a spa, aerobics class, a gym, or even at home. Chances are whatever activities you like and can do are on the list.

These awards are for regular people doing regular exercise—you do not have to be an Olympic athlete. You simply write to the address below and receive a sheet called the Personal Fitness Log. The sheet explains which activities are included and what you must do to be granted the award. You fill out the sheet as you exercise, send it in, and receive a handsome Personalized Certificate of Achievement with your name and qualifying sport, suitable for framing. You can also receive a nice lapel pin, and can win as many awards in as many sports as you would like. To receive the information on the award, just send a stamped, self-addressed envelope to:

Presidential Sports Award
President's Council on Physical Fitness and Sports
200 Independence SW, Suite 738H
Washington, DC 20201
Telephone (202) 690-9000

To show how these awards are truly achievable, I will list the criteria for earning awards in the "Fitness Walking" and "Tennis" categories. For Fitness Walking, a person must do the following within a four-month pe-

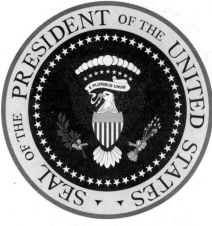

The Presidential Sports Award

riod: 1) Walk a minimum of 125 miles; 2) Each walk must be continuous, without pauses for rest, and the pace must be at least four m.p.h. (15 min. per mile); and 3) No more than two and one-half miles in any one day may be credited to the total. For tennis, one must: 1) Play tennis a minimum of 50 hours; 2) No more than one and one-half hours in any one day may be credited to the total; and 3) Total must include at least 25 sets of singles and/or doubles.

These examples show that the awards *can* be won, even by someone struggling with their weight. Some effort will be required, but then effort is just what we want, right? In my experience, this program can be very motivating. You may or may not be up to the required amount of exercise now, but you probably will be before long. So, write now! You may win the award before you know it.

A walking partnership

This is a good time to introduce the "R" (Relationships) part of the LEARN approach. Since we are focusing on walking, we can discuss its social aspects. Some people like to walk with others while some like to go solo. You are the best judge of what is right for you.

Walking with another person can be a powerful way to make walking more enjoyable. The company is a nice distraction because you can talk about politics, speculate about the stock market, bet on ball games, or best of all, gossip! A partner can also help by establishing a regular time for walking. There may be days when you would stay home, but knowing that a partner is waiting is just the stimulus you need to get out and get going.

Having a partner is not for everyone. Walking can be a nice time to enjoy yourself, to reflect, and to think about important matters. Don't feel pressured to have a partner, because going it alone may be best for you. Think about the advantages of walking with a partner or walking alone. You might try it both ways to see which you like.

Cravings versus hunger

Here is the place where your mind and body deceive each other, and where the "A" (Attitudes) part of The LEARN Program comes to the fore. When you eat, are you responding to physical hunger or to psychological cravings? Take the Cravings and Hunger Quiz here to find out. Which is the mind and which is the body?

Situations 1, 3, and 5 usually indicate psychological cravings. Situations 2 and 4 signal physical hunger. Situation 6 could be either. It is important to distinguish cravings from hunger. Once you can distinguish the cravings, we will work on special anti-craving techniques.

You can identify cravings by paying careful attention to when you want to eat. Does something stimulate the urge beside actual hunger? Does someone offer you food? Does something make you think about food? Do you have bad feelings that food would help satisfy? You can make note of these cravings on your Food Diary. This will remind you of the situations in which food will be hard to resist. Information on conquering the cravings is in the next lesson.

The mighty calorie

Lesson Two explained what a calorie is. We eat at least a half-million calories each year. You might wonder, therefore, what difference a few calories can make. They can make a *big* difference.

Cravings and Hunger Quiz

Answer each question below by circling either T for true or F for false.

T   F   Even after a large meal, I still want dessert.

T F 2. I often have a gnawing feeling in my stomach.

T F 3. When someone mentions a food I love, I feel like eating.

T F 4. I feel lightheaded after not eating for hours.

T F 5. When I drive by a fast-food restaurant, I want to eat.

T F 6. There is a time every day when I feel hungry.

As I mentioned earlier, 3500 calories will translate into a pound of body weight. If you consume 7000 calories more than your body uses, you will gain two pounds. These are rough estimates, and people vary greatly in the precise number of calories needed to gain or lose weight. What *is* clear is that calories *do* count. Let's examine the effects of adding an innocent ten calories per day to your total.

If you add ten calories per day to what you ordinarily eat, you will gain an extra pound in a year. Added over a decade or two, this is 10–20 pounds; and all from ten crummy calories per day! If the difference each day were 100 calories, this would be 10 pounds per year and 100 pounds for ten years! Let's look at the 10 calorie difference for the moment. This chart shows you how little you have to eat to get ten extra calories.

Think how easy it is to have an extra teaspoon of ketchup, one bite of an orange, or less

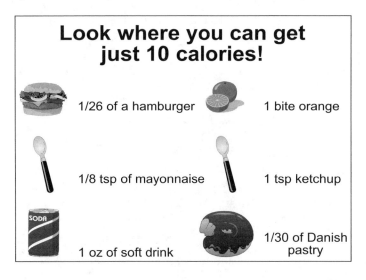

Look where you can get just 10 calories!

1/26 of a hamburger   1 bite orange

1/8 tsp of mayonnaise   1 tsp ketchup

1 oz of soft drink   1/30 of Danish pastry

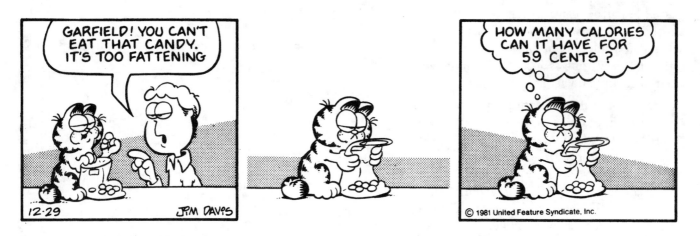

than one ounce of Pepsi. This shows the need for careful calculation of calories in your Food Diary and a vigilant attitude about foods.

You can also take a positive outlook on this calorie equation. Cutting out ten calories each day will save you a pound each year. You certainly won't miss the ten calories, but you can easily do without the pound.

Parties, holidays, and special events: a note

Many people find that their greatest challenge lies in how they handle holidays, parties, and special events. Loads of tempting food is usually available, hosts want and expect you to eat, and let's face it, celebrating just doesn't seem the same when you have to forego the special foods. Eating out at restaurants can be similarly challenging.

There are ways of being clever that can help you enjoy yourself while keeping control. Since we face so many of these events during a year, being prepared with the necessary skills can be a big help. I deal with these issues in detail in Lesson Fifteen in the section called "Holidays, Parties, and Special Events," and in Lesson Eleven in the section on "Eating Away from Home." Feel free to read these sections as needed to help with problems you may anticipate.

Assignment for this lesson

The main activity for this week is to begin your walking program. Walk as many days as

possible by using the guidelines provided in this lesson. Continue to use the Expanded Food Diary. It will be helpful to have more experience in identifying patterns and triggers. Remember what you learned from keeping the Expanded Diary in Lesson Two, and see if you can develop even more insight into the situations which place you at high-risk for overeating. Last, keep track of cravings and hunger and try to examine the situations in which cravings occur.

Self-assessment questionnaire

Lesson Three

T F 12. Walking one mile burns almost as many calories as running the mile.

T F 13. Expensive exercise suits are worth the money because the special materials help the body.

T F 14. Everyone should walk with a partner because the company increases pleasure.

T F 15. Overweight people do not experience hunger, only psychological cravings for food.

T F 16. Eating an extra ten calories per day will add one pound of weight over a year.

(Answers in Appendix C)

Expanded Food Diary—Lesson Three

Today's Date _____

Description	Time	Feelings	Activity	Calories
Breakfast				
Total calories from this meal				
Lunch				
Total calories from this meal				
Dinner				
Total calories from this meal				
Snacks				
Total calories from snacks				
Total calories for the day				

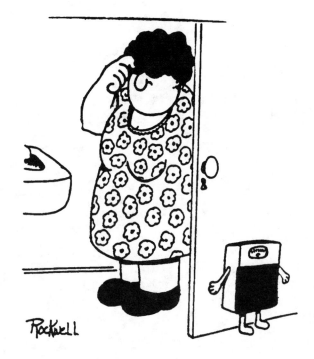

In this lesson we will cover ways to make walking fun. We will also discuss a new approach to lifestyle change—the ABC's of behavior, along with techniques to conquer food cravings and to set realistic goals. The possibility of a weight-loss partnership will be raised. Finally, I will introduce the Food Guide Pyramid and describe methods of following a balanced diet.

The ABC's of behavior

As we progress through the program, you will learn ways to change your behavior. We will use the ABC approach. The letters stand for Antecedents, Behavior, and Consequences.

Antecedents

These are the events, feelings, and situations which occur *before* eating. These usually occur together in a series of steps called the Behavior Chain, which will be discussed in Lesson Twelve.

Behavior

This refers to eating itself and to the related events and feelings. The relevant factors are the speed of eating, rate of chewing, taste of food, and the events *during* eating.

Consequences

These are the events, feelings, and attitudes which follow eating. These factors happen *after* eating and can determine whether the eating will occur again.

You can see each aspect of the ABC approach in the case of Steve. He was home on the weekend watching a football game. Steve was excited by the game because he bet $20 with his neighbor. He went to the kitchen to get his favorite TV snack, cheese curls. He ate the cheese curls rapidly and did not taste each one. He ate until he was very full and then felt guilty about eating so much.

The antecedents were being at home, watching the football game, being excited, and having the cheese curls available. The behavior was eating rapidly until very full. Steve did not taste all the cheese curls. The consequences were the unpleasant full feeling in the stomach and the guilt about overeating.

This analysis gives us many ideas about reducing Steve's chances for overeating. Steve could alter the antecedents by doing something other than watching the game, which is a high-risk situation, or by not having the cheese curls in the house. The behavior could be changed by eating slowly and savoring every bite. The consequences could change if he had different attitudes and could prevent the guilt and self-doubt that might stimulate more eating.

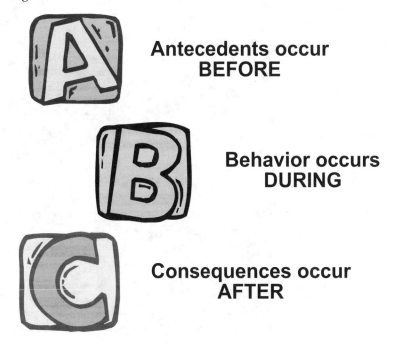

**Antecedents occur
BEFORE**

**Behavior occurs
DURING**

**Consequences occur
AFTER**

We will use the ABC approach in upcoming lessons. You can prepare yourself by thinking about the antecedents, behavior, and consequences of your eating. Do this by reviewing your Food Diaries for the past two lessons. You have been discovering patterns and triggers, and can now break down the situations further into each of the A, B, and C components. In Lesson Five, we will cover ways of controlling the situations (antecedents) which control eating.

Perfecting your walking program

How are you doing with your walking program? Do you feel good about this positive activity? It may still be too early to know how you will like it, but if your initial reactions are positive, then you are on the right track.

Maximizing the pleasure of walking

Walking can be lots of fun if you consider a few facts. The more fun you have, the more you will walk. Making the exercise a permanent habit is one key to success in this program.

◆ **Pay attention.** There are many interesting things to see wherever you walk. Look at the style of the houses or buildings you pass, or how your neighbors landscape their yards. What sort of cars go by and what type of people do you see? This is a good way to take advantage of what has always been available.

◆ **Bring entertainment.** Some walkers like to carry portable radios and cassette players. It is fine to listen to the news or music. Decide whether you want to enjoy the outside world or drown it out.

◆ **Don't overdo it.** A sure way to undermine an exercise program is to do too much too soon. You will be sore, frustrated, and discouraged. Beware of the tendency to increase your exercise too fast, even though you may be enjoying it.

◆ **Take a gradual approach.** *Gradual* is a key word in this program. Start exercise at the level you need, not what some book or video tape tells you. Work your way up from there, but do it sensibly. This is the principle of *shaping* discussed later in this lesson.

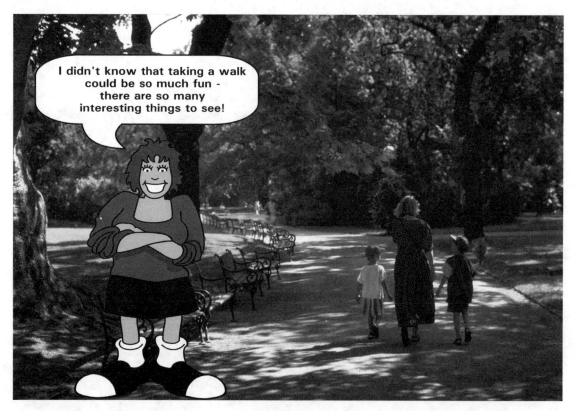

I didn't know that taking a walk could be so much fun - there are so many interesting things to see!

Increasing your walking

In Lesson Three, I recommended that your walking program begin with 15 minutes each day. If you can do this comfortably, increase the time. Again, your judgment must prevail. Do no more than you can handle, but try to make it a routine part of your day.

I recommend that you add five minutes of walking each day until you reach our goal of one hour of walking each day. As you add time, stop when you feel tired or uncomfortable. For example, you may feel fine when increasing from 15 to 20 minutes, but may feel fatigue or discomfort when going to 25 minutes.

Back up to the 20- minute *comfort level* and stay there until you are ready to move ahead. Some people will stay at one level for many weeks before moving ahead while others can progress more rapidly. It is important to tailor these guidelines to *your* needs.

Shaping the right attitudes

Conquering the Cravings

In Lesson Three, we learned to separate food cravings from physical hunger. Once you can spot the cravings, there are two ways to deal with them: distraction and confrontation.

The *distraction* approach involves ignoring the cravings. When you know a craving is about to engulf you, do something else. Think about something wonderful, plan a dream vacation, or do anything to take your attention away from the urge to eat. The craving will usually pass.

The distraction method works best for people who have a good imagination or can change activities or thoughts at an instant's notice. You only have to do these things for a few moments, because cravings generally pass within minutes or even seconds. If you are bombarded by cravings throughout the day, confronting the cravings may be most effective.

The *confrontation* approach pits you against the craving. Let's say you want to raid the refrigerator for ice cream. You could pretend the urge is another person trying to convince you to eat the ice cream. Argue with this person and say why you will not give in to the urge. Another approach is to visualize the ice cream container beckoning to you and tempting you with promises of fulfillment. Imagine how silly it is to let the ice cream get the best of you.

A typical confrontation scene might be as follows. You get the urge to stop for a snack while driving home from work. You recognize the craving and decide to get the best of it. You say, "You nasty craving! You want me to stop for Peanut Butter Cups when I'm not really hungry. I'll show you who's boss. I am in charge of my own life and my weight."

Think of these two approaches now and decide which will work for you. If you are in doubt, experiment with both. Try to arrive at a strategy as soon as possible, be it distraction or confrontation. This will prepare you in advance for the inevitable cravings you will face. Do your best not to give in.

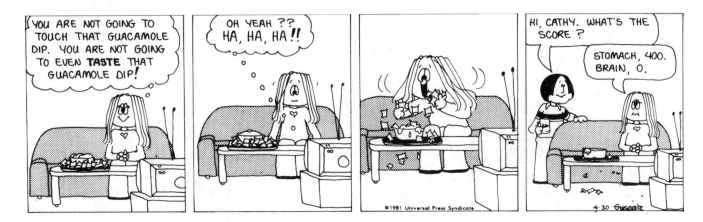

My Goals for this Program

Goal 1:

Is this reasonable? _____

Goal 2:

Is this reasonable? _____

Goal 3:

Is this reasonable? _____

Goal 4:

Is this reasonable? _____

Goal setting

One common attitude problem is having unrealistic goals. Some individuals do not recognize they are setting unattainable goals, but they do so nonetheless. Examples of this are starting a program in May for swimsuit season when there are 50 pounds to lose. Having fantasies of being thin and having life improve immediately is another example. These things may happen, but not right away.

Think about your goals for the program. Think of specific answers to these four questions:

❶ How much weight each week do you expect to lose?

❷ How soon do you expect to be thin?

❸ Will your life be different when you lose weight?

❹ Do you expect losing weight to be easy and quick?

These are just examples of some tricky areas. You are a sensible person and can formulate reasonable goals. Do you think your hidden or unconscious goals are not realistic? If so, remind yourself time and time again that setting unrealistic goals is a setup for trouble.

In the space to the left, list your four major goals for this program, and decide whether they are realistic. The goals may be specific weight-loss accomplishments (to lose one pound each week, or to lose 25 pounds in total) or other changes (clothes will fit better, look better for daughter's wedding).

The principle of shaping

Shaping refers to making gradual, step-by-step changes in your behavior. Two examples can highlight how this works. If your weakness is donuts and you begin every day with three of your favorite kind, dropping them completely may be difficult. You could start by cutting to two donuts, then one, and finally to none. Our approach to exercise is another example of shaping. We began with comfortable levels of walking with the goal of increasing in a gradual way to a final level.

You can see how the shaping principle applies to goal setting. Setting realistic goals means starting from a point you can master and then working up gradually to the level you desire. This will come through many times in the lessons that follow.

Following a balanced diet

There is no end to advice on nutrition. When I visit a bookstore or listen to radio talk shows, I am amazed at the half-baked schemes concocted by *experts*. One day it is apricot pits for cancer or papaya juice for obesity. The next day it is mega-doses of vitamins for heart disease and prune pulp for bad breath.

It is inviting to believe some of these nutty plans because they provide hope for difficult problems. But think back over the years. There was the *Scarsdale Diet, The Rotation Diet, The Beverly Hills Diet, The Carbohydrate Addicts Diet,* among many, many others. Each promised breakthroughs, grand solutions, and results that seemed guaranteed. Did you know anyone who lost weight and kept it off on one of those programs? Where are the programs now? How much would you bet that the miracle book that comes along next week, next month, or next year will be different than the rest—that it will deliver on what it promises and offer a final solution?

When it comes to nutrition, there is no magic, just common sense and rational eating. The key word to remember is *balanced*. This means eating a variety of foods from the different food groups. This may sound like what you learned in the sixth grade, but the message is just as important today.

The body needs a balance of nutrients. It does not function well with too little or too much of any nutrient. If your body needs a certain amount of Vitamin E each day, you will be worse off with one-half that amount or with 100 times more. This is similar to making your favorite cake. Each ingredient is important. One ingredient may give the cake a very good taste, but too much will ruin it.

Some clients in our clinic ask why nutrition is so important. The answer is simple. What we eat helps determine how healthy we are, which in turn influences how we cope with life both physically and psychologically. You could lose weight by eating nothing but grapefruit, but your body would suffer greatly from deficiencies in the nutrients grapefruit does not provide. How much you eat (calories) is only part of the answer. *How* you eat must also be considered.

You will notice that I say not a word about *forbidden* foods. I do not believe in prohibition for people losing weight. Such an approach is doomed to fail. If you like cheesecake, but feel it is illegal, you will eventually eat it and feel guilty. This will weaken your restraint even more. If you have the expectation that the first bite will send you into a frenzy and you will eat all the cheesecake in sight, you are setting yourself up to fall apart when you might otherwise have a little and be satisfied. It is fine to eat cheesecake, as long as it occurs within the guidelines for sensible nutrition.

The food guide pyramid

The pyramid is a graphic illustration of the research-based food guidance system developed jointly by the U.S. Department of Agriculture (USDA) and the Department of Health and Human Services (HHS). The following represent the dietary guidelines developed for Americans by the USDA and the HHS:

◆ **Eat a variety of foods.** Eating a variety of foods will help you to get the energy, protein, vitamins, minerals, and fiber you need for good health.

◆ **Maintain a healthy weight.** There are many studies that show maintaining a healthy weight will help reduce your chances of having high blood pressure, heart disease, certain cancers, a stroke, and the most common kind of diabetes.

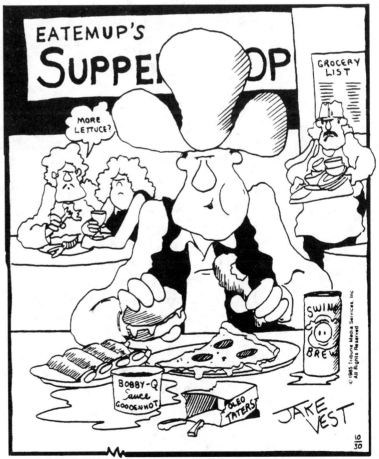

'A balanced meal has something from each of The Five Major Food Groups -- hamburgers, fried chicken, pizza, ribs and French fries.'

The Food Guide Pyramid

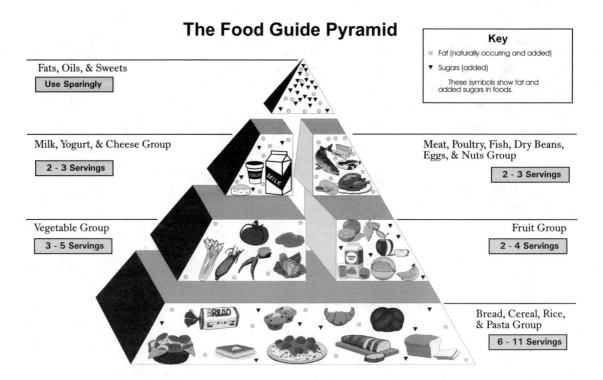

Key

○ Fat (naturally occuring and added)

▼ Sugars (added)

These symbols show fat and added sugars in foods.

Fats, Oils, & Sweets
Use Sparingly

Milk, Yogurt, & Cheese Group
2 - 3 Servings

Meat, Poultry, Fish, Dry Beans, Eggs, & Nuts Group
2 - 3 Servings

Vegetable Group
3 - 5 Servings

Fruit Group
2 - 4 Servings

Bread, Cereal, Rice, & Pasta Group
6 - 11 Servings

◆ **Choose a diet low in fat, saturated fat, and cholesterol.** Diets that are low in fat, saturated fat, and cholesterol may reduce your risk of heart attack and certain types of cancer. Fat contains more than twice the calories of an equal amount of carbohydrates or protein, so a diet low in fat can help you maintain a healthy weight.

◆ **Choose a diet with plenty of vegetables, fruits, and grain products.** These foods provide the essential vitamins, minerals, fiber, and complex carbohydrates. Since these foods are naturally low in dietary fat, they can help to lower your intake of fat.

◆ **Use sugars only in moderation.** A diet that includes high amounts of sugar has too many calories and may not provide the nutrients your body needs to be healthy. Too much sugar can also contribute to tooth decay.

◆ **Use salt in moderation.** A diet that is low in sodium can help reduce your risk of high blood pressure.

◆ **If you drink alcoholic beverages, do so in moderation.** Alcoholic beverages add calories, but provide little nutrition. Alcohol can also lead to many other health problems and may lead to addiction.

You can see from these dietary guidelines the key message is moderation. As we progress through the program these guidelines will become more and more familiar to you. Review each of the guidelines again and check to see how many you are now following. At this point in the program I want you to be familiar with the concepts and the guidelines so that you can be thinking of how they may apply to you and your eating habits.

A graphic illustration

The design of the Food Guide Pyramid divides foods into five separate groups as shown above. The pyramid also includes a category for fats, oils, and sweets. Each group in the pyramid includes suggested daily servings which are listed beside the groups. Small circles are used throughout the pyramid to identify food groups that contain high-fat foods, and triangles are used to identify foods that have added sugars.

At the top of the pyramid is the section containing foods that should be eaten sparingly. It should not be surprising that this smallest section consists of fats, oils, and sweets. As the food groups progress toward the bottom of the pyramid they become a larger part of your diet. For instance, the bread and cereal group is the largest section, and foods from this group should make up the largest portion of your daily diet.

Many things we eat are a mixture of foods from the five groups. Pizza, for example, has bread (dough), vegetables (tomatoes, peppers, etc.), cheese, and meat in some cases. A chicken pot pie has pastry, vegetables, meat, etc. You will become an expert at identifying the components of combination dishes.

In this lesson, I want you to become familiar with the five food groups in the pyramid. This graphic will become more familiar to you as you continue through the program. In the lessons that follow, I will describe in more detail each tier of the pyramid. At this point in the program do not be concerned with the number of servings you should be eating from the various food groups or how much food it takes to make one serving. I will discuss this and other information about each of the five food groups in later lessons. For now, be aware of the five different food groups and try to include each group into your diet. In your Monitoring Form this week, note whether you are eating foods from all five food groups.

The Food Guide Pyramid is a useful way to see that you get balanced nutrition, but it is possible to follow the guide and still take in too many calories to lose weight. Eating the recommended number of servings will generally help the average person maintain their weight, but you want to reduce, so the number of servings will have to be reduced. As you find the level of calories you need to lose weight, you will be able to adjust the number of servings from the pyramid.

In thinking about good nutrition while losing weight, both the Food Guide Pyramid and a means of counting calories are important.

Within the number of calories you budget for yourself each day, try to choose the right balance of servings across the food groups in the pyramid.

Selecting an eating plan: calorie counting vs. exchange plan

There are several available plans for eating nutritiously. One prevailing plan is to count calories while eating a specified number of servings in the five food groups. This approach is one many individuals are familiar with because counting calories is the way most people learn to judge how they are doing with a weight-loss plan. This is the approach used in this program. I introduce it in this lesson and then expand on it in the lessons that follow.

An excellent alternative eating plan is the Exchange Plan developed by the American Dietetic Association (ADA) and the American Diabetes Association. The exchange plan places food into six categories: starch/bread, meat and meat substitutes, vegetables, fruit, milk, and fat. Within each category, amounts of foods are provided so that in the amount listed, all foods have approximately the same carbohydrate, protein, fat, and calories. A food in a given category, therefore, can be exchanged with any other food in the same category. Copies of the exchange list guide are available for $1.50 each plus $4.95 shipping & handling. If you would like to receive a complete guide for the exchange plan, you can call 800-745-0775 or write to:

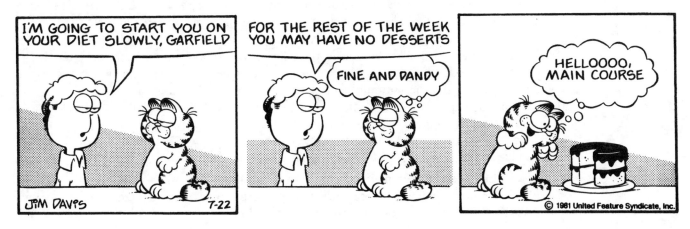

The American Dietetic Association

P.O. Box 97215

Chicago, IL 60678-7215

Both the calorie counting and exchange plans represent sound nutrition. If you are in a program run by a health professional, he or she may have a preference, so both plans are provided here. Otherwise, choose the plan you feel best meets your needs, and then follow it throughout the program. If you choose the exchange plan over the calorie counting approach, you can obtain a copy from the American Dietetic Association as outlined above.

Solo and social changing

Individuals come in many packages with many personalities. Some like to make changes on their own and do not want other people involved. Others like the aid and support they might get from family and friends. I call the first group *solo* changers and the other group social changers.

Solo changers like to travel the weight-loss path alone. They often do not tell others when they go on a program. They do not enjoy questions about their weight or their eating. No other person knows their weight. Social changers, on the other hand, like company. They talk with others about their program and are pleased when others notice their progress. They might join a program with a friend, or enlist someone in the family to exercise.

Being a social changer is fine. Being a solo changer is fine. What is important is to determine which type best fits you and to structure your program accordingly. There is much material in this manual about enlisting the aid of family and friends. This is likely to help the social person but not a solo type. Solo changers can be upset when others attempt to assist them, even when the assistance is offered for the right reasons.

Think about whether you are social or solo person. If you are social, the "Relationships" part of The LEARN Program may be helpful, starting with the information on partners in the next section. Think of support from oth-

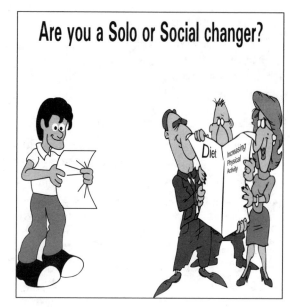

Are you a Solo or Social changer?

ers as a resource to be cultivated. If you are a solo person, decide exactly when and how you would like others to be involved. Support from others is a resource only if you find it helpful. There are many other resources at your disposal.

Would a partner help?

Program partnerships can be very powerful. They occur when a person enlists the aid of another. Sometimes the partner is also on a program, but fine partnerships can occur when the partner is thin. How can you tell if a partnership is for you?

First, there are different types of partnerships. The most logical one is with a spouse. A husband or wife can be a real aid, but not in all cases. Many of my clients have formed successful partnerships with co-workers, good friends, neighbors, or relatives.

You may already have a partner in mind. In Lesson Five, you can complete the Partnership Quiz to determine whether this person would be a good choice. In this lesson, you can decide whether your personality is best suited for a partnership or a solo program.

A program partnership is much like a friendship. It is based on give and take. All the support does not flow from the partner to you. You must reciprocate. There will be good times and bad. Some energy is required to keep the partnership intact, as with any relationship.

Do you think you would profit from a partnership? While you decide, let me explain what scientific studies have shown. There have been about 20 studies on partnership programs, including several that I have conducted with my colleagues. In some studies, working with a partner greatly increased weight loss. In others, there was no advantage to the partnership approach. I interpret these inconsistent findings to show that losing weight with a partner is helpful for some, but not for all.

Several examples may illustrate how others can help or hurt. Marjorie enlisted the aid of her husband in her program. He was supportive and showed his concern by walking with her and by not eating treats when she was around. This encouragement helped Marjorie.

Sharon's case was different. Her husband made fun of her and was bitter about her weight problem. He ate in front of her and was nearly always discouraging in his comments. It would have been destructive for Sharon to engage her husband in a partnership. Only you know whether this approach will work for you.

Think about having a weight-loss partner. Remember, this person does not have to be overweight. It is important that you feel comfortable with this person and that they are able to motivate you. Next, think about your own style and personality. Do you like to do things with others or alone? Can you confide in others or do you keep things to yourself? Could you discuss weight-control troubles with another person or would you rather not share them? Finally, what is your *gut* feeling? Do you think the partnership approach would work for you?

You will have time to ponder these important matters, because guidelines for starting a partnership will appear in the next lesson. Think about your own style and decide if a partnership would help. Sort through your friendships and form a pool of possible partners. The partnership may work for you. Do not feel guilty if you are a *solo* person. Many people do best this way.

Your target calorie level

Back in Lesson Two, you began experimenting with caloric intake to identify the level at which you will lose weight at the recommended rate (one to two pounds per week). Look back now to Lesson Two to see what calorie level you selected as your *best guess*.

Now that you are several lessons wiser and have had more experience with your body's response to making changes, it is time to select a more official Target Calorie Level. Enter this number in the space provided below. In the new Monitoring Form you will be using (see page 62), you will be recording whether you meet your calorie goal each day. The forms have a space for you to complete the following item: "Less than _____ Calories." The blank spaces are where you fill in your Target Calorie Level. Remember, this is to be the calorie level at which you will lose one to two pounds each week. The number can be modified as you progress through the program.

Introducing a new monitoring form

This lesson ushers in a new Monitoring Form. An example of a completed form appears at the end of this lesson. The new form has three sections. The section on the top is to record food intake, time, and calories, just as you have done with the Food Diary. There are no longer separate sections for breakfast, lunch, dinner, and snacks. List foods in the order you eat them. This will be a part of the Monitoring Form for the remainder of the program—that's how important it is.

The middle portion of the new form is for recording the behavior changes prescribed for each lesson. For this week, the prescribed activities are:

❶ Note the ABC's of eating
❷ Increase walking
❸ Set realistic goals
❹ Eat from the five food groups
❺ Eat less than _____ calories.

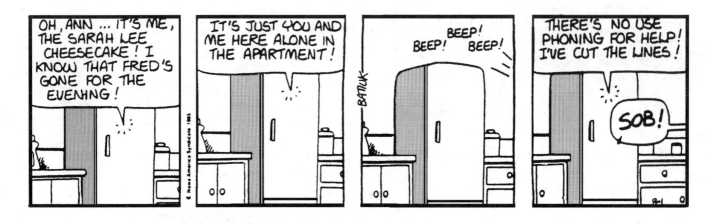

You simply mark down whether you follow the recommended behavior always, sometimes, or never. Different behaviors will be listed for each lesson.

Some of the techniques you will be trying will be listed under the *Always, Sometimes, or Never* part of the Monitoring Form, even though the behaviors do not fit neatly in these categories. For example, in Lesson Seven you will be encouraged to *shop from a list* to avoid impulse buying. However, most people do not shop for food each day, so it is difficult to note on the Monitoring Form each day whether you shopped from a list always, sometimes, or never. In cases like this, put NA (for Not Applicable), if *Always, Sometimes,* or *Never* do not apply.

The third section, on the bottom, is to keep a record of your physical activity and for keeping track of the number of servings you eat daily from the five food groups. The number of boxes by each food group is the daily recommended number of servings. In the lessons that follow, I will discuss the five food groups of The Food Guide Pyramid in more detail. There are also spaces for the type of exercise you do and the number of minutes you do it. This section will also be part of the form from now on. List everything here, like using stairs more than usual, working in the yard, walking, and playing sports.

Assignment for this lesson

This lesson covered several concepts. The first was the ABC approach of Antecedents, Behavior, and Consequences. Try to pinpoint each in preparation for techniques discussed in the next lesson. The second concept was shaping, which we applied by setting realistic goals. Make note of your goals and examine whether they are realistic. The time you spend walking can be increased by at least five minutes, unless you have difficulty. Use the procedures described in this lesson for making walking pleasurable. We also covered the essentials of a balanced diet and briefly discussed the five food groups from The Food Guide Pyramid. Use your monitoring form to learn whether you eat from the five food groups.

Self-assessment questionnaire

Lesson Four

T F 17. The ABC approach stands for Alternatives, Behavior, and Consciousness.

T F 18. Shaping refers to encouraging others to help you lose weight.

T F 19. The five food groups are Milk and Yogurt Products, Vegetables, Fruits, Meats and Proteins, and Breads and Cereals.

T F 20. Ice cream and several other high-sugar desserts are not allowed on this program.

(Answers in Appendix C)

Monitoring Form—Lesson Four *(sample)*   *Today's Date:*

Time	Food and Amount	Calories
7:15	Apple juice, ½ cup (4 oz)	58
	Special K cereal, 1 ⅓ cups (1 oz)	111
	Skim milk, 4 oz	43
12:30 pm	Club sandwich	590
	Orange, 1 med	65
	Coffee, black (4 oz)	0
6:30 pm	Broiled chicken breast, w/o skin (3 oz)	148
	Broccoli, steamed (1 cup)	46
	Butter, 1t	36
	French bread, 1 slice	81
	Ice tea	0
9:10 pm	Celery, 3 stalks	18
	Skim milk, 8 oz	86
	Total Daily Calories	*1,282*

Assignment this week		Always	Sometimes	Never
1.	Note ABCs of eating		✓	
2.	Increase walking	✓		
3.	Set realistic goals		✓	
4.	Eat from the five food groups		✓	
5.	Less than calories each day	✓		

Food Groups for Today		Physical Activity	Minutes
Milk, yogurt, and cheese	☑ ☑ ☐		
Meat, poultry, etc.	☑ ☑ ☐		
Fruits	☑ ☑ ☐ ☐		
Vegetables	☑ ☑ ☑ ☐ ☐		
Breads, cereals, etc.	☑ ☑ ☑ ☑ ☐ ☐ ☐ ☐ ☐		

Monitoring Form—Lesson Four

Today's Date:

Time	Food and Amount	Calories
Total Daily Calories		

Assignment this week	*Always*	*Sometimes*	*Never*
1. Note ABCs of eating			
2. Increase walking			
3. Set realistic goals			
4. Eat from the five food groups			
5. Less than _____ calories each day			

Food Groups for Today	*Physical Activity*	*Minutes*
Milk, yogurt, and cheese ❑ ❑ ❑		
Meat, poultry, etc. ❑ ❑ ❑		
Fruits ❑ ❑ ❑ ❑		
Vegetables ❑ ❑ ❑ ❑ ❑		
Breads, cereals, etc. ❑ ❑ ❑ ❑ ❑ ❑ ❑ ❑ ❑		

Wℯ now move to a discussion of the situations which control eating. We will discuss physical activities that can become part of your routine, and I will give you a chart showing the number of calories you burn for various activities. The issue of food fantasies will be covered, and you will be able to take the Partnership Quiz to determine who would be a good weight-loss program partner. Finally, I will cover more about eating a balanced diet using the food guide pyramid and discuss what makes up a serving from each of the five food groups.

Taking control of your eating

The Monitoring Forms have helped you discover patterns in your eating, but you have probably had your fill of discovery and would like to do something! Your patience will be rewarded, because we are about to cover several of the classic steps in behavior modification.

Many people have situations, times, or activities that stimulate eating. These events become *paired* with eating so that the event can make you feel hungry. Here are a few examples. You may read the paper every day at breakfast. You may watch television every evening and have a snack. You may always eat when you sit in a certain chair. If eating is paired repeatedly with these events, the events can make you feel like eating. If you sit in your chair, watch TV, or read the morning paper, you will feel like eating, irrespective of physical hunger.

It is important to separate eating from other activities. This will remove the ability of these activities to stimulate eating, freeing you to respond to actual hunger. There are several ways to make this happen. I will present four such techniques below.

Do nothing else while eating

You may be one of those individuals who does other things while eating. It could be working on a hobby, talking on the phone, writing letters, watching TV, reading a maga-zine, and so forth. This has two disadvantages. The first is mentioned above; eating can become paired with other activities. Second, the activity distracts you from eating, so you get all the calories and only part of the pleasure.

Calories should be tasted, not wasted

Many a monitoring form shows people who eat half a bag of popcorn, 45 Fritos, 22 pretzels, or three-quarters of a pound of mixed nuts. Many of the calories are wasted, not tasted. The following rule will actually help you enjoy food more.

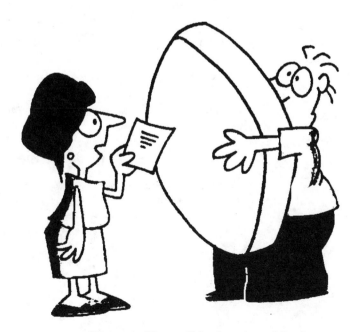

"It says, 'One pill before breakfast controls your appetite all day.'"

Do nothing else while eating,
and taste every bite.
Remember—calories
should be tasted, not wasted!

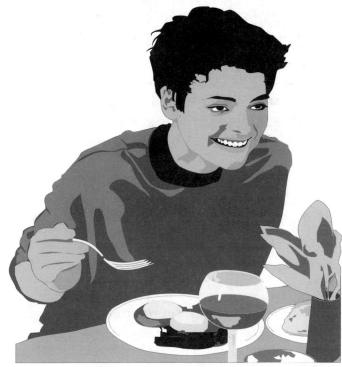

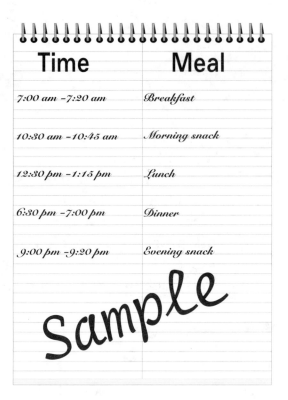

Time	Meal
7:00 am – 7:20 am	Breakfast
10:30 am – 10:45 am	Morning snack
12:30 pm – 1:15 pm	Lunch
6:30 pm – 7:00 pm	Dinner
9:00 pm – 9:20 pm	Evening snack

Sample

Do nothing else while eating

This means reading the paper at another time, eating before or after you watch TV, waiting to read the book, etc. Eating should be a pure experience. Don't contaminate it with extraneous activities. If this seems awkward, it is a sure sign that you are hooked on the association of eating with other activities. The more this technique bothers you, the more you need it.

Follow an eating schedule

You may have uncovered *time* patterns from your Monitoring Forms. If you eat many times each day, and if you always feel like eating at those times, a schedule will help. This does not necessarily mean three meals a day at conventional times. It does mean finding a schedule that is convenient for you.

Plan a schedule for your eating. If you eat breakfast at 7:00 a.m., put it in. If you have a mid-evening snack, add it (if necessary). Keep the number of times you eat under control.

This may involve eating three conventional meals, but remember to choose a plan you can tolerate.

Following a schedule will help you eat less and think more. You might have a snack planned at 9:00 p.m. If you feel like eating at 8:15, you can wait out the urge, and then see if you are still hungry at 9:00. You may get by with no snack at all! Above is an example of an eating schedule made by Judy, one of my clients.

The space on the next page contains blanks for you to plan your eating schedule. List the times and meals you can live with, and do your best to stick with the schedule. There will, of course, be times when you violate your schedule, but do your best. When you feel like eating at times other than your schedule permits, think carefully about whether you are hungry or are responding to associations of eating and other factors.

Eat in one place

There are some people who eat *anywhere*. They eat standing up, sitting down, at the kitchen counter, in an easy chair, lying in bed, or driving the car. They eat in the den, living room, bedroom, basement, and bathroom. One of my former clients even tied Oreo cookies in a bag and hung them with a rope out the window into the shrubs. She could eat with her head hanging out the window! Places can also be associated with eating, so it is important to limit the places you eat.

Here is a hypothetical example I use with my clients. Let's say that for the next ten years you came to my clinic every day to eat a delicious meal while seated in a yellow chair. At the same time, we would have a chair in your home where no eating would occur. After the ten years and 3650 meals, your response to the two chairs would be quite different. You would feel hungry in the yellow chair even after eating. This would not happen in the chair at home.

Select one place in your home where you will eat. Do *all* your eating there, but *do nothing else.* Do not use the place to play chess, pay the bills, or plot a way to beat the stock market or win the lottery.

Do not clean your plate

It is time to turn the tables on your plate. Until now, you may have been a slave to the rule issued by every mother, "Clean Your Plate!" It is nice to avoid wasting food, but think for a minute of the folly in cleaning your plate.

When you eat everything on the plate, you are at the mercy of the person doing the serving. Unless the person has mystical powers and knows your body's energy requirements, you will be served too much or too little. Given our cultural tendency to overdo it, you will usually be served more than enough. If you clean your plate, you are responding to the *sight* of food, and eating stops only when no more food is in sight. When you serve yourself, remember that you do so *before* you

My Eating Schedule	
Time	**Meal**

have eaten, so you might be inclined to serve large amounts.

You can exert control by breaking the habit of cleaning your plate. Try to leave some food on your plate each time you eat. Leave only small portions if you like (two peas or one bite of mashed potatoes), but leave a bit of everything. You can ask for second servings, but only if you are really hungry. This puts *you* in control of what you eat, not the chef.

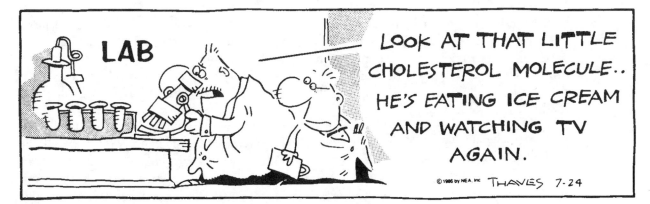

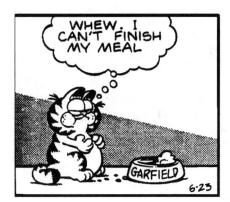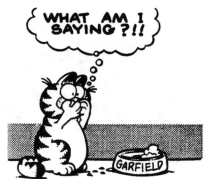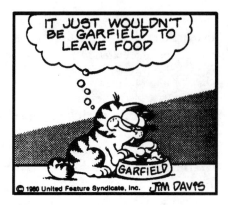

Making physical activity count

It is time to distinguish between *lifestyle* and *programmed* activity. Lifestyle activity is simple and can be done in your day-to-day routine. An example would be using stairs rather than an elevator when you go to work. Programmed activity is a traditional exercise regimen of jogging, biking, aerobics, racquetball, and so forth. I will discuss programmed activities beginning with Lesson Six. For now, let us consider lifestyle activities.

Lifestyle activity

You can imagine the virtues of lifestyle activity. It is easy, takes little time, does not hurt, does not require special clothes or equipment, and can become habit with little effort. It makes you feel better both psychologically and physically.

The idea here is to sneak in activity whenever possible. The suggestions that follow may help you get started with another part of the assignment for this lesson—*Increase Your Lifestyle Activity*.

Use stairs

Stairs can be a good friend because they are so readily available. Climbing stairs burns more calories per minute than rigorous activities like jogging and cycling. If you work on the fifth floor of a building, take the elevator to the fourth floor and walk the remaining flight. As your condition improves, get off on lower floors. One of my favorite examples is a client who lived in a two-story house with bathrooms on each floor. She decided to use the bathroom on the floor where she wasn't located, which gave her several extra trips per day up and down the stairs.

Park further

When you drive to the mall, don't circle around like a vulture in search of a spot by the door. Park where only the people with new cars pull in—away from the crowd.

Walk more

If you take the bus downtown, get off one or two stops early and walk the extra distance. If someone gives you a ride to the store, have them drop you off a few blocks away. At home, take things up the stairs in several trips instead of letting them accumulate for one trip.

Make it count

Count everything you do as exercise. When you do housework, turn on a timer and keep moving. Use the vacuum an extra day each week. Time yourself as you wash the car, rake the leaves, or mow the lawn. You will be surprised how fast the minutes go by, and you will accomplish another task as well.

The beauty of these small bouts of activity is that each one provides an opportunity for you to feel virtuous—to be reinforced for doing something positive. And this is not just a trick—you really are doing something positive. Anything you do to be more active is beneficial and you should acknowledge it as such. You deserve a pat on the back whenever you make an effort to do something good, and you're the closest one around to do it. My hope is that you will count yourself among the ranks of people who consider themselves exercisers. This can build on itself to the point where you are feeling much better about your body and your physical condition. It doesn't take much to notice improvement.

These are just examples of the general *principle* of increasing lifestyle activity. Think of more methods to fit your own routine. The section that follows, on the calorie values of exercise, may give you more ideas. Be sure to record your lifestyle activities on your Monitoring Form. You deserve credit for doing these activities, so they should show up in your records.

Tracking your progress with activity

When you are making positive changes, it is important to *feel* like you are making progress and to reinforce yourself accordingly. To do this, it can help to have a way of assessing how you are doing. The activity section on the monitoring forms at the end of each lesson are an excellent place to begin, but some people like to do more.

Some people like to keep a graph or a log of when they are active. Either could include the number of minutes being active, how fast you do some activity (like walking a certain distance), or how far the activity takes you (distance). Another helpful index of progress can be to use a pedometer. These are available in sporting goods stores and have been refined in the last several years to be much more accurate than earlier models. Some devices measure how far you walk and others give the number of steps you take. The ones with the number of steps are nice because you can see evidence of even small increases in activity.

There are individuals I have worked with who set up reward systems for themselves by making a contract. The contract states that certain rewards (e.g., a movie, a new CD, clothing, etc.) will be rewards for attaining a certain level of activity. These are fine, but whether or not you have a reward system, it is important to track your activity so you have a sense of how much you are improving. This helps you feel virtuous when you deserve it.

The calorie values of physical activity

How many calories do you burn when you wash the dishes? Is it more than when you rake leaves? Is it easier to burn calories by swimming, jogging, or cycling? Your questions will be answered in the table on the next page.

Several important points are highlighted by the calorie chart. First, *any* activity uses energy (calories), so any increase in activity can help. Sitting uses approximately 15 calories per ten minutes, while standing uses 17, and walking briskly uses 60. Even something as simple as standing rather than sitting can use a few extra calories. Second, heavier people burn more calories than other people while doing the same activity, because more energy is required to move the extra weight. Third, several routine activities like using stairs and walking are useful methods of burning calories.

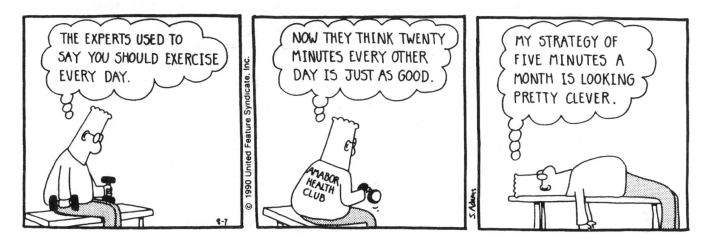

67

Calorie Values for 10 Minutes of Activity

Activity	Body Weight 125 Pounds	175 Pounds	250 Pounds	Activity	Body Weight 125 Pounds	175 Pounds	250 Pounds
Personal Necessities				*Light Work*			
Sleeping	10	14	20	Assembly line	20	28	40
Sitting (watching TV)	10	14	18	Auto repair	35	48	69
Sitting (talking)	15	21	30	Carpentry	32	44	64
Dressing or washing	26	37	53	Bricklaying	28	40	57
Standing	12	16	24	Framing chores	32	44	64
Locomotion				House painting	29	40	58
Walking downstairs	56	78	111	*Heavy Work*			
Walking upstairs	146	202	288	Pick & shovel work	56	78	110
Walking at 2 mph	29	40	58	Chopping wood	60	84	121
Walking at 4 mph	52	72	102	Dragging logs	158	220	315
Running at 5.5 mph	90	125	178	Drilling coal	79	111	159
Running at 7 mph	118	164	232	*Recreation*			
Running at 12 mph	164	228	326	Badminton	43	65	94
Cycling at 5.5 mph	42	58	83	Baseball	39	54	78
Cycling at 13 mph	89	124	178	Basketball	58	82	117
Housework				Bowling (nonstop)	56	78	111
Making beds	32	46	65	Canoeing (4 mph)	90	128	182
Washing floors	38	53	75	Dancing (moderate)	35	48	69
Washing windows	35	48	69	Dancing (vigorous)	48	66	94
Dusting	22	31	44	Football	69	96	137
Preparing a Meal	32	46	65	Golfing	33	48	68
Shoveling snow	65	89	130	Horseback riding	56	78	112
Light gardening	30	42	59	Ping-Pong	32	45	64
Weeding garden	49	68	98	Racquetball	75	104	144
Mowing grass (power)	34	47	67	Skiing (alpine)	80	112	160
Mowing grass (manual)	38	52	74	Skiing (cross country)	98	138	194
Sedentary Occupation				Skiing (water)	60	88	130
Sitting (writing)	15	21	30	Squash	75	104	144
Light office work	25	34	50	Swimming (backstroke)	32	45	64
Standing, light activity	20	28	40	Swimming (crawl)	40	56	80
Typing (electric)	19	27	39	Tennis	56	80	115
				Volleyball	43	65	94

Several facts must be considered when viewing these calorie figures. One is that calorie expenditures vary enormously for many activities, depending on their intensity. Two people shoveling snow may differ greatly in how quickly they shovel, how much snow is lifted with each shovel, and how much they move around while shoveling. Similar differences can occur with skiing, tennis, yard work, and so forth. Therefore, the figures in the tables are only averages.

The second fact is that the table shows the calories burned for ten minutes of continuous activity. If you do an activity for five minutes, divide the value in the table by two. If you are active for 30 minutes, multiply the value by three.

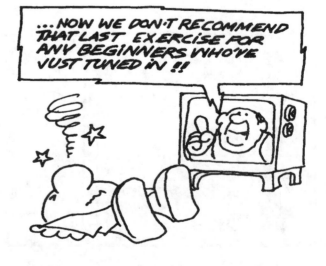

...NOW WE DON'T RECOMMEND THAT LAST EXERCISE FOR ANY BEGINNERS WHO'VE JUST TUNED IN !!

The word *continuous* is important to understanding the table. The table shows that a 125 pound person burns 56 calories for ten minutes of bowling. This is ten minutes of nonstop bowling and does not include time to keep score, chat with friends, polish your ball, or visit the snack bar. The ten minutes for skiing would not include time waiting in the lift line, marveling at the scenery, or falling down! So, to calculate the calories you burn for a given activity, add the time you are truly active, and then use the table on the previous page as a guide.

Food and weight fantasies

Many individuals have fantasies of foods. It is common, for example, to fantasize about having a *celebration* or *letting go* meal when the program ends. Some people even think about specific foods or the ability to eat large quantities again. There are also common weight fantasies. These usually are visions of a sleek body and huge weight losses.

Food or weight fantasies are a sign of unrealistic expectations. Weight loss is not easy, and pounds do not fly off as we'd like. Food fantasies reveal an expectation that the rigors of going through a program will end some magic day and that old eating habits will return.

We must keep up what we learn. You can eat your favorite foods now and will be able to eat them later. You will not, however, be able to return to uncontrolled eating. Identify what you want to eat, and eat a small quantity in a controlled manner. Most of all, *enjoy it*. By not overeating, you will not feel guilty, and by eating a small portion you will not feel resentful.

A quiz for choosing a partner

I promised in the last lesson to give you a quiz for evaluating whether a person would make a good partner to go through the program with you. Your job was to think of possible partners and then to use the quiz to make a final decision.

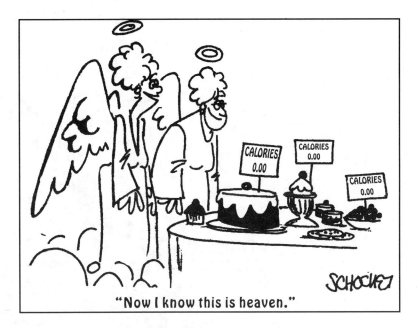

"Now I know this is heaven."

Partnership Quiz

____ 1. It is easy to talk to my partner about weight.
         True—5   False—1

____ 2. My partner has always been thin and does not understand my weight problem.
         True—1   False—3

____ 3. My partner offers me food when he or she knows I am trying to lose weight.
         True—1   False—5

____ 4. My partner never says critical things about my weight.
         True—3   False—1

____ 5. My partner is always there when I need a friend.
         True—4   False—1

____ 6. When I lose weight and look better, my partner will be jealous.
         True—1   False—3

____ 7. My partner will be genuinely interested in helping me with my weight.
         True—6   False—1

____ 8. I could talk to my partner even if I was doing poorly.
         True—5   False—1

If you scored between 30 and 34, you may have found the perfect partner. A score in this range indicates that you and this person are comfortable with one another and can work together.

If you scored between 25 and 29, your friend is potentially a good partner, but there are a few areas of concern. Try asking the partner to take the quiz and predict how you answered the questions. This may help you make a decision.

If you scored between 17 and 24, there are potential areas of conflict, and a program partnership with this person could encounter stormy going. Think of another partner.

The Food Guide Pyramid

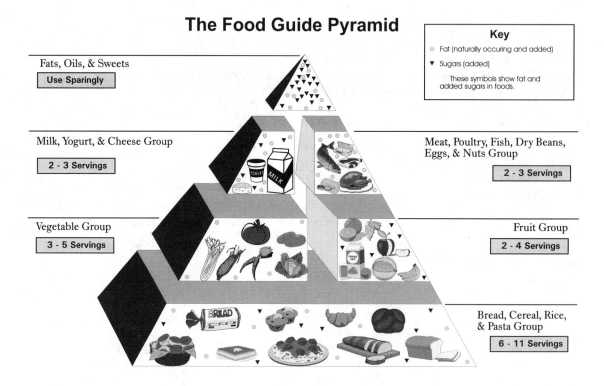

Key
- Fat (naturally occuring and added)
- ▼ Sugars (added)

These symbols show fat and added sugars in foods.

Fats, Oils, & Sweets
Use Sparingly

Milk, Yogurt, & Cheese Group
2 - 3 Servings

Meat, Poultry, Fish, Dry Beans, Eggs, & Nuts Group
2 - 3 Servings

Vegetable Group
3 - 5 Servings

Fruit Group
2 - 4 Servings

Bread, Cereal, Rice, & Pasta Group
6 - 11 Servings

To take this quiz, think of the person you would have as a partner, and answer the questions honestly. First, answer each question either true or false. Beside each of your answers is a number. Write this number in the space provided immediately before each question number. Add the numbers of your responses, then use the scoring guide at the bottom of the quiz.

These guidelines should help in choosing a partner. Once you have done so, discuss the possibility with the person you have in mind. The next lesson will bring specific suggestions on how to proceed.

Let me stress again that you need not have a partner. The decision is left to you. If you do decide on the partner approach, these questions could help in selecting a supportive partner. If you are uncertain about proceeding with a partner, even after taking the quiz, experiment with it. Use what you learn about partnerships to see if you profit from the aid of another person. If not, consider yourself a solo changer and move ahead.

Servings from the five food groups

The five food groups of the food guide pyramid were introduced in Lesson Four. One of your assignments for Lesson Four was to note whether you are eating foods from the five groups. We can now be more specific about the number of servings to have every day. First, we need to know what constitutes a serving. A serving from each group can be defined as the amount shown on the next page.

It is important to select the correct number of servings from each group to insure the right mix of nutrients. Look again at the graphic illustration of the Food Guide Pyramid (see next page). As we continue through the program, the pyramid will become a familiar friend. The average number of servings per day recommended for *adults* are listed in the graph. Use this as a guide to structure your diet. Do your best to eat the recommended number of servings every day. We will focus on each of the groups in latter lessons, and I will provide you with lists of servings from each group.

The Food Guide Pyramid

Milk, Yogurt, and Cheese

☞ 1 cup of milk or yogurt

☞ 1½ ounces of natural cheese

☞ 2 ounces of process cheese

Meat, Poultry, Fish, Dry Beans, Eggs, and Nuts

☞ 2–3 ounces of cooked lean meat, poultry, or fish (a 3-ounce piece of meat is about the size of an average hamburger, or the amount of meat on a medium chicken breast half)

☞ Count ½ cup of cooked dry beans, 1 egg, or 2 tablespoons of peanut butter as 1 ounce of meat (about ⅓ serving)

Vegetables

☞ 1 cup of raw leafy vegetables ½ cup of other vegetables, cooked or chopped, raw

☞ ¾ cup of vegetable juice

Fruits

☞ A medium apple, banana, or orange ½ cup of chopped, cooked, or canned fruit

☞ ¾ cup of fruit juice

Bread, Cereal, Rice, and Pasta

☞ 1 slice of bread

☞ 1 ounce of ready-to-eat cereal

☞ ½ cup of cooked cereal, rice, or pasta

Assignment for this lesson

Your Monitoring Form lists your assignments for this lesson. These are:

❶ Do nothing else while eating
❷ Eat on a planned schedule
❸ Eat in one place
❹ Leave some food on your plate
❺ Increase your lifestyle activity
❻ Eat the specified number of servings from the five food groups of the Food Guide Pyramid

Self-assessment questionnaire

Lesson Five

T F 21. Cleaning your plate is harmful because the server decides how much you will eat.

T F 22. Climbing stairs requires more energy per minute than many traditional exercises like swimming and jogging.

T F 23. If you eat an equal number of servings from the five food groups of the Food Guide Pyramid, you will have a balanced diet.

T F 24. Eating on a schedule is not advisable because it is too regimented.

(Answers in Appendix C)

Monitoring Form—Lesson Five   *Today's Date:*

Time	Food and Amount	Calories
	Total Daily Calories	

Assignment this week	Always	Sometimes	Never
1. Nothing else while eating			
2. Follow an eating schedule			
3. Eat in one place			
4. Leave food on your plate			
5. Record lifestyle activity			
6. Servings from the five food groups			
7. Less than _____ calories each day			

Food Groups for Today	Physical Activity	Minutes
Milk, yogurt, and cheese ❑ ❑ ❑		
Meat, poultry, etc. ❑ ❑ ❑		
Fruits ❑ ❑ ❑ ❑		
Vegetables ❑ ❑ ❑ ❑ ❑		
Breads, cereals, etc. ❑ ❑ ❑ ❑ ❑ ❑ ❑ ❑ ❑		

You have had a thorough introduction to the five components of the LEARN program. We continue on our path by dealing with your speed of eating, more on lifestyle activity, communication with a partner, and the role of fat in your diet.

Slowing your eating rate

Could you qualify for the Olympic speed eating trials? Many people, both heavy and thin, eat so fast that their taste buds see only a blur as the food speeds by. This minimizes the enjoyment of food. More importantly, eating rapidly can fool your body's defense against eating too much.

Your body has an internal satiety (fullness) mechanism. When you have eaten enough, the mechanism sends out signals saying "Enough is enough!" We think this takes about 20 minutes, although this is a very complex process involving the stomach, hormones in the small intestine, brain chemicals, and other factors. If you eat rapidly, you will consume too much food before the mechanism kicks in. You will outpace your body's internal controls.

Slowing down eating can be like halting a runaway freight train. You have had many meals in your life, so the habit of eating fast can be practiced thousands of times. Be patient and practice the following techniques until the old patterns are replaced by new ones.

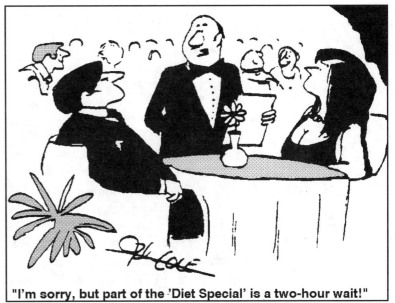

"I'm sorry, but part of the 'Diet Special' is a two-hour wait!"

Techniques to slow your eating

There are two main ways to slow your eating. Both can help put the brakes on eating and can increase the enjoyment of food.

Put your fork down between bites. When you take a bite of food, put your fork down, chew the food completely, swallow, and then pick up the fork for another bite. Do the same with a spoon, and if you are eating finger foods like a sandwich, put the food down between bites.

Pause during the meal. Take a break during your meal. Start with a brief pause, of perhaps 30 seconds. Gradually increase the time to one, then two, and finally three minutes. This pause gives you time to reflect on what you have eaten, so you can make a conscious decision to proceed with more. This may also help you eat less. One study with animals found that interrupting the meal led to fewer total calories, even though the animals could eat all they wanted after the break.

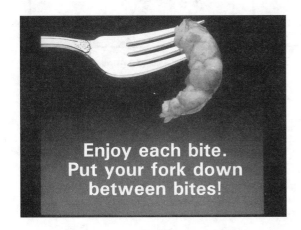

Enjoy each bite.
Put your fork down
between bites!

An impressive reason to be active

Previously, I mentioned that people who are regularly active tend to lose weight better *over the long-term*. Scientists have used nearly every known psychological and medical test to predict who will lose weight and keep it off. The most consistent finding is that exercise is associated with weight maintenance.

An impressive example of the research on this topic is a study by Kayman, Bruvold, and Stern published in the *American Journal of Clinical Nutrition*. They studied people in a large Health Maintenance Organization who had taken part in a weight-loss program. Many months after the program, the individuals were contacted to see what distinguished those who had maintained their weight losses from those who regained.

As the graph on the following page shows, exercise was a key factor. Of those who maintained their weight loss, 92 percent were getting regular physical activity. Only 34 percent of the regainers were exercising.

The effect of physical activity on weight maintenance could be occurring for many reasons. There may be physical effects on metabolism or other factors, but almost certainly the psychological advantages of activity are operating. When we are active, even in a modest way, we are doing something positive—we are making a statement to ourselves that we are committed to lifestyle change. This goes a long way in making a person feel good and in boosting confidence for weight control. So, if you are in this for the long run, regular physical activity is one of the best companions you can have.

Continuing walking and lifestyle activity

Let's review your progress with walking and lifestyle activity. This is a good time to look back at the section on the "Benefits of Exercise" from Lesson Two. As you may recall, being active brings many physical and emotional benefits. Two of the most important benefits, at this stage of your program, are that exercise may help control appetite and may bolster self-confidence.

Remember that exercise is one predictor of who will keep weight off over the long-run. On average, people who exercise are more likely to maintain their weight loss long after a program ends. There are exceptions, however.

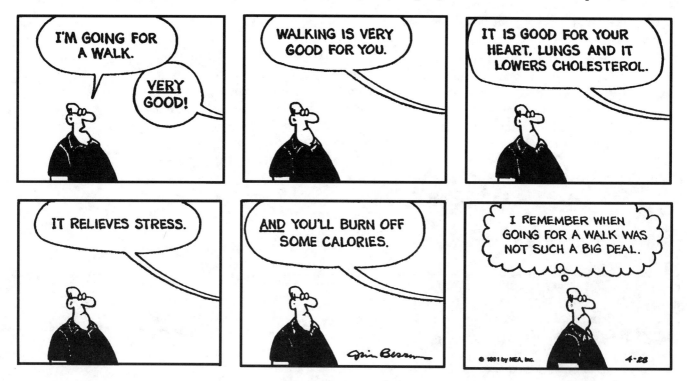

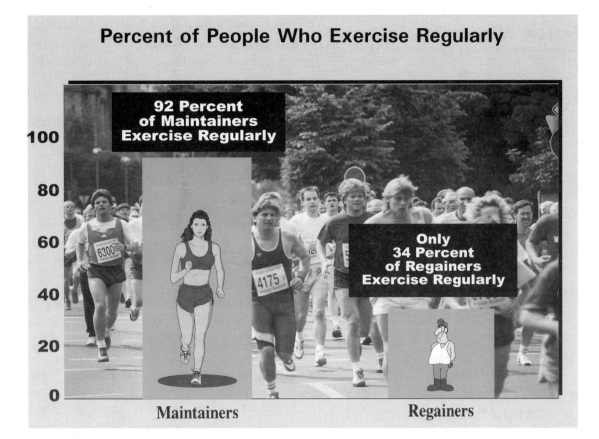

Percent of People Who Exercise Regularly

92 Percent of Maintainers Exercise Regularly

Only 34 Percent of Regainers Exercise Regularly

Maintainers   Regainers

Some people exercise and do not lose weight, and others lose weight without exercising. Where you fit in this scheme may not be evident for many months, but increasing your activity now may pay nice dividends later.

How much are you walking, and do you enjoy it? Lesson Four contained ideas for making walking pleasurable, so please review that material if you feel the ideas would help. You should be walking between 15 and 60 minutes each day. It is best to walk as much as possible without feeling discomfort. If you tire from walking, take several short walks rather than one long one. Having two brisk 30-minute walks or four 15-minute walks can help you as much as an hour walk in a single bout.

What types of lifestyle activities have you been doing? Have you found opportunities to use stairs, to park some distance from your destination, to do some extra walking? These lifestyle activities are nice because they remind us that we are doing something positive.

One reason I use the term *lifestyle* activity is the hope of developing permanent habits. Each trip up the stairs does not a pound lose, but summed over many days, months, or years, the effect can be powerful. New habits can be difficult to acquire, so it is important to practice, and then practice some more. Some of my clients say they now search out stairs wherever they go and feel that an opportunity is missed when they must use an elevator or escalator.

A pulse test for positive feedback

The Pulse Test is a simple means of feedback on your progress with exercise. The directions on the following page explain how to take your pulse and how to estimate your heart rate. Doing this every few weeks can reveal one important physical change due to exercise —a lower heart rate.

Your pulse, or heart rate, is the number of times your heart beats to supply the body with blood. A high pulse means that your heart must beat many times to do its job. A low pulse means the heart is in better condition and can do its job with less effort (fewer beats).

An example can illustrate the benefits of lowering your heart rate. Consider a woman whose resting heart rate is 75 beats per minute.

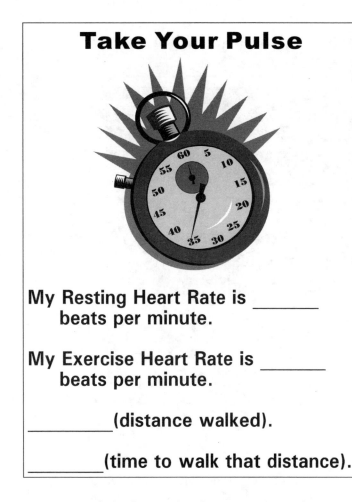

Take Your Pulse

My Resting Heart Rate is _____ beats per minute.

My Exercise Heart Rate is _____ beats per minute.

_____ (distance walked).

_____ (time to walk that distance).

If she lowers her heart rate to 70 beats per minute, her heart has five fewer beats to make each minute. This is 300 fewer beats per hour and 7200 fewer per day! By taking your pulse periodically, you can estimate the positive changes you make.

Before we move on to the actual Pulse Test, a few facts are important to mention. First, this is not a sophisticated exercise fitness evaluation that a cardiologist or exercise specialist would do. The numbers you estimate for your heart rate cannot be used to judge your overall fitness or your cardiovascular condition.

Second, some people improve their fitness in leaps and bounds but the Pulse Test shows no change in heart rate. This is particularly true of people who exercise regularly and/or have low heart rates. Beta-blocker drugs, which are prescribed for hypertension, lower heart rate so only small changes may be possible with exercise. Do not get discouraged if you walk like a real trooper and your pulse stays the same. You will be able to feel your

improvement in many other ways. For most people, however, the Pulse Test will detect changes in heart rate as their condition improves.

Steps for taking your pulse

❶ Select either wrist.

❷ Wrap fingers of other hand around back of the wrist.

❸ Press the index and middle fingers on the upturned wrist until you feel the regular pulsing of the blood through the vessel.

❹ Count the number of beats (pulses) in exactly 15 seconds.

❺ Multiply the number by four to calculate your beats per minute.

There are two times to take your pulse. The first is when you are at rest. Be still for at least five minutes, then take your pulse. The second time is during exercise. Do this during your walking program. Walk for at least three to four minutes at a comfortable pace. Stop walking, and take your pulse immediately. How rapidly your heart rate *recovers* to its resting level is one index of fitness. Write down the distance you walked, how long it took, and record your pulse rate.

Take your resting and exercise pulse rates as soon as possible, and write them in the spaces provided above. You can refer back to these figures as your condition improves. For the exercise figures, you should find improvements in the time it takes to walk a given distance, in heart rate, or in both. Take your pulse and write it down every two weeks. This will show your improvement over time.

Communicating with your partner

The Partnership Quiz from Lesson Five was designed to help you decide whether a partnership would help you, and if so, how to select an able partner. If you selected someone and have discussed the program with them, we can move to the next step.

In later lessons we will discuss methods for dealing with family and friends. This is different than a partnership where someone can be very involved with your program. With the family, there are more ways that support can be provided, and sabotage can be prevented. If you feel your family is a problem or can be a useful resource now, it may be helpful to read Lesson Ten. In the meantime, let's discuss partnerships.

Here are specific ideas for starting a program partnership. Communicating is the first and most important step. If you and your partner can communicate effectively, you are on the way to a successful partnership. Here are some ideas for making this happen.

It is essential that you and your partner talk together. Sit down and have a friendly talk with the person you have chosen as a partner. Discuss the topics below in an open and honest way.

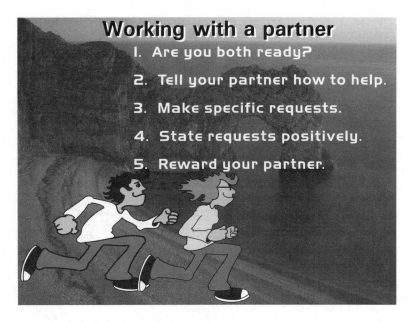

Working with a partner

1. Are you both ready?
2. Tell your partner how to help.
3. Make specific requests.
4. State requests positively.
5. Reward your partner.

- **Are you both ready for a partnership?** Is your partner ready to listen to requests for help and make the required effort? Is he or she ready to help you during good times and bad? Are you ready to help your partner in return? Some degree of commitment is necessary from both of you.

- **Tell your partner how to help.** A common and crucial mistake is to expect your partner to read your mind. If it is your spouse, you may think he or she should know what you want and need. Most people are not good mind readers, so leave nothing to chance. Tell your partner what he or she can do. Do you want to be praised when you do well or scolded when you do poorly? Should the person avoid eating in your presence? Can your partner help by exercising with you?

- **Make specific requests.** The more specific your requests, the easier it will be for your partner to comply. If your request is vague and general, like "Be nice," your partner is at a disadvantage. A more specific request is better, such as "Please tell me you love me when I lose weight." Instead of saying, "Don't eat in front of me," say "It helps me when you

eat your evening bowl of ice cream in the other room." Replace a general statement like, "Exercise with me" with "Please take a half-hour walk with me each morning."

- **State your requests positively.** It is better to ask for something positive than to criticize something negative. Clever changes of words can help. If your partner nags, you can say "It really helps me when you say nice things." If your partner offers you food, you can say "I appreciate the times when you don't offer me food. It is easier to control my eating then." Human nature responds well to the chance to do something positive, so try this approach with your partner.

- **Reward your partner.** For your partner to help you, you must help your partner. One-way relationships don't last long. If you are going through this program together, you can work out weight-control-related ways of helping. If your partner is not on a program, be forward, and ask what you can do in return. Remember, being a partner can be draining, so you need to acknowledge your partner's help.

Use these techniques to start the ball rolling with your partner. Upcoming lessons will give you more ideas for working with your partner. It is important to lay this ground work first.

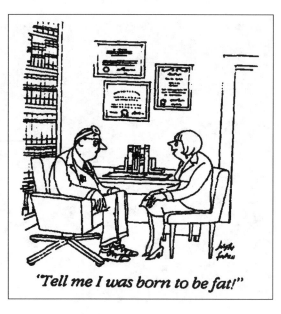

"Tell me I was born to be fat!"

The role of fat in your diet

Fat is what it's all about, right? You want to eat less fat and get rid of body fat. How are dietary fat and body fat different, and what role should fat play in your diet? You might think that fat is just what we see on meats and that it goes right to our store of body fat. The picture is more complex and is very interesting.

The importance of fat

Fat plays an important role in everyone's diet and has received a lot of attention lately due to its associations with heart disease and cancer. Dietary fat provides *essential* fatty acids that carry fat soluble vitamins (A,D,E, and K) throughout the body and a *semi-essential* fatty acid that helps to prevent growth deficiencies and build the membranes of cell walls. Fat in your body protects vital organs and prevents excessive heat loss. Fat is also a valuable source of energy, particularly for endurance activities; carbohydrate is used for quick energy. Fat also provides flavoring to many of the foods that we eat.

Our bodies can manufacture many of the essential fatty acids we need from carbohydrates or protein, however, there are some that it cannot make—these must be included in the food that we eat. The fat we eat is a combination of fatty acids and glycerol. All fats in foods are mixtures of three types of fatty acids: saturated, monounsaturated, and polyunsaturated. The fatty acids consist of carbon atoms that are attached to oxygen and hydrogen atoms. Each carbon atom has four possible binding sites. When the hydrogen/oxygen atoms are attached to all four binding sites, the fatty acid is *saturated* (i.e., the carbon atom is saturated with the maximum number of hydrogen/oxygen atoms). When the hydrogen/oxygen atoms are attached to less than all four binding sites, the fatty acid is said to be *unsaturated.* You can visually identify saturated fats because they are usually solid at room temperature and come primarily from meat and dairy products, although they are also found in some vegetable fats, such as coconut, palm and palm kernel oils.

When two nearby carbon atoms are each missing one molecule from one of their four binding sites, a double bond can be formed between the two atoms. When this happens the fat is considered to be *monounsaturated.* Monounsaturated fats are found mainly in olive, peanut, and canola oils. If more than one double bond is formed, the fat is said to be *polyunsaturated.* Polyunsaturated fats are generally liquid or soft at room temperature and are found mainly in safflower, sunflower, corn, soybean, and cottonseed oils and some fish.

This distinction between saturated and unsaturated fats is important for health reasons. Again, the saturated fats are easy to distinguish because they are usually solid at room temperature and come primarily from animal sources (butter, lard, meat). High consumption of these fats has been associated with heart disease and is likely related to risk for colon and breast cancers.

On the other hand, polyunsaturated fats are usually liquid or soft at room temperature and are from vegetable sources (vegetable oils, margarine). These are healthier than the saturated fats. This is why so many people have switched from butter to margarine, reduced their intake of high-fat meats like beef and pork, and cook more with vegetable oils. The best unsaturated oils are corn, soy, sunflower, and safflower (the most highly unsaturated oil). A noteworthy point is that all fats contain the same number of calories.

How much fat should I eat?

There are three basic facts to remember for your diet. The first is that fat provides a lot of energy, which is bad news for a person trying to lose weight. Fat contains twice the calories (nine per gram) than either protein or carbohydrate. You will get more calories from the fat on a single steak than from an equal amount of pure sugar.

Second, the amount of fat you eat is associated with risk for several serious diseases. The average American gets close to 40 percent of total calories from fat. It is recommended that this be reduced to no more than 30 percent. Saturated fat should be limited to less that 10 percent of calories, or about one-third of total fat intake. Reducing your fat intake should help with weight and with general health.

Third, I mentioned earlier that fat calories are more easily converted to body fat than are calories from other sources. Therefore, keeping fat intake under control can go a long way toward helping you reduce your weight.

To calculate the amount of fat you should eat each day, begin with your total daily calorie goal. Multiply this number by 30 percent to determine your daily calories from fat. Since each gram of fat contains nine calories, divide your daily calories from fat by nine to determine your daily grams of fat. See the example in Calculating My Daily Fat Intake. Use the blank chart at the bottom of this page to calculate your daily fat gram goal.

Sources of fat

We generally don't realize how much fat we eat. About 60 percent of the fat we eat cannot be seen (hidden fat) because it is contained

How many grams of fat can I have each day?

If your daily calorie intake is:	These are the grams of fat to be 30% of total calories
1100	36
1200	40
1300	43
1400	46
1500	50
1600	53
1700	56
1800	60
1900	63
2000	66
2100	70
2200	73
2300	76
2400	80
2500	83

in other food products, such as meat, cheese, nuts, breads, etc. In determining the amount of fat in your diet, it is important to account for both types of dietary fat.

Calculating My Daily Fat Intake (*Example*)

Total Daily Caloric Intake (calories)		1500
Target Percentage of Total Calories	x	30%
Daily Calories from Fat		450
Number of Calories in One Gram of Fat	÷	9
Daily Grams of Fat		50

Calculating My Daily Fat Intake

Total Daily Caloric Intake (calories)		_____
Target Percentage of Total Calories	x	30%
Daily Calories from Fat		_____
Number of Calories in One Gram of Fat	÷	9
Daily Grams of Fat		_____

Food Group Choices

Foods	Servings	Grams of Fat

Fats, Oils, and Sweets

Foods	Servings	Grams of Fat
Butter, margarine, 1t	–	4
Mayonnaise, 1T	–	11
Salad dressing, 1T	–	7
Reduced calorie salad dressing, 1T	–	A
Sour cream, 2T	–	6
Cream cheese, 1 oz	–	10
Sugar, jam, jelly, 1t	–	0
Cola, 12 fl. oz	–	0
Fruit drink, 12 fl oz	–	0
Chocolate bar, 1 oz	–	9
Sherbet, ½ cup	–	2
Fruit sorbet, ½ cup	–	0
Gelatin dessert, ½ cup	–	0

Milk, Yogurt, and Cheese Group

Foods	Servings	Grams of Fat
Skim milk, 1 cup	1	Trace
nonfat yogurt, plain, 8 oz	1	Trace
Low-fat milk, 2 percent, 1 cup	1	5
Whole milk, 1 cup	1	8
Chocolate milk, 2 percent, 1 cup	1	4
Low-fat yogurt, plain, 8 oz	1	4
Low-fat yogurt, fruit, 8 oz	1	3
Natural cheddar cheese, 1 ½ oz	1	14
Process cheese, 2 oz	1	18
Mozzarella, part skim, 1 ½ oz	1	10
Cottage cheese, 4 percent fat, ½ cup	¼	5
Ice cream, ½ cup	⅓	7
Ice milk, ½ cup	⅓	3
Frozen yogurt, ½ cup	½	2

Meat, Poultry, Fish, Dry Beans, Eggs, and Nuts Group

Foods	Servings	Grams of Fat
Lean meat, poultry, fish, cooked,	3 oz	6
Ground beef, lean, cooked	3 oz[B]	16
Chicken, with skin, fried	3 oz[B]	13
Bologna, 2 slices	1 oz[B]	16
Egg, 1,	1 oz[B]	5
Dry beans and peas, cooked, ½ cup	1 oz[B]	Trace
Peanut butter, 2T	1 oz[B]	16
Nuts, ⅓ cup	1 oz[B]	22

Vegetable Group

Foods	Servings	Grams of Fat
Vegetables, cooked, ½ cup	1	Trace
Vegetables, leafy, raw, 1 cup	1	Trace
Vegetables, non leafy, raw, chopped, ½ cup	1	Trace
Potatoes, scalloped, ½ cup	1	4
Potato salad, ½ cup	1	8
French fries, 10	1	8

Fruit Group

Foods	Servings	Grams of Fat
Whole fruit: medium apple, orange, banana	1	Trace
Fruit, raw or canned, ½ cup	1	Trace
Fruit juice, unsweetened, ¾ cup	1	Trace
Avocado, ¼ whole	1	9

Bread, Cereal, Rice, and Pasta Group

Foods	Servings	Grams of Fat
Bread, 1 slice	1	1
Hamburger roll, bagel, English muffin, 1	2	2
Tortilla, 1	1	3
Rice, pasta, cooked, ½ cup	1	Trace
Plain crackers, small, 3–4	1	3
Breakfast cereal, 1 oz	1	A
Pancakes, 4" diameter, 2	2	3
Croissant, 1 large (2 oz)	2	12
Doughnut, 1 medium (2 oz)	2	11
Danish, 1 medium (2 oz)	2	13
Cake, frosted, 1/16 average	1	13
Cookies, 2 medium	2	19
Pie, fruit, 2-crust, 1/6 8" pie	2	19

A Check product label.
B Serving sizes vary with the type of food and the meal.

Source: Adapted from Home and Garden Bulletin Number 252, U.S. Department of Agriculture, 1992.

The Food Guide Pyramid

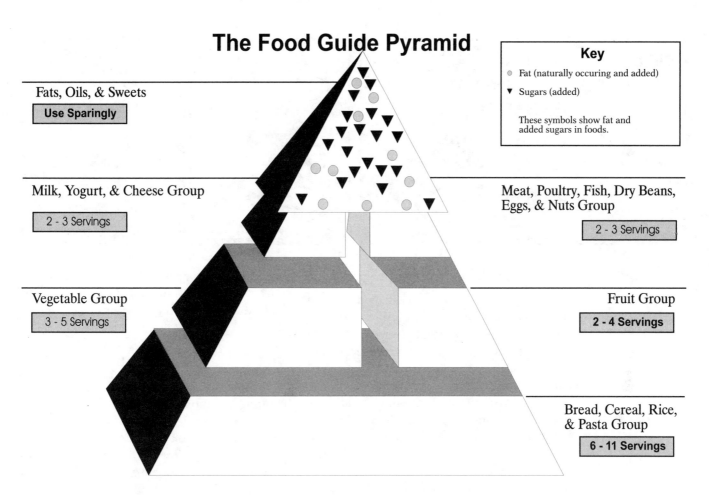

Key

- Fat (naturally occuring and added)
- ▼ Sugars (added)

These symbols show fat and added sugars in foods.

Fats, Oils, & Sweets
Use Sparingly

Milk, Yogurt, & Cheese Group
2 - 3 Servings

Meat, Poultry, Fish, Dry Beans, Eggs, & Nuts Group
2 - 3 Servings

Vegetable Group
3 - 5 Servings

Fruit Group
2 - 4 Servings

Bread, Cereal, Rice, & Pasta Group
6 - 11 Servings

The chart on the previous page provides you with a sampling of foods from the five food groups of the Food Guide Pyramid. This chart includes the number of servings of each food and the amount of fat for each. Use this chart along with the calorie guide in Appendix F to help you reduce your dietary fat.

Dietary fat adds up

The fat in some foods adds up quickly. You should keep in mind that fat contains more that twice the calories of protein or carbohydrates. One gram of fat has nine calories, whereas one gram of carbohydrates or protein has only four calories. One teaspoon (one pat) of butter or margarine has four grams of fat; that's 36 calories of fat for every teaspoon. It is important to watch out for those extras that contain high amounts of fat. For example, a bologna-and-cheese sandwich made with two slices (two oz) of bologna, two slices (1½ oz) of cheese, and two teaspoons of mayonnaise, counts up to about 36 grams of fat, approximately nine teaspoons. A similar sandwich, however, made with lean beef, lettuce, to-

mato, and low-fat mayonnaise, and served with a cup of nonfat milk instead of cheese, has only about six grams of fat.

Reducing the fat in your diet

There are many tips available for lowering the amount of dietary fat we eat every day. The first step is to determine a target intake of fat as we did in the calculation on page 79. Next, you should become aware of the fat content of the foods that you eat. In addition to reading food labels, there are many good books available that can help you. Here are some additional tips that will help you decrease the level of fat in your diet.

From the milk, yogurt, and cheese group

Use skim or low-fat milk (two grams of fat) instead of whole milk (16 grams of fat) for drinking as well as cooking. Also, use nonfat or low-fat fruit yogurt (two grams of fat) over whole-milk yogurt (seven grams of fat). Frozen yogurt or ice milk (two to three grams of fat per one-half cup) is a nice substitute for ice cream (seven grams).

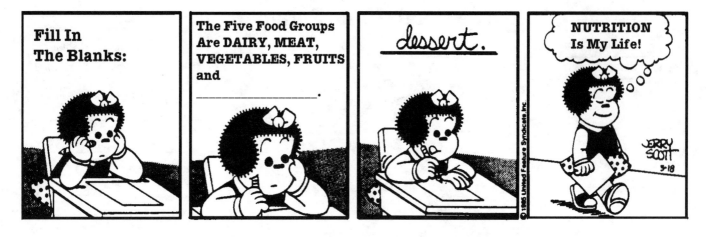

From the meat, poultry, and fish group

Eat modest portions of meat, poultry, and fish. Three cooked ounces is the recommended portion size. Choose lean cuts of meat, such as sirloin tip and round steak, and choose lean and extra lean ground beef, center cut ham, loin chops, and tenderloin. Limit your use of processed meats which tend to be high in fat. When in doubt, read the food label. If the fat content is not listed on the food product be extra cautious. If cholesterol is a problem, limit your use of organ meats (liver, kidneys, brains, etc.) and limit the number of egg yolks to three or less per week. Legumes (dried beans and peas) are good alternative sources of protein and have little or no fat. Use them in mixed dishes instead of meat, or combine them with a small portion of meat or poultry.

From the vegetable and fruit groups

Fruits and vegetables provide a good supply of fiber, vitamins, and minerals—all with low fat and no cholesterol. Use them generously at mealtime and for snacks. For both cooked and fresh vegetables (including salads) try seasonings and substitute flavorings, such as herbs, spices, or a splash of lemon instead of butter or salad dressings. Remember, there are four grams of fat in each teaspoon of butter, margarine, or mayonnaise. Cutting out the salad dressing can save up to nine grams of fat for each tablespoon.

From the bread, cereal, and rice group

Use rice, pasta, and other grain products as the mainstay of a low-fat eating plan. Small portions of meat, fish, and poultry go a long way when combined with grain products. Eating whole grain products will help you maximize your intake of fiber and other nutrients. Choose a dinner roll (two grams of fat) rather than a croissant (12 grams of fat).

Cooking tips

Trim away all visible fat from meat before cooking. Remove skin and fat from chicken and turkey before cooking. Use nonstick pans and sprays for cooking. In sauces, salads, and soups, substitute low-fat or nonfat plain yogurt for sour cream or mayonnaise. Broil or bake meats instead of frying.

Snacks and desserts

Eat plenty of fresh fruit and vegetables every day. Pop popcorn in a microwave or air popper. To add flavor, spray the popcorn lightly with hot vegetable oil or vegetable spray and add seasoning salts. Sorbet, flavored ice, and frozen fruit bars are a nice snack. Danish, doughnuts, cookies, and frosted cakes are high in fat and should be eaten sparingly. Also, potato chips and other crunchy snacks are high in dietary fat. Be sure to read the food label for the fat content of these foods.

Warning: alcohol and calories

As you will see from the table provided on the next page, alcohol is packed with calories. A can of light beer will have 100 calories; the tab for regular beer is 150 calories, about the same as a can of Coke or Pepsi. Mixed drinks and cordials are higher yet. Think of a daiquiri with more than 200 calories and a pina colada over 250.

Watch out for all those calories in alcohol

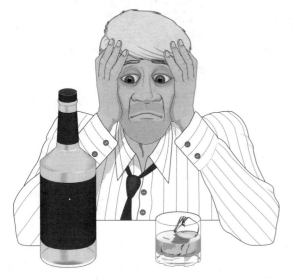

Some people can have a pretty successful time with weight loss simply by eliminating or greatly reducing their alcohol intake. Many just decide the pleasure they derive from the drinks does not justify all the calories. Remember that you get plenty of calories and no nutrition with alcohol, so if you use up part of your day's allotment of calories with drinks, there will not be much room in the remaining calories to pack in the nutrients you need for healthy living. If the drinks are important to you, use the skills you are learning to help keep the amount under control. Pour small amounts, taste every bit (calories should be tasted, not wasted), be certain to drink only things that are special to you, and don't drink out of habit and continue taking in calories just because you have done so in the past.

One other factor to be alert for is the "disinhibiting" effect of alcohol. Alcohol releases inhibitions in some people and they do things they might not do when not drinking. You are working to inhibit your calorie intake, and drinking may make you vulnerable to the "what the heck" phenomenon in which you relax your guard and eat more than you might like.

Calorie Costs of Alcohol

Beverage	Serving Size (oz)	Calories
Beer or ale	12	140–160
Beer, light	12	100
Bloody Mary	5	116
Bourbon & soda	4	105
Brandy or cognac	1	65–80
Champagne	4	90
Coffee-flavored creme liqueur	1.5	154
Cold Duck	4	120
Cordials and liqueurs, 34 to 72 proof	1	102–125
Creme de Menthe	1.5	186
Daiquiri—with lime	4	222
Distilled spirits:		
Gin, vodka, rum, whiskey; 80 to 100 proof	1.5	95–124
Gin and tonic	7.5	171
Manhattan	2	128
Martini	2.5	156
Pina colada (canned)	4.5	346
Screwdriver	7	174
Sherry	3	125
Tequila sunrise	5.5	89
Tom collins	7.5	121
Vermouth, dry	1	32
Vermouth, sweet	1	45
Wine, dry white	4	79
Wine, red	4	85
Wine, dessert (sweet)	4	181
Wine, light	4	52
Wine, nonalcoholic	6	60
Wine cooler	12	220

Note: The calorie values here are approximations only and may vary depending on a drink's proof, specific sweetness, age, and amount of ice used.

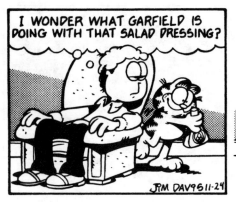
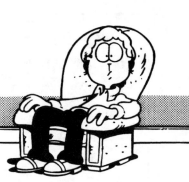
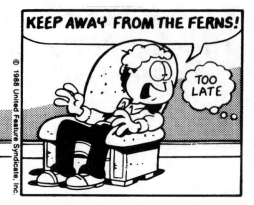

Planning healthy meals

Many excellent resources are available for planning healthy meals. These include cookbooks and guides for buying, preparing, and serving healthy foods. These are handy aids because losing weight conjures up impressions of deprivation and boring food. A trip to the bookstore can help prevent this boredom. The following books are filled with ideas and recipes that can help you eat delicious foods while reducing calories, fat, sodium, cholesterol, and increasing fiber. Get those tastebuds ready!

American Heart Association Quick and Easy Cookbook. New York: McKay, 1997.

Better Homes and Gardens Eat & Stay Slim. Des Moines, Iowa: Meredith, 1997.

Better Homes and Gardens Eating Well With the Food Guide Pyramid. Des Moines, Iowa: Meredith, 1996.

Better Homes and Gardens Family Favorites Made lighter. Des Moines, Iowa: Meredith, 1992.

Better Homes and Gardens Healthy Family cookbook. Des Moines, Iowa: Meredith, 1996.

Better Homes and Gardens Healthy Meals Fast. Des Moines, Iowa: Meredith, 1996.

Better Homes and Gardens Low-Fat Meals. Des Moines, Iowa: Meredith, 1996.

Betty Crocker's New Choices Cookbook. New York: Prentice-Hall, 1993.

CookingLight Five Star Recipes. Birmingham, AL: Oxmoor House, 1996. 1-800-633-4910 to order.

EatRight Lose Weight: 7 Simple Steps. Bermingham, AL: Oxmoor House, Inc., 1997. 1-800-633-4910 to order.

Low-Fat Ways To Lose Weight. Birmingham, AL: Oxmoor House, 1996. 1-800-633-4910 to order.

Low-Fat Ways To Cook Vegetarian. Birmingham, AL: Oxmoor House, 1996. 1-800-633-4910 to order.

Light Chinese Dishes. New York: HPBooks, 1995.

Secrets of Low-Fat Cooking. New York: Eating Well Books, 1997.

SouthernLiving Soup & Stew Recipes. Birmingham, AL: Oxmoor House, 1996. 1-800-633-4910 to order.

SouthernLiving Best Recipes Made Lighter. Birmingham, AL: Oxmoor House, 1997. 1-800-633-4910 to order.

30-Minute Vegetarian Recipes. Des Moines, Iowa: Meredith, 1995.

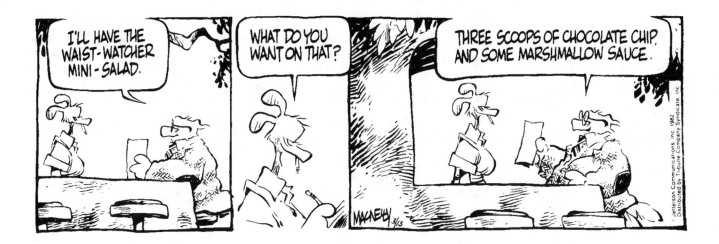

Assignment for this lesson

There are two behavioral techniques to practice: putting your fork down between bites and pausing during the meal. Try to increase your lifestyle activity, and have a candid and specific talk with your partner if you decide the partnership approach is for you. Check the amount of fat in your diet, and establish a target level of daily fat grams. Try to keep your fat intake to 30 percent or lower of total calories.

Self-assessment questionnaire

Lesson Six

T F 25. Eating rapidly helps you enjoy food *more* because the taste buds get more stimulation.

T F 26. Pausing during a meal increases food intake because the body digests food and sends out signals to eat more.

T F 27. Your resting pulse will increase as you lose weight and get in better condition.

T F 28. You should tell your program partner in specific terms how he or she can help.

T F 29. Since too much dietary fat has been linked to heart disease and other health-related risks, it's best to eliminate all fat from your diet.

T F 30. The recommended daily intake of dietary fat is 30 percent or less of total calories.

T F 31. One gram of fat contains more than twice the calories of one gram of carbohydrate or protein.

T F 32. Saturated fat is usually solid at room temperature and is found only in animal foods, such as meats and dairy products made from whole milk or cream.

T F 33. Since all fruits and vegetables have only small amounts of fats, it is not as important to count the amount of fat in these foods as it is to count the dietary fat from meat and dairy products.

(Answers in Appendix C)

Monitoring Form—Lesson Six

Today's Date:

Time	Food and Amount	Calories
	Total Daily Calories	

Assignment this week	Always	Sometimes	Never
1. Fork down between bites			
2. Pause during meal			
3. Increase lifestyle activity			
4. Talk with a program partner			
5. Keep fat intake to 30 percent or less of total calories			
6. Less than _____ calories each day			
7. Less than _____ grams of fat each day			

Food Groups for Today	Physical Activity	Minutes
Milk, yogurt, and cheese ❑ ❑ ❑		
Meat, poultry, etc. ❑ ❑ ❑		
Fruits ❑ ❑ ❑ ❑		
Vegetables ❑ ❑ ❑ ❑ ❑		
Breads, cereals, etc. ❑ ❑ ❑ ❑ ❑ ❑ ❑ ❑ ❑		

We are nearly to the halfway point of the LEARN program. This is a good time to reflect on what you have learned, the behaviors you have practiced, and the new outlook on your dietary habits and lifestyle changes we have been discussing. Have some of the techniques become habits? Is this a program you can live with? These are the key questions we must consider for the long-term outlook.

In this lesson, we will cover shopping for food and will take up the issue of programmed activity. You will also learn a model of how we think and feel and methods for making your partnership work. We will also discuss the importance of food, and you will learn all about the Milk, Yogurt, and Cheese Group of the Food Guide Pyramid.

Shopping for food

Let's look back on the ABC approach introduced in Lesson Four. The "A" refers to the antecedents that set the stage for eating. One important antecedent is shopping for food. If you buy good foods, you will eat good foods. This may sound obvious, but too few people plan their shopping accordingly.

Having problem foods available in the house, office, car, briefcase, purse, or pocket can be asking for trouble, even if you vow to "eat only a little." If something threatens your restraint, say fatigue or boredom, you can pay a dear price for a decision to buy the food made hours or days earlier. On the other hand, if your refrigerator resembles a salad bar because of wise shopping, weakened restraint can inflict only minor damage. There are several clever methods you can use while shopping to make prudent food choices.

◆ **Shop on a full stomach.** It is easy to buy impulsively when you are hungry because everything looks appetizing. An innocent trip to the store to *buy a few essentials* can become an eating excursion. The supermarket to a hungry person is like water to someone stranded in the Sahara. The stores are made to tempt you. Your restraint is high when you first walk in, but little good it does when you are in the produce section! As you move through the store, you get worked up just as you pass the cookie aisle. Desire reaches its peak as you travel down Dessert Lane (the frozen food and ice cream section). Shop only after you have eaten. You will be surprised how much grief this can prevent.

◆ **Shop from a list.** Prepare a shopping list before you leave the house, and shop only from the list. Decide what to buy *before* you are tempted by the foods in the store. Make the list when you are not hungry.

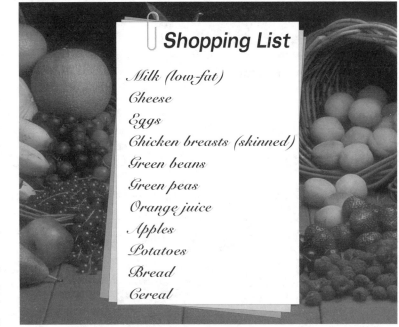

Shopping List

Milk (low-fat)
Cheese
Eggs
Chicken breasts (skinned)
Green beans
Green peas
Orange juice
Apples
Potatoes
Bread
Cereal

◆ **Buy foods that require preparation.** With this age of prepackaged foods, microwave ovens, and fast food restaurants, you can eat at an instant's notice. Eating requires little thought and can be done impulsively. Buying foods that require preparation can halt this process.

Let's use an example of a common food. If you have a hankering for fried chicken, you could visit the Colonel and procure 1000 calories in an extra crispy three-piece dinner. Little time would separate craving and consumption. If you chose the preparation route, you would buy a whole chicken, cut it, prepare it, then fry it. You could think about how much you wanted the chicken and might eat less (if you eat it at all). In addition, preparing the chicken yourself would give you the option of baking it, which would bring far fewer calories than deep frying.

Introducing programmed activity

We have focused on lifestyle activity, particularly walking. This is where most overweight individuals should start. By now, however, you may feel more comfortable with being physically active and may be ready for more. It is time to introduce the topic of regular, programmed exercise.

I expect that about half of the people who read this manual will be ready for more rigorous activity. The others must continue walking and lose more weight before taking on programmed activity. If you are in this category, read this section for its information, and remember to refer back to it when you are

ready to increase your activity. In the meantime, continue to increase your walking by adding time or by increasing the speed with which you walk.

As I mentioned earlier, programmed activities include jogging, walking, aerobics, racquetball, swimming, cycling, or any regular activity. Selecting the right activity is something of an art and will be discussed later. For now, I want to address the issue of how much exercise is necessary.

Great news about activity

For many people, exercise is a major factor in their long-term prospects for weight control. It is true that many people lose weight without exercise, but for others, exercise makes an enormous difference. Do you remember the graph in Lesson Six that showed the difference between the maintainers and the regainers?

Exercise helps people lose weight for both physical and psychological reasons. It burns calories and may boost your metabolic rate. Perhaps as important are the ways exercise makes us feel good. Each time we exercise, we are sending a signal to ourselves that we are making positive changes. The exercise may reduce stress and may give us more energy for life's other activities (like planning our weekly diet). Some people find exercise especially helpful by scheduling it at times they are most likely to eat.

One bit of very good news about exercise comes from work by Dr. Steven Blair and his colleagues at The Cooper Institute of Aerobics Research in Dallas, Texas. These researchers studied physical fitness and health in 10,224 men and 3,120 women. Each person in the

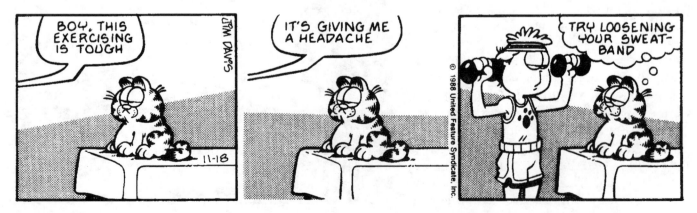

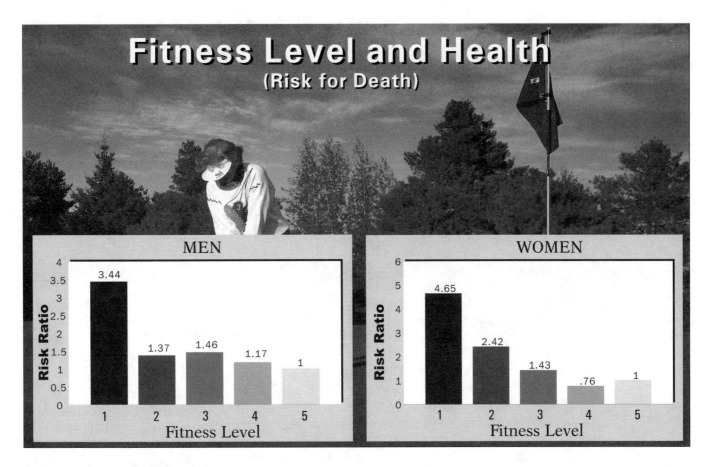

Fitness Level and Health
(Risk for Death)

MEN

Risk Ratio

Fitness Level	Value
1	3.44
2	1.37
3	1.46
4	1.17
5	1

WOMEN

Risk Ratio

Fitness Level	Value
1	4.65
2	2.42
3	1.43
4	.76
5	1

study had undergone a detailed medical exam that included a maximal stress test on a treadmill. The people were grouped into categories of physical fitness based upon their performance on the treadmill test. They were then followed for an average of eight years.

Dr. Blair and his colleagues placed these people into five categories of fitness, ranging from the very unfit (Fitness Level 1) to the very fit (Fitness Level 5). The graphs shown here give the risk ratio (which represents the death rate) for both men and women depending on their level of fitness. The risk for the most fit people is given a value of one, and then risks for the other categories are given in reference to that number. For instance, in the figure showing risk rates for men, the men in Fitness Level 5 (the most fit) have a risk factor of one. The risk increases to 1.17 (a 17 percent increase) for men in Fitness Level 4 and to 1.46 (a 46 percent increase) for men in Fitness Level 3.

There are several striking aspects to this study. First, it is yet another piece to the puzzle showing that people who exercise and are physically active live longer. For our pur-

poses, however, the important news is that even modest levels of fitness are associated with greatly reduced risk. Look at the figure showing numbers for the men. Men in the lowest level of fitness (Fitness Level 1) have a risk ratio of 3.44 compared to a ratio of 1.37 in Fitness Level 2. There is a **substantial** decline in risk by moving from the least fit group to the next group. There are certainly gains made by increasing fitness further, but the big drop occurs as people go from being completely sedentary to moderately active. The figure for women shows much the same pattern.

The moral to this story is that you do not have to kill yourself to keep from dying. Even small amounts of exercise are likely to have a big impact on health and will certainly be helpful in losing weight. In the Blair study, one only had to do regular walking at a moderate pace to be fit enough to be in Level 2, which had about half the risk of the group who were least fit. How much exercise should you do? You should do as much as you can and still have fun. Don't worry so much about how much or what type, just try to do it regularly.

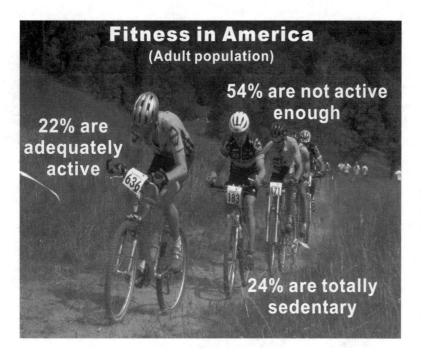

Fitness in America
(Adult population)

22% are adequately active

54% are not active enough

24% are totally sedentary

Remember, any type of activity should be considered *exercise*. If you take an extra flight of stairs, rake the leaves, walk an extra block, or chase the rabbits out of your vegetable garden, you have exercised and should say so in your own mind. You deserve to feel good about these activities and can feel confident that you are making progress.

A new activity formula for Americans

The work of Dr. Blair and other experts in the field has provided a growing body of evidence that regular, moderate intensity physical activity can result in substantial health benefits. One of the primary benefits is protection against coronary heart disease. Other health benefits may include protection against several other chronic diseases, such as adult-onset diabetes, hypertension, certain cancers, osteoporosis, and depression.

While most of us would readily agree that regular physical activity is beneficial, most of us are not physically active on a regular basis. Only about 22 percent of adults in this country engage in leisure time physical activity. About 24 percent of adults are completely sedentary, and the remaining 54 percent are inadequately active. They too would benefit from

more regular physical activity. With all of this scientific evidence, why are we a nation of inactivity? Two reasons come mind.

We live in a high-tech society. The more technologically advanced we become, the more inactive we become. Cars, garage-door openers, portable telephones, television, remote controls for most electrical devices, and many other labor saving gadgets have changed the way we work, take care of our homes, and use our leisure time. Technology almost entices us to be inactive. Further, our environment presents many obstacles and barriers to physical activity. Walking to the corner store is difficult if there are not adequate sidewalks, and riding a bicycle or walking to work is difficult because of the way suburbs have moved us farther away from where we work.

The second reason many people may be inactive is that they have a misconception about exercise. Many people have thought that the exercise prescription for cardiovascular training (I will discuss this in the next lesson) is **THE** prescription for *exercise*. **It is NOT!** This may have led many people to believing that if they couldn't follow the *prescription* then they may as well not exercise at all. The following new guidelines may help to dispel this old myth.

New guidelines for exercise

In July of 1993, The American College of Sports Medicine and the U.S. Centers for Disease Control and Prevention, in cooperation with the President's Council on Physical Fitness and Sports, released new exercise guidelines and recommendations for Americans. The new guidelines recommend 30 minutes or more of moderate intensity physical activity over the course of most days of the week (at least five days).

This is great news for many overweight individuals. Six five-minute walks counts as 30 minutes of activity. Activities that can also contribute to the 30-minute total include walking up stairs, gardening, cleaning house, raking leaves, and walking part or all of the way to and from work. The recommended 30 minutes of physical activity may also come from planned exercise or recreation, such as jogging, riding a bicycle, playing golf or tennis, or swimming. A brisk two-mile walk is another way to achieve 30 minutes of physical activity.

As you can see, there are many reasons to increase your physical activity. The best advise is to build physical activity into your daily routine—make it become part of your lifestyle just like eating, working, and sleeping. The physical and psychological aspects of a more active lifestyle can be quite rewarding.

Your body and your self-esteem

How we feel about our bodies can be central to how we feel about ourselves. Our view of our own body is called body image, and unfortunately, body image is negative in most people, especially women, and especially people who are overweight. This is not surprising considering the enormous pressure in our society to be thin and for women to be valued for how they look rather than for who they are as people. Many, many people internalize these social norms, find a major difference between they way they look and the way they think they should look, and then hurt themselves emotionally as a result. It really isn't fair, be-

cause the social norms present an ideal that is unrealistic and not even healthy.

Let's look at how this might work for a young woman; we'll call her Ann. As Ann approaches puberty, she is full of energy, is athletic, enjoys being active, has fun, and takes pleasure in what her body can do for her. Yet, she is increasingly aware of the need to be thin. She is not prepared for this pressure to be so intense at the very time puberty causes her body to deposit more fat. Instead of accepting and enjoying the changes in her body, she feels her body is betraying her. Natural processes like eating and exercise become a battleground. She must restrict what she eats and must now exercise, not for fun, but for the purpose of losing weight. Ann may enter into a fight with her own body that will never end.

As Ann enters her 20s and then passes the 30, 40, and 50 benchmarks, two things are likely to happen. One is that she will be dissatisfied with her body. She will overlook its virtues—that it allows her to be active, to move places, to feel both sensual and sexual pleasure. Instead she will focus on the disparity between ideal and actual and will feel it is her fault that she does not look perfect.

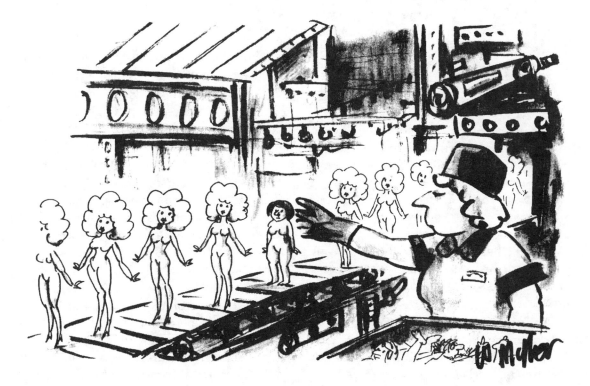

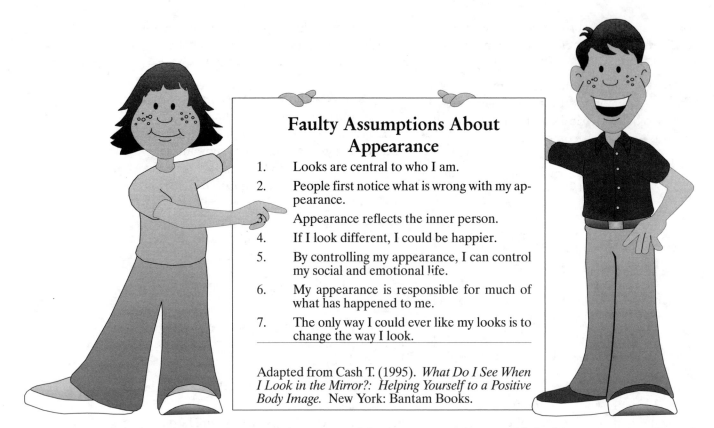

Faulty Assumptions About Appearance

1. Looks are central to who I am.
2. People first notice what is wrong with my appearance.
3. Appearance reflects the inner person.
4. If I look different, I could be happier.
5. By controlling my appearance, I can control my social and emotional life.
6. My appearance is responsible for much of what has happened to me.
7. The only way I could ever like my looks is to change the way I look.

Adapted from Cash T. (1995). *What Do I See When I Look in the Mirror?: Helping Yourself to a Positive Body Image.* New York: Bantam Books.

The second event is that Ann will let her body image have too much impact on her self-esteem. Our self-esteem is made up of how we evaluate ourselves on many dimensions (as a parent, child, brother or sister, employer or employee, friend, etc.). Our looks influence us all, but for some people, appearance creeps to the heart of self-esteem. It can crowd out other positive influences, so that no matter how good we are at other things, there is always this looming matter of how we look.

Having a positive body image

Having a positive view of our body, no matter how imperfect, is really important. If you dislike how you look, and accept society's unrealistic beauty standards, you will be unhappy with what you accomplish in this program or any other. The risk is that you will make very positive changes in eating, activity, and weight, but feel you are still far from your goal, and therefore will despair over your lack of success. This is a setup for disappointment, frustration, and giving up.

An excellent book on this topic written for the general public is by Dr. Thomas F. Cash and is called *What Do I See When I Look in the Mirror?: Helping Yourself to a Positive Body Im-age.* This is published by Bantam Books and can be purchased or ordered in a bookstore. The book contains many good ideas for evaluating how we feel about our bodies, how this affects how we feel about ourselves in general, and how we can respond.

In his book, Cash discusses fundamental assumptions people make about their appearance and their lives. Some of these are shown here in the accompanying table entitled, "Faulty Assumptions About Appearance."

These assumptions lead to overestimation of how appearance governs one's life and to overemphasis on changing appearance to improve well-being. With these assumptions, which are very common, a person is always dissatisfied and no weight loss is enough.

So, what can we do to be happier about the way we look? The book by Cash mentioned above has some excellent ideas, complete with exercises and means for evaluating whether your body image is changing. Here are some ideas that may be helpful.

- ◆ **Get accustomed to seeing our bodies.** Most people who do not like their bodies do everything they can to avoid looking. Mirrors, especially full-length mirrors, store windows, and other places are avoided. Stop avoiding and find a way to believe that your body can be your friend.

- ◆ **Challenge the faulty assumptions about appearance and life.** To equate appearance with happiness is to give the body much more power than it deserves. You can be a smashing success at many things in life (most notably being a good person) irrespective of appearance. Appearance is only one aspect of our lives, and for many, it means little.

- ◆ **Confront what is realistic for us as individuals.** Given what you have looked like during your adult life, given how your parents looked, and given how difficult it might be for you to lose to "ideal" weight, be realistic and stare in the face of how you might realistically look. Perhaps you can do more, but perhaps not.

- ◆ **Uncouple body image from self-esteem**. The assumption that how you look is who you are can be very damaging.

- ◆ **Focus on how our body is a gift.** The body can do many fine things for us. It allows us to live, to move, to accomplish what we'd like, not to mention how good it feels when we relax, work out, and engage in sensual activities with another person. The body gives us many gifts of living, and therefore is a gift. If we focus on the virtues of our bodies, it becomes less an adversary. Being friends with your body is central to your long-term happiness.

None of these will be easy because how you feel about yourself is the product of years and years of experiences, thoughts, attitudes, and feelings. Just vowing to be happier with the way we look is not enough. We must challenge the faulty assumptions constantly. We must make a concerted effort to reward ourselves for looking good, and then practice this new way of thinking for days, weeks, and months. It takes a lot to undo the powerful messages we have been exposed to, so please keep at it. You deserve to feel good about yourself, no matter what you weigh.

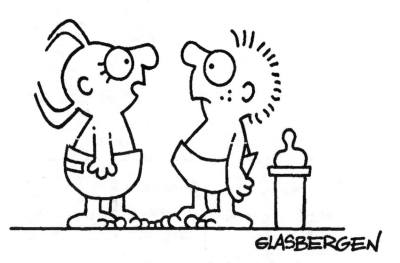

"*Be honest with me . . . do disposable diapers make my hips look too big?*"

Striving for perfection

We would all like to be perfect—it is human nature. However, this desire can never be consummated. Although this is obvious to most people, many people on weight loss programs expect more than can be delivered.

Your thinking process

We discussed goal setting in Lesson Four and concluded that setting unrealistic goals can halt your progress. It is time to explore this matter further. We set goals for everything we do. Although we do not articulate a goal for every activity, hidden within our mind are expectations of how well we should perform. If you mow the lawn, write a letter, buy clothes, or simply talk to a friend, you expect a certain level of performance. If you scalped the lawn, wrote an unintelligible letter, bought gaudy clothes, or said insensitive things to your friend, you would be upset because you expected more—you did not satisfy your internal standard.

You can see how difficult life would be if your goals were absurdly out-of-reach. If you expected *Better Homes and Gardens* to lust after your lawn, for the National Archives to enshrine your letter, for the President's wife to wear your clothes to the Inaugural Ball, or for your friend to memorialize your words in a book of quotes, you would be crushed by what

Measuring Up to Your Own Goals

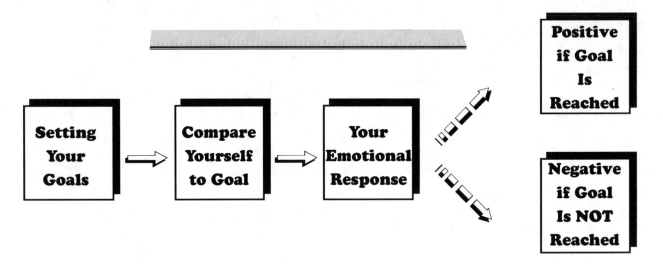

is otherwise an acceptable performance. Unfortunately, it is just such out-of-reach goals that people losing weight tend to set for themselves about their eating, exercise, and weight loss. When the goals are not met, the negative emotional response can send your progress into a tailspin.

This occurs in a three-part process. Setting the goals comes first and is often unconscious. You then compare actual performance to that goal. Finally, there is a positive emotional reaction if the goal is achieved and a negative one if it is not. The model above shows this three-step process.

Below are a few examples of how this process pertains to weight loss goals. These are common examples, so while you are reading, think if these or similar situations occur with you.

This emotional response is what worries me. Many people have enough trouble controlling their eating and exercise without the extra burden of negative feelings and thoughts.

You can change the emotional response by altering the two steps that precede it, namely the goal setting and the comparison you make to the goals.

When you have negative feelings, examine them and trace them to the goals you set. If you feel guilty because you sneak a Snickers, think about your goal, which is probably something like, "I should never cheat on this program." You can examine the comparison to this goal by understanding that you or anyone else could never be satisfied with this as a standard. This will change the emotional response.

On the next page are the same situations with different goals, comparisons, and emotional responses.

Use these examples to analyze your own goals, comparisons, and responses. This can lift the weight of negative feelings from your shoulders.

Setting Goal	Comparing Performance	Emotional Response
Will never cheat on a program.	Cheating on program does occur.	Guilt and resignation.
Will be good at sports.	Others do better and look better.	Embarrassment.
Will lose weight each week.	Some weeks weight stays stable or goes up.	Discouragement and self-blame.

Setting Goal	Comparing Performance	Emotional Response
Will follow the program as much as possible.	Meet goal on most occasions.	Satisfaction and desire to do better.
Will increase level of exercise.	Increase is steady and substantial.	Pride in doing something positive.
Will lose weight most weeks.	Lose weight 10 out of 12 weeks.	Feel good about hard work.

The importance of food

In simple terms, food is energy; it is the fuel our body uses to enable us to carry on our daily activities. Like most energy sources, *quality* is as important as *quantity*, and having the right mixture of nutrients at the right time is also important. Some nutrients have energy (calories) and others do not, but both are critical to our bodies. The nutrient needs of our bodies are comparable to the different needs of our automobiles. Gasoline and diesel fuel provide fuel or energy. Oil, water, transmission fluid, and other lubricants are also critical to a car's operation, but they do not provide energy.

There are over 45 different nutrients that our bodies need every day. They are essential for our health and must be provided in the food that we eat. There are six classes of these nutrients, and they can be divided into two categories:

❶ Nutrients with energy (calories) and

❷ Nutrients without energy

Nutrients with energy include carbohydrates, proteins, and fats. In Lesson Six we discussed the role of fat in your diet; proteins and carbohydrates will be covered in later lessons. The nutrients without energy include minerals, vitamins, and water.

Nutrients without energy

There are three classes of nutrients that are essential to our bodies, are contained in the food that we eat, and provide no energy or calories. These nutrients include minerals, vitamins, and water.

Minerals

Our bodies contain over 60 different minerals, of which about 22 are essential. The amount or quantity needed of the different minerals varies greatly. The 22 essential minerals are classified by their presence in the body as either *Macronutrients* (those having a greater presence) and *Micronutrients* (those of lesser quantity). It is important to remember that this classification is based upon presence

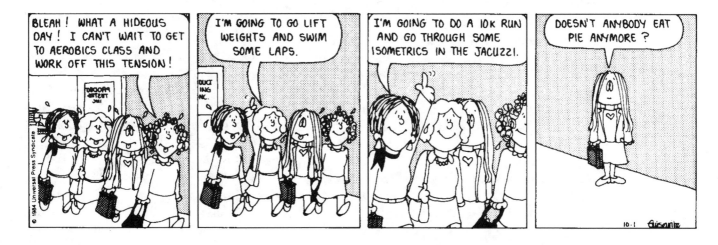

The Six Classes of Nutrients

Nutrients with Energy (Calories)

1. **Carbohydrates**—starches, sugar, and fiber.
2. **Protein**—includes 22 amino acids.
3. **Fats**—saturated, monounsaturated, and polyunsaturated fatty acids.

Nutrients Without Energy

4. **Minerals**—22 in total

7 Macronutrients	15 Micronutrients	
calcium	arsenic	manganese
chlorine	boron	molybdenum
magnesium	cobalt	nickel
phosphorus	copper	selenium
potassium	chromium	silicon
sodium	fluorine	vanadium
sulfur	iodine	zinc
	iron	

5. **Vitamins**

   Fat Soluble
   Water Soluble

Vitamin A-RDA 5000 IU	Vitamin C-RDA 60 mg
Vitamin D-RDA 400 IU	Vitamin B$_1$ (thiamine)-RDA 1.5 mg
Vitamin E-RDA 30 IU	Vitamin B$_2$ (riboflavin)-RDA 1.7 mg
Vitamin K	Vitamin B$_3$ (niacin)-RDA 19 mg
	Vitamin B$_6$ (pyridoxine)-RDA 2.0 mg
	Vitamin B$_{12}$ (cobalamin)-RDA 6 micrograms
	Folicin-RDA 400 micrograms

6. **Water**

in the body and not on importance. For example, a deficiency in cobalt, which comprises only two parts per trillion of body weight, can have more damaging effects that a deficiency in calcium, which accounts for two percent of body weight.

Minerals serve many functions. They help to aid in the growth of body tissue, transmit nerve impulses, regulate muscle contraction, maintain water balance in the body, form parts of essential body compounds, maintain the acid-base balance in the cells, and facilitate many biological reactions. Minerals are found together in the foods we eat and interact with each other as well as with other nutrients in the body. Because of this interaction and combination, certain foods are considered better sources than others.

Vitamins

Vitamins are also essential nutrients that are needed to sustain life. They are required for the regulation of the body's metabolism and for the transformation of energy (protein, carbohydrates, and fat) in the body. Some vitamins help to form important enzymes, and others act as catalysts to speed certain chemical reactions. There are two types of vitamins:

❶ Fat soluble
❷ Water soluble

Fat soluble vitamins

The four fat soluble vitamins are A, D, E, and K. These vitamins are found in dietary fat and are stored in the body's fat tissue if consumed in excess amounts. Since these vitamins are stored, toxic doses can be an important issue. You should be cautious of people who promote large quantities of these vitamins. No more than the Recommended Daily Allowance (RDA) is suggested.

Vitamin A is essential for the growth of skin, bones, and teeth. It is also important in vision. The RDA for vitamin A is 5000 International Units. Vitamin D is essential for bone and tooth development. In addition, it helps the body utilize calcium and phosphorus. The RDA for vitamin D is 400 International Units. Vitamin E is essential for the functioning of red blood cells and helps the body utilize the essential fatty acids. The RDA for Vitamin E is 30 International Units. Vitamin K is used by the liver to produce prothrombin, a factor in blood plasma that combines with calcium to help in blood clotting. An RDA has not been established for vitamin K.

Water soluble vitamins

Water soluble vitamins consist of seven primary vitamins: Vitamin C and the B complex vitamins that include vitamin B$_1$ (thiamine), vitamin B$_2$ (riboflavin), vitamin B$_3$ (niacin), vitamin B$_6$ (pyridoxine), folacin, and vitamin B$_{12}$ (cobalamin). Unlike the fat soluble vitamins, these are absorbed in the body's water, and excess amounts are usually excreted.

Vitamin C is used by the body for teeth, bones, cells, and blood vessels; it is essential for good heath. The RDA for vitamin C is 60 mg.

Vitamin B₁ is essential for the heart and nervous system and plays an important role in carbohydrate metabolism. A deficiency of this vitamin can result in beriberi and certain nervous disorders. The RDA for vitamin B₁ is 1.5 mg. Vitamin B₂ is also important in carbohydrate metabolism and body tissue repair. It is necessary for the skin and helps prevent light sensitivity in the eyes. A deficiency of this vitamin in the diet can lead to stunted growth and loss of hair. The RDA for vitamin B₂ is 1.7 mg. Vitamin B₃ (more commonly known as niacin) is important for metabolism and absorption of carbohydrates in the body and plays an important role in converting food to usable energy. The RDA for vitamin B₃ is 19 mg. Vitamin B₆ aids in the metabolism of protein, carbohydrate, and fat. The RDA for vitamin B₆ is 2.0 mg. Vitamin B₁₂ is essential for normal growth and neurological function. This vitamin also helps prevent anemia. The RDA for vitamin B₁₂ is 6 micrograms. Folacin is also important and helps the body metabolize food and is useful in preventing certain anemias. The RDA for folacin is 400 micrograms.

As a general rule, nutrition experts believe that people in the U.S. receive an adequate supply of minerals and vitamins if they eat a balanced diet. Following the dietary guidelines of the Food Guide Pyramid will help insure a balanced diet. Therefore, most people do not need or benefit from mineral or vitamin supplements, much less the mega-doses promoted by some people, including seemingly credible nutrition stores.

Water

Many people overlook the importance of water in their diets, not realizing that water is an essential nutrient. Considering that water makes up about 60 percent of our body and that water is needed by every cell in our body, water is indeed an important nutrient. Most people in the U.S. do not consume enough water, albeit in abundant supply. It *should* be consumed generously. As a rule of thumb, about four cups of water should be consumed for every 1000 calories eaten. For most adults, this is equivalent to about ten cups (2½ quarts) of water each day.

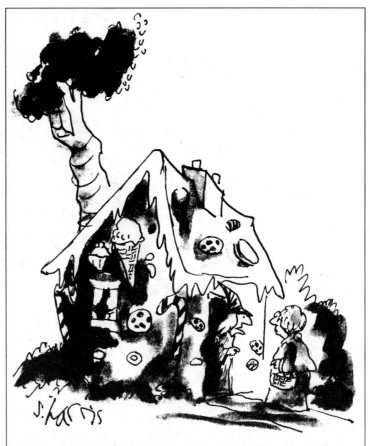

"It's a good thing I built this place when I did. The new zoning law prevents any house from going over 75,000 calories."

Milk, yogurt, and cheese in your diet

The second tier of the Food Guide Pyramid represents foods that come essentially from animal sources—milk, yogurt, and cheese; and meat, poultry, fish, dry beans, eggs, and nuts. The focus in this lesson will be on the Milk, Yogurt, and Cheese Group.

Food items in this group include milk, yogurt, and cheese. These foods are good sources of protein and carbohydrate, but can provide large amounts of unwanted dietary fat (see the food list on page 99). In addition, foods from the Milk Group are good sources of Vitamin A, Vitamin D, and calcium. Vitamins A and D are essential for the growth and development of skin, bones, and teeth. Calcium is an essential mineral for good health. Approximately 2 percent of the body is calcium, most of which is teeth and bones. Food items from the Milk Group are the best source of calcium and generally supply the greatest amount of calcium in

The Food Guide Pyramid

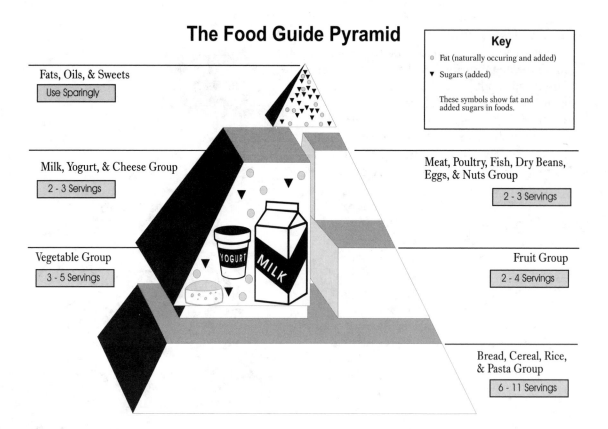

Key
- Fat (naturally occuring and added)
- ▼ Sugars (added)

These symbols show fat and added sugars in foods.

Fats, Oils, & Sweets
Use Sparingly

Milk, Yogurt, & Cheese Group
2 - 3 Servings

Meat, Poultry, Fish, Dry Beans, Eggs, & Nuts Group
2 - 3 Servings

Vegetable Group
3 - 5 Servings

Fruit Group
2 - 4 Servings

Bread, Cereal, Rice, & Pasta Group
6 - 11 Servings

---

our diet. One cup of milk (8 fl oz), for example provides 500 IUs of Vitamin A (i.e., 10 percent of the 5000 RDA) and 100 IUs of Vitamin D (i.e., 25 percent of the 400 RDA). The same cup of milk also provides about 313 mg of calcium (i.e., 40 percent of the 800 mg RDA).

Cheese items have proportionally more calories from protein than carbohydrate. Milk and yogurt, on the other hand, provide more carbohydrates per serving than protein.

How many servings?

The Food Guide Pyramid suggests two to three servings per day from the Milk Group. For most people, two servings from this group is sufficient; however, for teenagers, young adults, and women who are pregnant or breast feeding, three servings per day is recommended. It is important to know what makes up a serving size. Many people may know that servings from this group are important, yet most do not know how many servings are optimal.

How much is a serving?

The guide here lists single serving portions for many common food items from this group. The following items count as a single serving:

- ☑ 2 oz processed cheese
- ☑ 1 cup (8 oz) milk
- ☑ 1 cup (8 oz) yogurt
- ☑ 1½ oz natural cheese
- ☑ 1½ cups (12 oz) ice cream
- ☑ 2 cups (16 oz) cottage cheese

Eating food items from the Milk Group should be balanced during the day. In other words, it is best not to eat all of the required servings at the same time. An example of balance would be to have a cup of milk at breakfast (with cereal or in a glass), cheese or yogurt for lunch, and a serving of milk, yogurt, cheese, or ice cream for dinner.

Watch out for fat

Most products from the Milk Group come from animal sources. As such, these food items also contain cholesterol and fat. The fat content as well as the number of calories in each serving can vary greatly. For instance, one serving of skim milk (8 oz) has 86 total calories, compared to one serving of ice cream (12 oz) which can have as many as 524 calories.

Milk, Yogurt, and Cheese

Each of the following counts as one serving.

Description	Calories	Protein (g)	Carbo. (g)	Fat (g)
Milk, skim—1 cup (8 oz)	86	8.4	11.9	Trace
Milk, 1%—1 cup (8 oz)	104	8.5	12.2	2.4
Milk, 2%—1 cup (8 oz)	125	8.5	12.2	4.7
Milk, whole—1 cup (8 oz)	150	8.0	11.0	8.0
Yogurt, non-fat—8 oz	90	10.0	13.0	Trace
Yogurt, light—8 oz	100	9.0	17.0	Trace
Yogurt, low-fat—8 oz	144	11.9	16.0	3.5
Yogurt, skim—8 oz	127	13.0	17.4	Trace
Yogurt, whole—8 oz	139	7.9	10.6	7.4
Yogurt, frozen 1 cup (8 oz)	210	6.2	33.2	6.2
Ice cream, 10% fat—1½ cup (12 oz)	404	7.2	48.0	21.5
Ice cream, 16% fat—1½ cup (12 oz)	524	6.2	48.0	35.6
Ice milk, vanilla—1½ cup (12 oz)	276	7.8	43.5	8.4
Ice milk, soft serve—1½ cup (12 oz)	335	12.0	57.6	6.9
Cheese, American processed—2 oz	212	12.6	1.0	17.8
Cheese, cheddar—1½ oz	171	10.6	.6	14.1
Cheese, colby—1½ oz	168	10.0	1.0	13.7
Cheese, cottage, creamed—2 cups (16 oz)	434	52.4	11.2	19.0
Cheese, cream—1½ oz	149	3.2	1.2	14.9
Cheese, mozzarella—1½ oz	120	8.3	.9	7.2
Cheese, mozzarella part skim—1½ oz	108	10.4	1.2	6.8
Cheese, ricotta whole milk—½ cup (4 oz)	216	14.0	3.8	16.1
Cheese, ricotta part skim— ½ cup (4 oz)	171	14.1	6.4	9.8

Note: This table should be used as a guide for the foods listed. Since food values vary by brand name it is important to read the food labels for these foods.

Moreover, the one serving of skim milk has only a trace (less than one percent) of fat. Compare this to the ice cream with 35.6 grams of fat—that is 61 percent of total calories from fat!

Assignment for this lesson

Your Monitoring Form contains entries for the new behaviors discussed above. The first three relate to lifestyle changes with shopping: shop on a full stomach, shop from a list, and buy foods that require preparation. Begin thinking about a programmed activity. This is also the time to examine your goals and emotional responses. Refer to the model in this lesson to discover the relationship between the goals you set and your feelings and emotions.

When you spot unrealistic goals, replace them with more rational goals. Finally, use the upcoming days to experiment with a shopping partnership and to decrease the amount of fat in your diet. And finally, plan your diet to include the required number of servings from the Milk, Yogurt, and Cheese Group.

Self-assessment questionnaire

Lesson Seven

T F 34. It is wise to shop for food when you are hungry to test the new restraint you have learned.

T F 35. Buying foods that require preparation can increase your awareness of eating and help you eat less.

T F 36. Most people get enough exercise to realize the many health benefits of an active lifestyle.

T F 37. Exercise must be done in specific amounts for it to aid you with weight loss.

T F 38. Thirty minutes of moderate—intensity physical activity is now recommended for Americans.

T F 39. All nutrients that we eat contain calories.

T F 40. The recommended number of daily servings from the Milk, Yogurt, and Cheese Group is two to three.

T F 41. Eating yogurt everyday can help you lose weight.

(Answers in Appendix C)

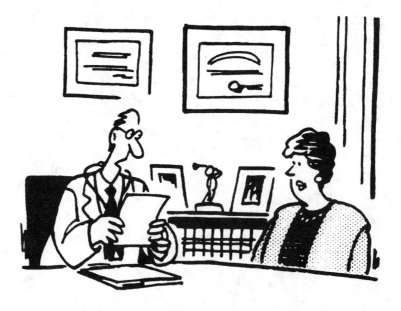

© 1987 by NEA inc   1-8

"I see you've slipped off the program. You tested positive for ICE CREAM USE."

Monitoring Form—Lesson Seven

Today's Date:

Time	Food and Amount	Calories
Total Daily Calories		

Assignment this week		*Always*	*Sometimes*	*Never*
1.	Shop on a full stomach			
2.	Shop from a list			
3.	Eat foods that require preparation			
4.	Examine goals and emotions			
5.	Daily servings from the Milk Group			
6.	Less than _____ calories each day			
7.	Less than _____ grams of fat each day			

Food Groups for Today	*Physical Activity*	*Minutes*
Milk, yogurt, and cheese ❑ ❑ ❑		
Meat, poultry, etc. ❑ ❑ ❑		
Fruits ❑ ❑ ❑ ❑		
Vegetables ❑ ❑ ❑ ❑ ❑		
Breads, cereals, etc. ❑ ❑ ❑ ❑ ❑ ❑ ❑ ❑ ❑ ❑		

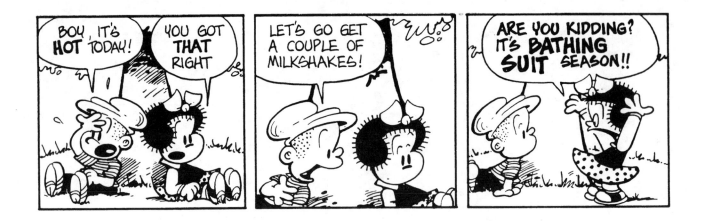

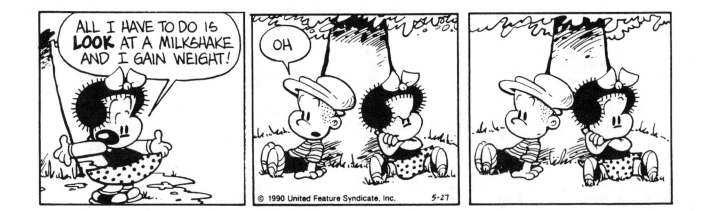

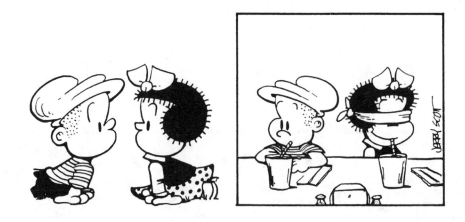

It is time to expand our discussion of behavior modification (lifestyle) techniques to storing food and to further discuss programmed activity. You will learn about attitude traps, and I will introduce one of the five categories of problem thinking—dichotomous thinking. The importance of protein in the diet will be covered, and you will learn all about the Meat, Poultry, Fish, Dry Beans, Egg, and Nut Group of the Food Guide Pyramid.

Storing foods (out of sight, out of mouth)

The less you see and think about food, the easier it will be to control eating. Where and how you store food can influence what and how much you eat.

Let's examine two approaches to the same problem to illustrate this point. Suppose salted nuts are your passion and you bring home a one pound bag from Tiny's Nut House. You could make the nuts a constant temptation by keeping them in an open dish, using the classic dodge that, "I need them in case someone drops by."

Another approach would be to keep the nuts out of sight. This would put some effort between the nuts and you. You could lock them in a safe which is stored in your attic behind 24 boxes of old papers and books. In which case would you eat more nuts?

The attic example is far-fetched, but it does show how the accessibility of food can influence whether you eat. Storing food wisely and keeping it out of sight can be helpful. Here are some ways to follow through.

♦ **Hide the high-calorie foods.** High-calorie impulse foods should be stored out of sight. Put the ice cream under the frozen peas and behind the chicken breasts so you won't see it each time you open the door. Store the cookies on a high shelf behind the seldom-used guest dishes, and put the potato chips on a low shelf behind the colander.

This leads back to Antecedents (discussed in Lesson Four). Bringing problem foods in the house and having them available are steps that precede eating. It would, of course, be preferable to intervene at the earliest step and not buy the foods at all. If you do buy the foods, keeping them out of the way is the next logical step.

Keeping food out of sight serves two purposes. If you don't see it, you may not be stimulated to eat. Also, putting some effort between you and the food stops automatic eating and gives you time to change your mind. You can help the cause even more by storing foods in opaque containers. Keeping

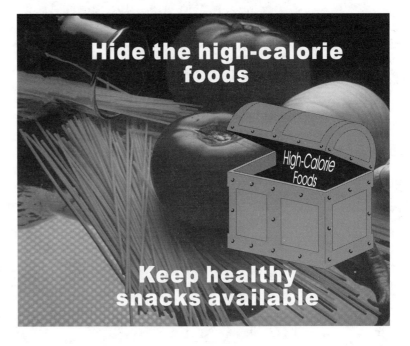

Hide the high-calorie foods

High-Calorie Foods

Keep healthy snacks available

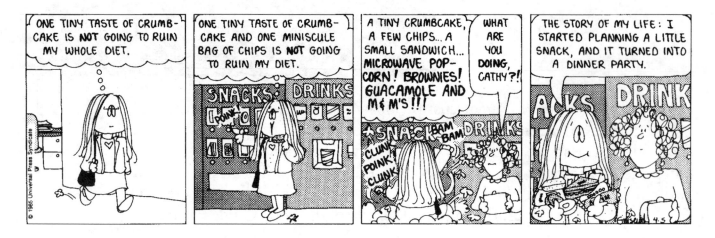

the brownies in a plastic bowl will make them less tempting than having them in a clear cookie jar.

- ◆ **Keep healthy snacks available.** Since Sherlock Holmes would now have trouble finding the high-calorie foods in your house, you can use the space vacated by goodies to store healthy foods. If you get an urge to eat, reach for the celery, carrot sticks, raisins, apples, cauliflower, vegetable soup, and oranges.

Compulsive eating and binge eating

There is increasing awareness that some people with weight problems struggle with episodes of eating large amounts of food and feeling out of control. Overeaters Anonymous popularized the most widely used term for this problem— compulsive overeating. Researchers have called this binge eating.

The official definition of binge eating has two features. The first is eating what others would consider a large amount of food and the second is feeling out of control. When this happens with sufficient frequency (two times a week or more) and over a sufficient period of time (six months) a person can qualify for a diagnosis called Binge Eating Disorder. I hasten to add that some people have binges many more times than this, and some people have fewer or less frequent binges but still have a troubling problem.

In the early stages of research on binge eating, some experts felt that individuals who ate compulsively needed treatment for this type of

eating disorder in addition to whatever help they needed for weight. More recently, research has shown that individuals who participate in a program like *The LEARN Program* stop binge eating as well as people who get a program focused specifically on the binge eating, but in addition, lose more weight. Therefore, if you have a problem with binge eating, you may find that this program helps with both the control over eating and with weight loss.

There will be some people who need additional help. If by this time in the program you are having problems with eating compulsively, you might examine whether additional resources would be helpful. I can suggest three approaches.

The first approach is to use a book entitled *Overcoming Binge Eating* written by Dr. Christopher Fairburn, a leading authority from Oxford University in England. The book is an excellent guide that has been tested thoroughly and brings the best of science to the reader in a useable and friendly format. The book is published by Guilford Press in New York and can be ordered by calling 1-800-736-7323. This is the best such guide of its type in the world today.

The second, but more expensive alternative, is to seek counseling. If you choose this course, try to see someone with special experience in treating eating disorders. Several organizations can provide the names of professionals in your area who have experience with eating disorders, although there is no guarantee that such professionals are truly skilled. These organizations are listed in the table here. The two approaches that have been proven effective for binge eating are cognitive behavior therapy and interpersonal psychotherapy, so you might ask if the professional you contact offers one of these.

A final approach is to consider help from Overeaters Anonymous (OA). While OA has not been evaluated, it does offer strong support and a focus on compulsive eating. For some people, the support, the around-the-clock help available from a sponsor, and the group meetings can be quite helpful.

Selecting and starting a programmed activity

It is time to choose your programmed activity. What follows are guidelines for making your selection, along with simple exercises for warming up and cooling down. I'll also discuss cardiovascular training.

Choosing the best activity

There are many activities to choose from. Several possibilities will be discussed below. There are four factors to consider in making your decision.

- **Select something you can do.** Consider your current physical condition when choosing an activity. Basketball is strenuous and is not advisable if you are not in tiptop condition. Pick something where you can move at your own pace. Walking, cycling, and swimming are good examples.

- **Select something you would like to do.** Hiking may be something that always caught your fancy, so go ahead and try. If you are turned off by swimming, don't do it just because you think you should. It helps to like the activities you choose.

- **Select a solo or social activity.** We covered this earlier in our discussion of walking. In your choice of an activity, consider whether you would like to exercise alone (jogging, swimming, cycling) or with other people (tennis, golf, aerobics class). If you are a social

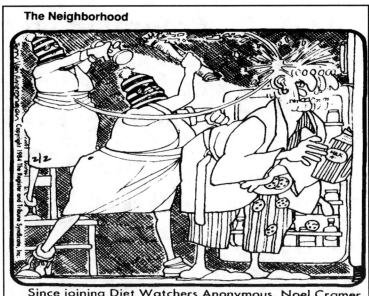

The Neighborhood

Since joining Diet Watchers Anonymous, Noel Cramer continues to be surprised at just how comprehensive the group's services are.

Support Organizations for Eating Disorders
(Potential Help for Compulsive Eating/Binge Eating)

United States

National Eating Disorders Organization
445 E. Granville Road
Worthington, OH 43085-3195
614-436-1112

American Anorexia/Bulimia Association
418 E. 76th Street
New York, NY 10021
212-734-1114

National Association of Anorexia Nervosa and Related Diseases
Box 7
Highland Park, IL 60035
708-831-3438

Anorexia Nervosa and Related Eating Disorders
P.O. Box 5102
Eugene, OR 97405
503-344-1144

Canada

National Eating Disorder Information Centre
200 Elizabeth Street
College Way
Toronto, Ontario M5G 2C4
416-340-4156

Bulimia, Anorexia Association
3640 Wells Street
Windsor, Ontario N9C 1T9
519-253-7545

United Kingdom

Eating Disorders Association
Sackville Place
44 Magdalen Street
Norwich
Norfolk NR3 1J3
01603-621414

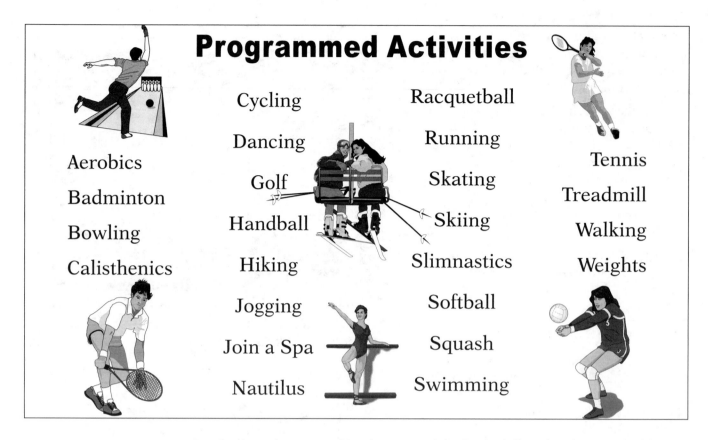

Programmed Activities

Aerobics

Badminton

Bowling

Calisthenics

Cycling

Dancing

Golf

Handball

Hiking

Jogging

Join a Spa

Nautilus

Racquetball

Running

Skating

Skiing

Slimnastics

Softball

Squash

Swimming

Tennis

Treadmill

Walking

Weights

---

person, having others around can be an incentive to participate.

♦ **Do not be embarrassed.** This is easier said than done. Many heavy people avoid exercise completely, or avoid it when they can be seen by others. They are embarrassed about their bodies, their clothes, and their poor physical condition. Try to put this aside. Take a deep breath, and ask yourself which is more important, avoiding embarrassment or losing weight.

A helpful tip

Let me pass along a tip drawn from my own experience. I exercise regularly and try to have a number of activities to choose from. I run, ride a bike, play tennis, and do strength training. Mixing up these activities provides me with choice and variety, both of which help minimize boredom. I can watch TV, listen to music, or both while doing some of these things, so I sometimes "save" the exercise when I know there is something I might like to see on the television.

Most people can probably find more than one activity as a possibility. If an outside activity is not possible, then an inside alternative might fit the bill. They key is whether you will still be active months or years from now. Whether this occurs depends in large part on whether you enjoy it, and whether *I* enjoy it depends in large part on variety and the presence of other interesting things.

Warming up and cooling down

It is important to warm up before exercise and to cool down afterwards. This will help stretch your muscles to avoid strains and pulls. It will also help your heart and circulatory system make the transition from rest to exercise and then back to rest. You should warm up and cool down at least five minutes for a 30-minute bout of exercise.

In general, a good warm-up for most activities is the same activity performed at lower intensity. Walking slowly is a good warm-up for brisk walking, and brisk walking can serve as a warm-up for running. Here are several additional exercises to warm up. Please note that some exercises may be problematic if you have certain conditions. Trunk twists may create difficulty if you have back problems. Check with your physician or a sports medicine specialist if you have such problems.

- **Trunk Twists.** Stand with your feet shoulder width apart. Extend your arms to the side so they are horizontal. Twist your trunk to the right as if you are trying to look over your right shoulder. Then reverse directions and move your trunk so your left arm extends to your right. This exercise should be done slowly or as a held stretch to avoid jerking of the muscles.

- **Toe Touches.** Stand with your feet a little more than shoulder width apart. Bend at the waist, and slowly attempt to touch your toes with your finger tips. Keep your knees *bent* and do not bounce the upper body. Hold the stretch for a few seconds. Return to the standing position and then repeat. If you have back problems, the sit and reach exercise may present fewer difficulties.

- **Sit and Reach.** Sit on the floor with your legs straight out in front of you. Slowly reach to touch your toes, and hold the reach for a few seconds. As with the toe touches, keeping the legs bent is important to avoid strain on the knees and back.

- **Arm Circles.** In the standing position, hold your arms out to the side of your body in a horizontal position. Roll your arms up, back, and then down to produce backward circles.

When you begin your programmed activity, be it cycling, swimming, walking, or anything, begin slowly and gradually increase your pace. To end your exercise session, gradually decrease the pace, and then finish with some combination of the exercises described above. The warming up and cooling down activities are worth the little extra time they take. They can prevent nagging injuries that could keep you away from exercise for a long time.

Cardiovascular training

Exercise physiologists have done extensive research to show how much exercise is necessary to improve cardiovascular condition. This refers to the efficiency of your heart, blood vessels, and general circulatory and res-

piratory systems. From this research was born a formula known to millions of people. This three-part formula deals with *how much*, *how often*, and *how long* you must exercise to get this training effect. Keep in mind that this formula for cardiovascular training is much different than the activity needed to reach a moderate level of fitness as I discussed in Lesson Seven.

This is what aerobics is all about. An activity is *aerobic* if the body uses large amounts of oxygen (i.e., if the heart, lungs, and blood vessels are working hard). As a result of this hard work, these parts of the body become conditioned. This conditioning is associated with greater life expectancy, lowered risk of heart disease, and other positive effects.

What about the FIT approach?

The question then is "How much and what type of activity should I do?" The answer to this question comes from the American College of Sports Medicine (ACSM), an authoritative organization of professionals in exercise physiology and sports medicine.

The ACSM has published a position paper entitled, "The Recommended Quantity and Quality of Exercise for Developing and Maintaining Cardiorespiratory and Muscular Fitness in Adults." *Cardiorespiratory* fitness refers to the condition of your heart (cardio) and lungs (respiratory).

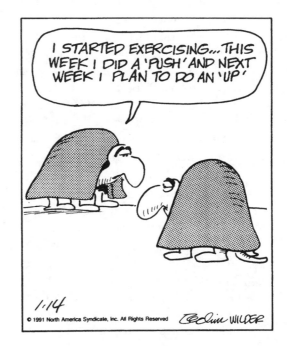

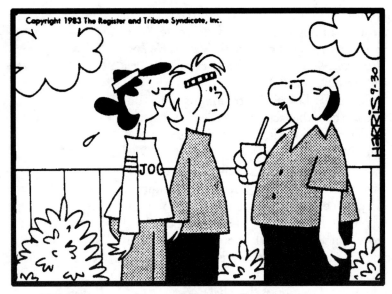

"Stanley exercises religiously. Does one push-up and thanks God it didn't kill him."

The ACSM document focuses on the F.I.T. principle (Frequency, Intensity, and Time). These are important for cardiovascular conditioning, while frequency and the number of repetitions is important for increasing muscular strength. There are five main components to the ACSM guidelines:

❶ Frequency of Training

Exercising 3–5 days per week is recommended.

❷ Intensity of Training

During a bout of exercise, your heart rate should be 60–90 percent of maximum. You can estimate your maximum heart rate by subtracting your age from 220. For instance, for a person who is 40 years old, maximum heart rate would be 180 beats per minute (220-40). During a workout, this person would want the heart to beat 108–162 times per minute (this is 60–90 percent of the maximum of 180 beats per minute).

❸ Duration of Training

The recommended duration of activity is 20–60 minutes of continuous aerobic activity. High intensity activities require less duration. The ACSM notes that *total fitness* can be attained with longer duration programs, and that lower intensity exercise over a longer time is easier to sustain.

❹ Type of Activity

Recommended activities are those that use large muscle groups, are rhythmic and aerobic, and can be maintained continuously. Examples are walking, hiking, running, jogging, cycling, cross country skiing, dancing, skipping rope, rowing, swimming, stair climbing, skating, and endurance game activities.

❺ Resistance Training

To improve muscle strength, 8–12 repetitions of 8–10 exercises that focus on the major muscle groups are recommended for a minimum of two days per week.

If you are sufficiently fit to focus on these issues, these guidelines should be helpful. If not, it is important to emphasize small and gradual changes in physical activity, remembering that *any* activity is helpful.

Do you need this?

It takes vigorous activity to get your heart rate to this target zone of 60–90 percent of maximum. Keeping it there for 20 minutes can be difficult for some people. Take your pulse the next time you go for a walk. Use the procedure described in Lesson Six to take your pulse, except take the pulse immediately after you stop walking. Count the beats in ten seconds, then multiply by six for the number of beats per minute. The level is probably below the 60–90 percent demanded by the formula.

The important question is, "Do you need to do this much?" The answer is "yes" if you want to get the training effect. The answer is an emphatic "no" if you are exercising to boost your weight loss or to reach the moderate level of fitness discussed in Lesson Seven. *Any exercise is better than no exercise.* Low levels of activity can help, so you may be best off ignoring the formula. I presented it here to clarify the numbers that are widely cited. Exercise in any amount carries many benefits, so do not be discouraged if you do not meet the standards set by the formula.

It is also essential to remember that the high level of exercise needed to improve cardiorespiratory fitness is not necessary to lower risk. You may recall information from the Blair study (see the graph on page 89) showing that the greatest benefit to health occurs between people in the least fit (completely sedentary) and the next group (people who are only moderately active). Hence, we must match our activity to our goals, and to improve health and lose weight, small amounts of physical activity may be very helpful.

Remember to be cautious when beginning an exercise program. Guidelines for deciding whether you need medical screening are listed in Lesson Three. Review the guidelines and consult a physician if these or any other factors suggest any problems. Most people without a specific health problem can safely begin a program of at least brisk walking.

It is essential that you warm up and cool down before and after exercise. The body does not like abrupt changes, so you must warm up to prepare it for vigorous activity and cool down in the transition from exercise to rest. You may want to review the section about warming up and cooling down that I presented earlier in this lesson.

Danger! An exercise threshold attitude

Many people on weight-loss programs labor under the insidious influence of a dangerous attitude—the exercise threshold. They feel they must do a magic amount of exercise for it to have any value. One client asked me, "Is it enough that I walked around the block after dinner last night?" Implicit in this word *enough* is that exercising below this threshold has no value. You must banish this concept from your mind!

The threshold concept was born from the cardiovascular training idea discussed above. If you will forgive me for stating it again: *Any exercise is better than no exercise.* Walking

around the block is not as impressive as running a marathon, but it's a far sight better than watching reruns of Gilligan's Island and munching on corn chips. If you walk two blocks, it is better than one block, but not as good as three blocks. Do *anything* to be active. Remember, small amounts of exercise add up, so do not feel you must strain to accomplish some arbitrary level.

Internal attitude traps

Each of us holds internal conversations. We discussed this earlier regarding goal setting and emotions. How you view your lifestyle changes can help or hinder you greatly. There are several common traps you may encounter. If you are prepared with counter thoughts and attitudes, your job will be easier.

Countering the traps

You might visualize the part of yourself that pressures you to eat. You can be more than a match for this part, but only if you are conscientious and face the problem directly. What follows are some common traps, called *fat thoughts*. I will give you material for possible counter measures.

Internal Trap #1
"The diet is the key."

Fat Thought: The diet and this program are the only reasons I lose weight. When the diet is over, I will have real trouble keeping the weight off.

Counter: I am losing weight because of my own efforts. Just because the program ends

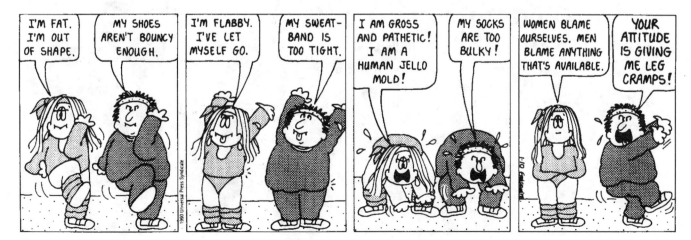

does not mean my new habits will vanish. The program helps me along, but I get the credit.

Internal Trap #2
"Is this worth the effort?"

Fat Thought: I have been on my program for weeks and I still have lots of weight to lose. I can't wait till this program ends so I can get back to normal.

Counter: Stop this right now! Who said this would be easy? It took a long time to gain the weight, and it will take a long time to lose it. I would like to lose fast and easy, but facts are facts. I don't want to let down now and waste the effort. I *can* stick with it.

Internal Trap #3
"I have done this before."

Fat Thought: I have heard this nutrition stuff before, and we covered behavior modification in Weight Watchers. It didn't help me then and will not help me now.

Counter: I have never been taught these things in such a concentrated way, and my motivation to learn may be different now. I know deep down this is the only way to get permanent results, so putting down the approach just means I have trouble doing the work. Only I can do it, so I must forge ahead.

Try to recognize these and other internal traps. The *fat thoughts* you have lived with for years will do their best to control your attitudes and eating. Now you can blast them with a counterattack.

Dichotomous (light bulb) thinking

This is the classic attitude problem that plagues many people on weight-loss programs. It involves viewing the world and losing weight as either right or wrong, perfect or terrible, good or bad, friend or foe, legal or illegal. I see this in nearly every client I work with.

Here are some examples. You might have six straight days in which you meet your calorie level and then splurge the seventh day by eating cake and boosting your calorie total to 2000. The common response would be "I really blew it now. I am off my program."

Notice the phrase "off my program." This is the dichotomous view that you are either perfect or terrible, that you are either on or off a program. This is where the term *Light Bulb Thinking* was born, because a light bulb is either on or off.

The danger is the despair that you feel about making inevitable mistakes. Having 2000 calories is insignificant in your total calories for a week, month, or year. However, your *reaction* to those calories can be devastating. If you feel guilty and depressed, the likely response to soothe the feelings is eating.

Another example is the tendency for people to classify foods as good or bad, dietetic or fattening, and legal or illegal. The specific foods that are good or bad vary from person to person. For you, ice cream might be the illegal food, but for another person it might be corn chips, beer, donuts, potato chips, or fast food. Dichotomous thinking occurs when you slip and feel you have blown the program. A slight transgression can send you into a tailspin.

It is essential that you be aware of your dichotomous thoughts. Have you made internal rules about foods that you can and cannot eat, a calorie level you *must* maintain, things you must do to stay "on the program," or what

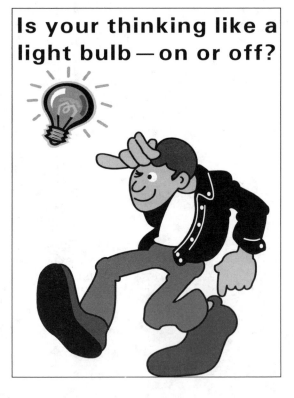
Is your thinking like a light bulb — on or off?

constitutes proper dietary behavior? Notice how you feel when you violate the rules. Negative feelings usually indicate dichotomous thinking.

You can contend with dichotomous thinking by talking back to yourself. You realize how illogical it is to feel terrible about one slip or to make rules where eating some food throws you off your program.

Please realize that attitudes are habits just like any other. Simply reading this material and knowing that attitudes might be hindering your progress is not enough. It will help to practice the new thinking and then to practice again. Try not to be a passive recipient of my advice. Be active and search for these thoughts, and be poised to counter them when they occur.

In the spaces below, write down your most common dichotomous thoughts and write a counter statement for each. You can then be prepared in advance when the fat thoughts occur.

The importance of protein

Protein is a popular topic of conversation. We hear about high-protein diets and low-protein diets. We know about liquid protein, protein bread, and protein supplements. What is this fuss about?

Protein is the most abundant material in the body aside from water. It has many functions and is found in all cells. It plays many roles:

- Protein is contained in hemoglobin, which carries oxygen in the blood.
- Protein is related to DNA (deoxyribonucleic acid), which provides the genes with the code to transmit heredity.
- Protein is used to build muscle and all other body tissue.
- Protein is an important part of insulin, which regulates blood sugar.
- Protein is used to build the enzymes that digest our food.

What is protein?

Proteins are built from approximately 20 amino acids which are put together in long chains. Protein can be synthesized or manufactured by the body, but only if the *essential* amino acids are present at the same time. Of the 20 different amino acids, nine are considered *essential* and cannot be made by the body. Therefore, they must be provided in the foods that we eat. The protein our body uses best contains these amino acids. The 11 *nonessential* amino acids can be synthesized by the body, but only if the building blocks are present. These building blocks include the nine essential amino acids, nitrogen, and calories.

You may have heard about *high-quality* and *low-quality* proteins. When the dangers of the liquid protein diet became clear in the mid and late 1970s, the use of low-quality protein in the liquid formulas was cited as one of the hazards.

Countering Dichotomous (Light Bulb) Thinking	
My Fat Thoughts	*My Counter Statements*
1.	
2.	
3.	
4.	
5.	
6.	
7.	
8.	

High-quality proteins are those the body can use to function properly, because they contain all of the essential amino acids. Low-quality proteins have one or more essential amino acids missing.

Sources of protein

Meat and dairy products contain high-quality proteins and do not have to be supplemented with other proteins since they contain all nine of the essential amino acids. Plant proteins usually lack one or more of the essential amino acids, but can provide adequate amounts of the essential and nonessential amino acids. Vegetarian diets can provide adequate protein if the sources are reasonably varied and the caloric intake is enough to meet the individual's energy needs.

Eating a variety of legumes and grains will produce high-quality protein. Legumes include dried peas and beans, such as black-eyed peas, chick peas (garbanzo beans), kidney beans, lentils, lima beans, navy beans, and soybeans. Soy protein has been has been shown to be nutritionally equivalent in protein value to proteins of animal origin. Nuts are also in this category, but they contain high amounts of fat. Grains include barley, corn, oats, rice, sesame seeds, sunflower seeds, and wheat.

Protein rarely exists by itself (egg whites or albumin is the exception) and is most often ac-companied with mixtures of fat in foods like meat, fish, poultry, and milk products. Protein contains four (4) calories per gram; this is the same caloric content by weight as carbohydrates. One ounce (28 grams) of lean meat, fish, or poultry contains approximately seven (7) grams of protein and three (3) grams of fat (a total of 55 calories), whereas protein foods with higher fat content provide as much as 70 to 120 calories per ounce and 5 to 10 grams of fat per ounce.

How much protein should you eat?

Some health experts believe that Americans eat too much protein and that reduction would be desirable. A major benefit would be a reduction in total fat since the most popular protein foods (meat, fish, and poultry) also provide significant amounts of fat. We must remember, however, that protein in the diet is essential. Recommended amounts of protein range from 10 to 15 percent of total calories or approximately 50–75 grams of protein per day for adults. To see how your daily protein intake fits the guidelines for a healthy diet, multiply your target calorie level by 15 percent, the maximum recommended protein calories per day. For example, if your target caloric intake is 1200, 1200 x .15 = 180. Since there are 4 calories in every gram of protein, divide 180 by 4; 180 ÷ 4 = 45. You know that you need to eat about 45 grams of protein daily to meet the government's recommended guidelines.

The meat, poultry, fish, eggs, and nut group

The food items in this group include meat, poultry, fish, dry beans, eggs, and nuts. Meat, poultry, and fish provide good sources of protein, B vitamins, iron, and zinc. Dry beans, eggs, and nuts are similar to meats in providing protein and most vitamins and minerals.

How much is a serving?

As a general rule, two to three ounces of cooked lean meat, poultry, or fish count as one serving from the Meat and Protein Group. A

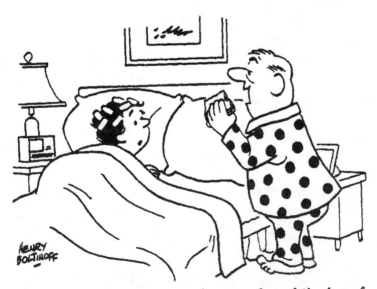

"I tried counting sheep, and remembered the leg of lamb."

The Food Guide Pyramid

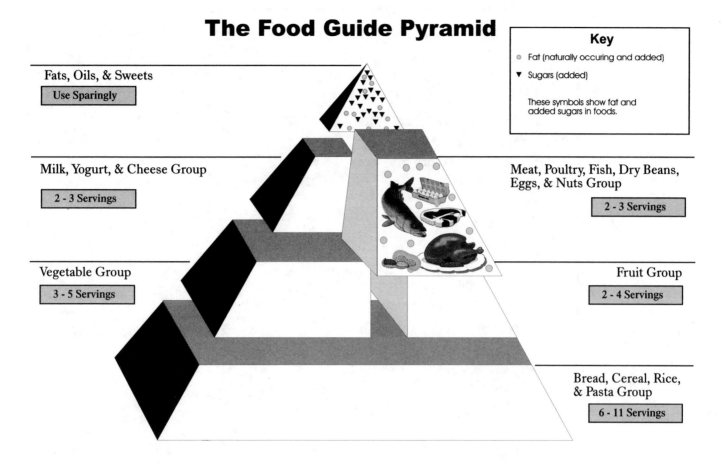

Key
- Fat (naturally occuring and added)
- ▼ Sugars (added)

These symbols show fat and added sugars in foods.

Fats, Oils, & Sweets
| Use Sparingly |

Milk, Yogurt, & Cheese Group
| 2 - 3 Servings |

Meat, Poultry, Fish, Dry Beans, Eggs, & Nuts Group
| 2 - 3 Servings |

Vegetable Group
| 3 - 5 Servings |

Fruit Group
| 2 - 4 Servings |

Bread, Cereal, Rice, & Pasta Group
| 6 - 11 Servings |

three-ounce piece of meat is about the size of an average hamburger, or the amount of meat on a medium chicken breast half. For other foods in this group, count ½ cup of cooked dry beans, two tablespoons of peanut butter, or one egg as one ounce of meat (i.e., 1/3 of a serving). As an example, six ounces for the day (two servings) may come from:

☑ 1 egg (counts as 1 oz of lean meat) for breakfast;

☑ 2 oz of sliced turkey in a sandwich at lunch;

☑ 3 oz cooked lean hamburger for dinner.

How many servings?

The Food Guide Pyramid suggests two to three servings per day from the Meat and Protein Group. The total from all servings should be the equivalent of between five and seven ounces of cooked lean meat, poultry, or fish per day. The chart on the following page shows items from this food group.

Watch out for fat

As mentioned earlier, the best sources of protein come from animal products, such as dairy, meat, poultry, fish, and eggs. However, these food sources can be high in saturated fat and cholesterol. These tips will help reduce fat in your diet:

◆ Choose lean meat, poultry without skin, fish, and dry beans and peas. These foods are the choices that are lowest in dietary fat.

◆ Prepare meats in lowfat ways; trim away all the visible fat and boil, roast, or broil these foods instead of frying them.

◆ Eat egg yolks sparingly; they are high in cholesterol. Use only one yolk per person in egg dishes and make larger portions by adding extra egg whites.

◆ Remember, nuts and seeds are high in fat, so they should be eaten in moderation.

◆ For beef, roasts & steaks of round, loin, sirloin, and chuck arm are lean choices.

Meat, Poultry, Fish, Dry Beans, Eggs, and Nuts

Description	Calories	Protein (g)	Carb. (g)	Fat (g)
Beef:				
Chuck arm, lean braised (3 oz)	191	28.0	0	7.9
Ground, lean broiled (3 oz)	231	21.0	0	15.7
Round, lean broiled (3 oz)	204	23.0	0	11.6
Sirloin, lean broiled (3 oz)	229	23.5	0	14.3
Chicken:				
Dark, w skin roasted (3 oz)	215	22.0	0	13.4
Dark, w/o skin roasted (3 oz)	174	23.3	0	8.3
Light, w skin roasted (3 oz)	189	24.7	0	9.2
Light, w/o skin roasted (3 oz)	147	26.3	0	3.8
Fish:				
Flounder/sole, baked (3 oz)	173	25.7	0	7.0
Haddock, baked (3 oz)	95	20.6	0	.8
Lobster, steamed (3 oz)	83	17.4	1.1	.5
Shrimp, breaded & fried (3 oz)	206	18.2	9.8	10.4
Shrimp, boiled (3 oz)	84	17.8	.0	.9
Trout, baked (3 oz)	129	22.4	.0	3.7
Tuna, canned in water (3 oz)	111	25.1	.0	.4
Pork:				
Chop, lean center broiled (3 oz)	190	16.0	0	13.0
Ham, cured roasted (3 oz)	239	17.4	0	18.2
Loin, lean braised (3 oz)	266	25.3	0	17.5
Black-eye peas, boiled (1½ cup)	297	19.8	53.3	1.4
Chick-peas, boiled (1½ cup)	403	21.8	67.5	6.5
Great northern beans, boiled (1½ cup)	315	22.2	55.9	1.2
Kidney beans, boiled (1½ cup)	338	23.1	60.6	1.4
Lima beans, boiled (1½ cup)	326	22.0	58.9	1.1
Navy beans, boiled (1½ cup)	389	23.7	71.9	1.5
Pink beans, boiled (1½ cup)	378	22.9	70.8	1.2
Pinto beans, boiled (1½ cup)	353	21.0	65.8	1.4
Pigeon peas, boiled (1½ cup)	306	17.1	58.6	.9
Split peas, boiled (1½ cup)	347	24.6	62.1	1.2
Egg, raw whole (3 eggs)	126	10.5	.9	8.4
Peanut butter (6 T)	564	23.1	20.7	48.0
Peanuts, dry roasted (1 cup)	814	23.7	34.7	70.5
Rice, long grain brown (1½ cup)	324	7.5	67.2	2.7
Rice, long grain white (1½ cup)	396	8.3	85.8	.9

Note: Each of the food items listed above counts as one serving. This table should be used as a guide for the foods listed. Since food values vary by brand name it is important to read the food labels for these foods.

- For pork, roasts & chops of tenderloin, center loin, and ham are the leaner choices.
- For veal, all cuts are generally lean, except for ground veal.
- Lamb roasts & chops of leg, loin, and fore shanks provide the lean cuts.
- Fish & shellfish are generally low in fat, however, those canned or marinated in oil are higher.
- For chicken and turkey, both light and dark meat are lean choices provided the skin has been removed.

Assignment for this lesson

This lesson covers behavior, attitudes, and nutrition, along with more emphasis on exercise. Make a sweep through your house and hide the high-calorie foods. Replace them with nutritious foods. Select a programmed activity and go to it! Be prepared to counter dichotomous (light bulb) thinking. Finally, be aware of the amount of protein you eat and check to make sure you are eating the required number of servings from the Meat Group of the Food Guide Pyramid.

Self-assessment questionnaire

Lesson Eight

T F 42. Keeping high-calorie foods stored out of sight can decrease impulsive eating.

T F 43. Warming up and stretching before exercise is to strengthen your muscles.

T F 44. To get a cardiovascular training effect, there must be the right combination of frequency, intensity, and time.

T F 45. Fat thoughts can hinder a person's efforts to lose weight.

T F 46. Light bulb or dichotomous thinking refers to your own *bright* ideas about losing weight.

(Answers in Appendix C)

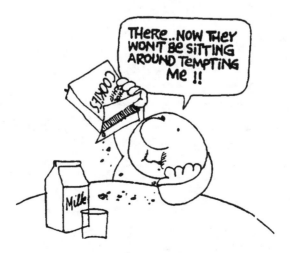

THERE..NOW THEY WON'T BE SITTING AROUND TEMPTING ME !!

Monitoring Form—Lesson Eight

Today's Date:

Time	Food and Amount	Calories
Total Daily Calories		

Assignment this week		Always	Sometimes	Never
1.	Hide high-calorie foods			
2.	Keep healthy foods in sight			
3.	Begin programmed activity			
4.	Counter dichotomous thinking			
5.	Daily servings from the Meat and Protein Group			
6.	Less than _____ calories each day			
7.	My diet has _____ grams of protein			

Food Groups for Today		Physical Activity	Minutes
Milk, yogurt, and cheese	❑ ❑ ❑		
Meat, poultry, etc.	❑ ❑ ❑		
Fruits	❑ ❑ ❑ ❑		
Vegetables	❑ ❑ ❑ ❑ ❑		
Breads, cereals, etc.	❑ ❑ ❑ ❑ ❑ ❑ ❑ ❑ ❑ ❑		

This lesson will continue our discussion of handling food. We have gone from shopping to storing, and will now discuss serving, displaying, and handling food. I will introduce another major attitude category, called the Impossible Dream. The Relationship area provides information to be read by partners. The Nutrition section will deal with more about vitamins, carbohydrates, and the Vegetable Group of the Food Guide Pyramid.

Serving and dispensing food

Here are five questions I like to ask to determine whether a person reacts to the site, smell, thought, or other stimulation from food.

❶ Do you feel like eating dessert when it looks appetizing even after eating a large meal?

❷ Is there always room for something you like?

❸ Do you get excited by a buffet?

❹ If you drive by a bakery or fast food place and smell the food, do you want to eat regardless of when you ate last?

❺ Do you feel like eating when you see a picture of a delicious dessert in a magazine?

If you answer "yes" to these questions, you may be high in externality. This means you are sensitive to external cues or signals, namely the sight, smell, or suggestion of food. If this describes you, join the crowd. There are millions like you, both heavy and thin. It can be very helpful for you to reduce your exposure to food. If this description does not fit you, read on anyway. These techniques may help you corral your desire to overeat.

The methods you learned earlier for buying and storing food were designed to reduce exposure to food. We have been moving forward in the sequence of antecedents. We began with the first step (shopping). We then moved a step closer to eating (storing food). We will now move even closer by discussing serving and dispensing food.

I will describe several techniques for storing food. All follow from a general *principle*, which is to interrupt the sequence of events associated with eating. Some techniques will apply to you more than others. You can use the principle to develop techniques of your own.

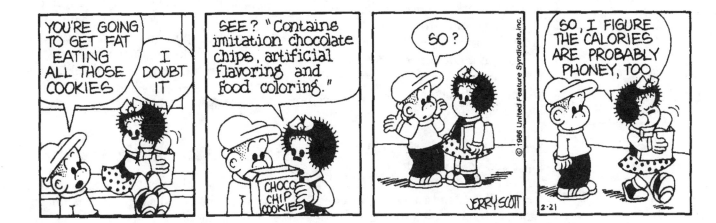

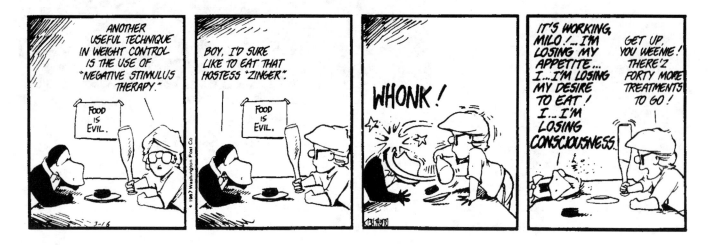

The following techniques are designed to help you control eating when your exposure to food signals is at its peak. The aim is to minimize your contact with these signals.

- **Remove serving dishes from the table.** After first servings have been made, remove the food dishes from the table. Having the food handy is asking for trouble. If the food dishes are in another room or on another table, you can *think* before taking more. This does not prohibit you from having seconds, but it does interrupt the automatic eating that occurs when your plate is a magnet for anything left on the serving dishes.

- **Leave the table after eating.** This may sound anti-social, but some people are helped by leaving the table after dinner. This reduces the time you are exposed to food and to the circumstances of eating. If you finish long before the others, you may be eating too fast, and slowing down would help. If not, perhaps the others can retire to another room with you for the post-meal chat. This technique can work in concert with the previous suggestion to remove serving dishes from the table. If *all* the dishes are gone, it is not necessary to leave the table because exposure to food signals will be low. If food remains, bid the table farewell and depart for safer surroundings.

- **Serve and eat one portion at a time.** Make and serve yourself only one portion of food. If you want two pieces of toast, make one and eat it before making another. If you want a container of yo-

gurt, put half in a bowl and return for the second half if you still want it. You might find yourself passing up the second portion because you are no longer hungry. Here again is a chance to interrupt that automatic eating. This can also help you separate hunger from habit. Because you have eaten one container of yogurt every morning for ten years does not mean your body is hungry for that amount every day.

- **Follow the five-minute rule.** Wait five minutes before going back for extra helpings. This will help you slow the rate of eating and will give you time to decide how much food you really need.

- **Avoid being a food dispenser.** Are you the gatekeeper for food in your house? Do the kids get their snacks from you? Do you prepare all the food? This is a disadvantage because your routine brings you in contact with food many times each day.

Drop the job of being a food dispenser. Have the children pack their own lunches if possible. Your spouse can manage snacks without you, and may be willing to help even more by taking on some of the responsibility you have for distributing food.

More on activity

We are now in Lesson Nine and have covered much of the introductory information on both lifestyle and routine activity. Much has been said about the importance and benefits of regular activity.

Are you being more active?

By this time in the program, my hope is that everybody is exercising daily. If this is possible for you, make it your goal, and do your best to make some time for exercise each day. Of course, missing a day here and there does not mean you have failed in your program. Daily activity is, however, a nice goal to strive for.

Look back over your Monitoring Forms, and see if your level of exercise has changed. Have you found something you like? Do you use this exercise regularly? Does it help you stick to your planned diet and lose weight?

If you are having trouble with the exercise, read over the exercise sections in Lessons One through Seven. Let me remind you that people who are still exercising a year or two after they enter a program tend to be the ones who have lost weight and kept it off.

There are several good reasons why many people resist exercise. For some people the exercise is difficult to manage physically, and for others, strong negative feelings about sports and exercise present a psychological barrier. One common problem is the lack of time and the difficulty in budgeting an hour each day to physical activity.

These are all understandable reasons not to exercise. I hope you find the reasons in favor of exercise to be more compelling. It could mean a great deal to you, both now and in the future.

Consider this a pep talk. I really do feel exercise is important, and I would like to do whatever is possible to encourage you to be active.

Matching your activity to your goals

In the previous chapters we have discussed various reasons to be active. Some people aim to improve their cardiovascular fitness and choose aerobic activities. Some want to increase strength and improve their physique, so they work out with machines or use free weights. Others want to use the exercise to speed weight loss, so they do whatever they can to keep moving, usually with walking or jogging. Each type of activity is valuable, but for different purposes.

By now you have a good idea about what you hope to accomplish with exercise. The table presented on the next page entitled "The Benefits of Various Exercises" shows the strong and weak points of different activities. This may be helpful as you match your exercise to your goals.

It is apparent from the table that the activities useful for controlling body weight also earn high marks for cardiovascular fitness. This is because the movement activities like jogging and cycling require effort (calories) for a sustained time and also give the heart a workout.

Remember, however, that cardiovascular fitness improves only when the right combination of frequency, intensity, and duration are present (See Lesson Eight). To utter once

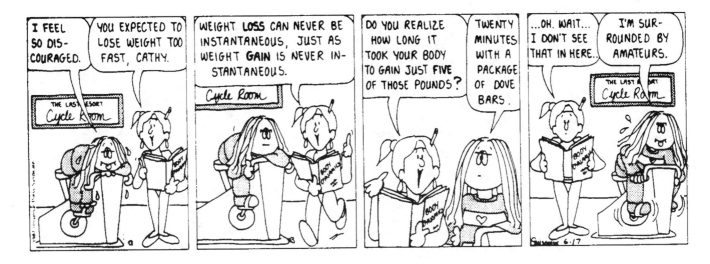

119

The Benefits of Various Exercises

	Developing Cardiovascular Fitness	Developing Developing Strength	Muscular Endurance	Developing Flexibility	Controlling Body Fat
Archery[1]	1	2	1	1	1
Badminton[1]	2	1	2	2	2
Baseball[1]	1	1	1	1	1
Basketball—					
half court[1,2]	2	1	2	1	2
vigorous[1,2]	4	1	3	1	4
Bowling[1]	1	1	1	1	1
Canoeing[1]	2	1	2	1	2
Fencing[2]	2	2	3	2	2
Football[2]	2	3	2	1	2
Golf (walking)[1]	2	1	1	2	2
Gymnastics[2]	2	4	4	4	2
Handball[1,2]	3–4	1	3	1	3–4
Horseback Riding[1]	1	1	1	1	1
Judo/Karate[1,2]	1	2	2	2	1
Mountain Climbing[1,2]	3	3	3	1	3
Pool/Billiards[1]	1	1	1	1	1
Racquetball[1,2]	3–4	1	3	1	3–4
Rowing, Crew	4	2	4	1	4
Sailing[1]	1	1	1	1	1
Skating—					
ice[1,2]	2–3	1	3	1	2–3
roller[1,2]	2–3	1	2	1	2–3
Skiing—					
cross-country[1,2]	4	2	3	1	4
downhill[1,2]	1	2	2	1	1
Soccer[2]	4	2	3	2	4
Softball[1,2]	1	1	1	1	1
Surfing[1,2]	2	1	3	2	2
Table Tennis[1]	1	1	1	1	1
Tennis[1,2]	2–3	1	2	1	2–3
Volleyball[1,2]	2	2	1	1	2
Waterskiing[1,2]	2	2	2	1	2

[1] Indicates lifetime sport.

[2] Indicates fitness needed to prevent injury.

4 = excellent   3 = good   2 = fair   1 = poor

Adapted from C.B. Corbin and R. Lindsey, *Fitness for Life (3rd ed.).* New York: Scott, Foresman & Co., 1993.

again the most oft-repeated sentence in this book: *Any exercise is better than no exercise!*

The myth of spot reducing

Many people would need a computer to count the number of sit-ups they have done to tighten the tummy, leg exercises to trim the thighs, and contortions of the neck to wipe out a double chin. The trouble is, these things don't work, yet millions still fall for slick advertisements or books that promise ways of reducing specific parts of the body.

Where your body stores fat depends on genetic and hormonal factors. Women tend to store fat below the waist, on their hips, thighs, and buttocks. When they become heavy, they also store it above the waist. Men tend to store fat above the waist, in the abdomen. When you lose weight, your body burns fat, but you have little control over where it happens.

Exercises *will* help you with muscle tone. This can improve appearance somewhat. Doing the sit-ups will tighten the muscles in your abdomen and will help you look a little less flabby, but they cannot force your body to take fat from there.

Impossible dream thinking

Along with Dichotomous Thinking, Impossible Dream Thinking ranks high as an attitude barrier to losing weight. This type of thinking occurs when you fantasize or dream about impossible accomplishments. You might have 100 pounds to lose on Thanksgiving and fantasize wearing a size nine to the office Christmas party.

Before you turn the page and skip to the next section, let me assure you that most people are not aware of these thoughts. Yet, after some reflection, most see it clearly. Maybe a few more examples will bring this home.

Impossible Dream thinking occurs when you daydream about how wonderful life will be after weight loss. It is common for those losing weight to imagine an improved marriage, better job, wonderful social life, intimate relationships, and other happy endings to their struggle to lose weight. These things may be possible, but it is unlikely that weight loss alone will make them happen.

This type of thinking also occurs when you imagine succeeding at a program without hard work. When most begin a program and fantasize about the future, they do not picture pain and puffing from exercise and the agony of passing up chocolate mousse.

It does no harm to hope for the best and aspire to improve your life. However, weight loss will usually not make a bad marriage good and will not shoot you to the top of the corporate ladder. Getting your weight down can ac-

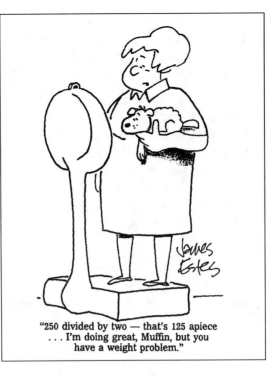

"250 divided by two — that's 125 apiece . . . I'm doing great, Muffin, but you have a weight problem."

tually be a disappointing experience if the fantasy is not fulfilled. This is what happened with one of my clients, Audrey.

Audrey was one of my first overweight clients. She was 28 years old and was working on an advanced degree in chemistry. She had been heavy since childhood and had been in no serious relationships. She was lonely and yearned to settle down with a stable and loving partner.

Audrey lost weight rapidly and seemed happy about her progress. She spoke often, but in a joking way, about how she would meet the person of her dreams when she got thin. I would spot it now, but at the time I did not realize how serious she was about this fantasy. When she reached her goal, she became steadily more depressed because no spectacular romance evolved. It was clear that there were problems other than weight that prevented the relationships from developing, but Audrey saw weight loss as her salvation. Fortunately, Audrey and I worked on these problems, and she did eventually find the romance she was seeking.

This is a dramatic example of Impossible Dream Thinking. This specific case may not parallel your situation, but think honestly about whether you are harboring impossible dreams.

Oh please, scale, say that I'm down to 110, so I'll look really good and I'll meet someone, and we'll fall in love and get married and I'll be happy for the rest of my life...

SIPRESS

For many people losing weight, life does change in dramatic and positive ways. I hope this happens for you and that what you hope will happen actually occurs. Please remember, however, that weight loss may not automatically change your life.

Here are four ways to deal with Impossible Dream thinking. They can help keep your spirits high.

- **Counter the dreams.** Pinpoint your Impossible Dreams and counter them with more rational expectations. Methods for developing counter statements were discussed in Lesson Eight in the section on Dichotomous Thinking.

- **Set short-term goals.** Concern yourself with what you will do today and tomorrow, not what life will be like when you lose weight. This gives you many chances to experience success because you will be making small accomplishments in route to a larger goal. It will also prevent unrealistic fantasies from dominating your program.

- **Focus on behavior, not weight.** Remember that your behavior must change before weight can change, so give yourself credit for following the program. You will have something to feel good about every day and will not be so discouraged by weight setbacks.

- **Set flexible goals.** If your goals don't work, set new ones. If you vowed to run three miles each day but cannot, run one or two miles every other day and work your way up. This puts the focus on short-term changes in behavior, so Impossible Dream Thinking will fade to the background.

Something for your partner to read

In earlier lessons, we discussed ways to select a partner and to ask for help. One way to help your partner help you is to make *specific* suggestions. I have often encountered partners who ask for guidance on what they can do. Most are genuinely interested in helping and need only suggestions.

This section is written for *you and your partner.* Have your partner read it and then discuss the material together. Decide on concrete ways your partner can help, and implement these right away.

- **Partners can model good eating habits.** A partner may help you immensely by doing what you are doing. Eating slowly is a good example. A partner can exercise with you, can help keep food out of sight, and can display a positive attitude. This will remind you to do the same and will be a visible sign that your partner is trying to help.

- **Partners can praise your efforts.** A pat on the back and a few kind words can go a long way. Your partner should not wait for weight loss to occur to be kind to you, and should not focus just on weight. When you make positive changes in eating or exercise, your partner can acknowledge it with supportive comments. Waiting for weight change misses many opportunities to help.

- **Partners can help with the weigh-in.** Not everyone on a program will want a partner to know their weight, but if the relationship can tolerate this knowledge, having your partner present at a regular weigh-in can help. This gives your partner an idea of how you are doing. You may like this additional motivation. The partner must be forewarned, however, that weight loss will not occur every week, and if the weigh-ins are more frequent than once per week, fluid shifts will give false indications about your progress in the program.

♦ **Partners can be rewarded in return.** I explained earlier that the person in the program must be kind to the partner in exchange for the partner's support. This is a basic rule of relationships. In fact, many people feel better knowing that they are doing something nice for their partner. I also explained how you should be frank with your partner in asking for support and should be specific in these requests. These same rules apply to the partner. Your partner should tell you in specific terms what he or she can do to be nice. An example of a specific request might be, "I would like you to go to the movies with me once each week."

More facts about vitamins

Do you take vitamins? Chances are the answer is yes. Do you need the vitamins you take? Chances are the answer is no. Pretty bold statement, right?

The amount of money made on vitamins is unbelievable. The amount of fraud and exploitation is intolerable. An example from my own experience shows this. I once stopped in a *health food* store hoping to find some fruit.

When I entered, the owner was prescribing an assortment of vitamins to a woman who had arthritis and heart disease. She seemed to have little money but was willing to risk it on the hope the fellow might be right. What he told her was not only false, but could have harmed her because he was prescribing high doses of fat soluble vitamins.

When I asked why he thought this would help the woman, he asked me if I could prove it would not. It was interesting that he felt the burden was on me to show that he was wrong. He then asked me if I had cancer, diabetes, poor vision, or impotence (!) and pointed me to shelves of vitamins that looked like alphabet soup.

This fellow was in his own small business, but similar hoaxes occur nationwide in chain stores. Many malls, shopping centers, and downtown shopping districts have such stores that seem official because of their fancy displays, nice signs, and wholesome appearance. Yet, they sell vitamins and other products most people don't need.

Perhaps some straightforward talk about vitamins will help clarify this confusing situation. Before I tell you what vitamins are and what they do, let me state my belief about vitamins and weight loss, a belief shared by every nutrition expert I have consulted:

> **THERE IS NO EVIDENCE THAT ANY VITAMIN OR COMBINATION OF VITAMINS HELPS PEOPLE LOSE WEIGHT**

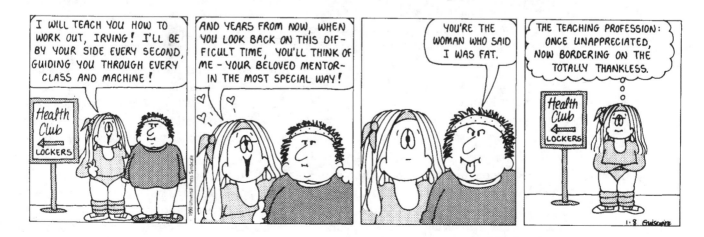

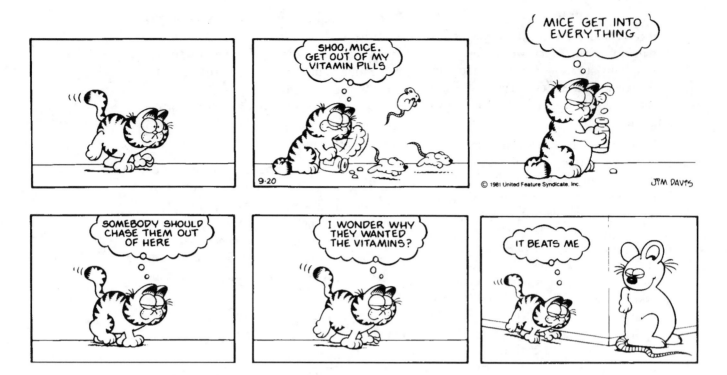

To review from Lesson Seven, vitamins are required for the transformation of energy in the body and for the regulation of metabolism. They do not produce energy themselves, but are crucial to the body's energy process. Some vitamins are needed to form important enzymes and others acts as catalysts (they speed chemical reactions).

There are two main types of vitamins: fat soluble and water soluble. The fat soluble vitamins are vitamins A, D, E, and K. They are absorbed in fat tissue and are not excreted by the body if you take too much. They can be toxic.

The water soluble vitamins are Vitamin C and the B complex vitamins which include thiamin, riboflavin, and niacin. These are absorbed in the body's water. Excess amounts can usually be excreted through the urine, so taking more than your body needs is wasting money because the vitamins simply pass through.

More information on specific vitamins is given throughout this manual. This includes the functions of each vitamin, their sources in foods, and facts about vitamins and health.

Nutrition experts feel, as a general rule, that most people in developed countries, particularly the U.S., receive adequate vitamins if they eat a balanced diet. Most people need no vitamin supplement at all, much less the mega-

doses prescribed by someone with unproven ideas.

Since you are exercising and eating less, taking a multiple vitamin each day will probably not hurt and may help remedy any deficiency created by the change in food intake. But again, if you are careful with the foods you choose, this may not be necessary.

Reading food labels

By now it should be apparent that one of the keys to eating right for weight loss is portion control (i.e., calories). Learning how to use and apply a calorie guide such as Appendix F in this manual is one way you can control the number of calories you eat each day. Another helpful tool is the food label. The U.S. government has passed legislation requiring almost all food products to include a standardized labeling system. Food labels can be very helpful, and you should know what they mean for you. The following discussion will help you understand how to read and use food labels.

Food label reform was enacted in 1990 to serve three primary purposes. The first is to help Americans choose a more healthful diet. The second is to decrease the confusion about

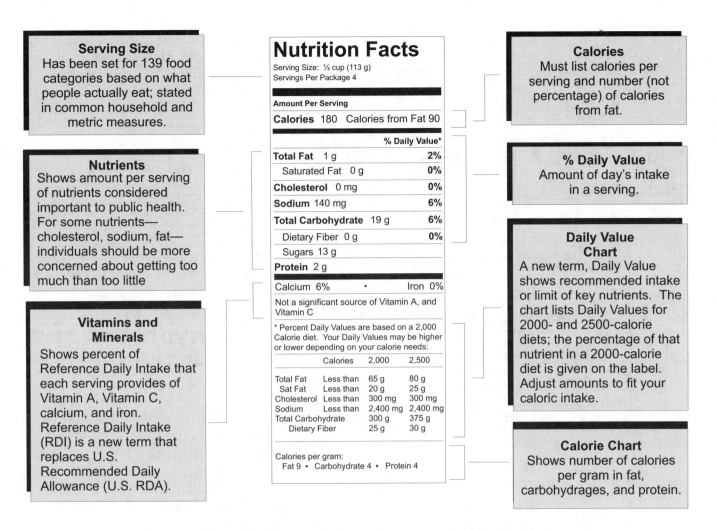

Serving Size
Has been set for 139 food categories based on what people actually eat; stated in common household and metric measures.

Nutrients
Shows amount per serving of nutrients considered important to public health. For some nutrients— cholesterol, sodium, fat— individuals should be more concerned about getting too much than too little

Vitamins and Minerals
Shows percent of Reference Daily Intake that each serving provides of Vitamin A, Vitamin C, calcium, and iron. Reference Daily Intake (RDI) is a new term that replaces U.S. Recommended Daily Allowance (U.S. RDA).

Nutrition Facts

Serving Size: ½ cup (113 g)
Servings Per Package 4

Amount Per Serving

Calories 180   Calories from Fat 90

	% Daily Value*
Total Fat 1 g	**2%**
Saturated Fat 0 g	**0%**
Cholesterol 0 mg	**0%**
Sodium 140 mg	**6%**
Total Carbohydrate 19 g	**6%**
Dietary Fiber 0 g	**0%**
Sugars 13 g	
Protein 2 g	

Calcium 6%	•	Iron 0%

Not a significant source of Vitamin A, and Vitamin C

* Percent Daily Values are based on a 2,000 Calorie diet. Your Daily Values may be higher or lower depending on your calorie needs:

		Calories	2,000	2,500
Total Fat	Less than		65 g	80 g
Sat Fat	Less than		20 g	25 g
Cholesterol	Less than		300 mg	300 mg
Sodium	Less than		2,400 mg	2,400 mg
Total Carbohydrate			300 g	375 g
Dietary Fiber			25 g	30 g

Calories per gram:
Fat 9 • Carbohydrate 4 • Protein 4

Calories
Must list calories per serving and number (not percentage) of calories from fat.

% Daily Value
Amount of day's intake in a serving.

Daily Value Chart
A new term, Daily Value shows recommended intake or limit of key nutrients. The chart lists Daily Values for 2000- and 2500-calorie diets; the percentage of that nutrient in a 2000-calorie diet is given on the label. Adjust amounts to fit your caloric intake.

Calorie Chart
Shows number of calories per gram in fat, carbohydrages, and protein.

---

advertising descriptors and other misleading information that has prevailed for years. Finally, the new labeling requirements offer an incentive for food companies to improve the nutritional quality of their products.

Under the new regulations, most foods now require nutrition labeling. Nutrition information is voluntary for many raw foods, including the 20 most frequently eaten fresh fruits and vegetables and raw fish. Although currently voluntary, the Nutrition Labeling and Education Act of 1990 (NLEA) states that if voluntary compliance is insufficient, nutrition information for such raw foods may become mandatory.

The nutrition facts panel

The new food label includes a revised nutrition facts panel as shown in the diagram here. The heading of the panel includes the new title "Nutrition Facts." This new title alerts consumers that the label meets the requirements of the new regulations. The panel includes cer-

tain items that are mandatory and other items that are voluntary. The panel includes new terms that may be unfamiliar to many people. References are made to Daily Values (DV) and comprise two new sets of dietary guidelines: Daily Reference Values (DRVs) and Reference Daily Intakes (RDIs). To help make the new label less confusing, however, only the Daily Reference Value term is used.

Daily reference value

Under the new regulations, DRVs have been introduced for those nutrients that contain energy (calories). These include fat, carbohydrate (including fiber), and protein. It is important to understand these percentages so that they are not mistaken as percentages of total calories. The DRVs are based on the number of calories consumed per day. As a common reference 2000 calories have been established as a daily intake. The DRVs for the energy nutrients are calculated in the following manner:

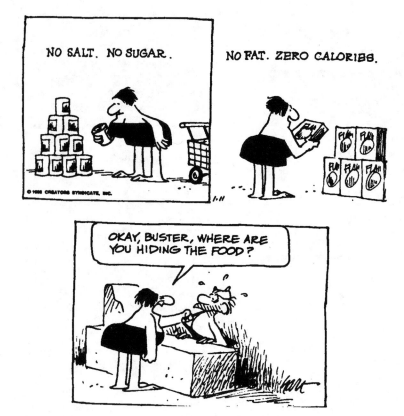

Ingredient list

The ingredients list of the food is required on the food label. Food components are listed in order by weight from the most to the least.

Take a few minutes to carefully read through the illustration of the food label on the previous page. Knowing how to read a food label can save you time in the grocery store isles plus many other benefits.

Carbohydrates and your diet

People like to blame carbohydrates for everything. Some people on weight-loss programs say that carbohydrates excite the binge center in their brain, and parents blame sugar when their kids misbehave. There is much talk about simple and complex carbohydrates, carbohydrate craving, and low-carbohydrate diets. You may be puzzled by all this, so let's clear the air.

What are carbohydrates?

Stated in technical terms, carbohydrates are a combination of hydrogen, oxygen, and carbon atoms, which assemble to make simple sugars, complex sugars, or starches. These sugars provide energy to the body. Complex sugars must first be broken down by the body into simple sugars to be utilized. This is why simple sugars (like sucrose) enter the body's energy supply more quickly than the complex sugars or starches in vegetables or cereals.

There are many sources of the simple sugars and starches. Simple sugars consist mainly of sucrose (table sugar), fructose (in fruit and honey), and lactose (in milk). The starches are in foods like cereals, pasta, rice, breads, and vegetables.

Carbohydrates, like protein, provide four calories per gram. In contrast, fat has more than twice the calories per gram. The major part of our diet is carbohydrate, and it is easy to eat too much. Many of the carbohydrate

- Fat is based on 30 percent of calories.
- Saturated fat is based on 10 percent of calories.
- Carbohydrate is based on 60 percent of calories.
- Protein is based on 10 percent of calories. The DRV for protein applies only for adults and children over four years of age. Protein for RDIs have been established for special groups.
- Fiber is based on 11.5 grams of fiber per 1000 calories.
- The DRVs also include sources for some non-energy nutrients, including cholesterol, sodium, and potassium. In addition, the DRVs for fats, cholesterol, and sodium represent the highest limits that are recommended. These values are as follows:
- Total fat: less than 65 gm
- Saturated fat: less that 20 gm
- Cholesterol: less than 300 mg
- Sodium: less than 2,400 mg
- Reference daily intakes

The new term Reference Daily Intakes (RDI) replaces the familiar term U.S. Recom-

The Food Guide Pyramid

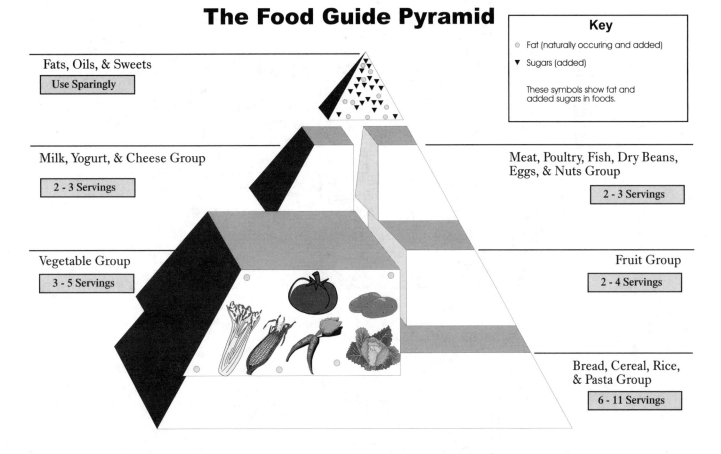

Fats, Oils, & Sweets
Use Sparingly

Milk, Yogurt, & Cheese Group
2 - 3 Servings

Vegetable Group
3 - 5 Servings

Key
○ Fat (naturally occuring and added)
▼ Sugars (added)

These symbols show fat and
added sugars in foods.

**Meat, Poultry, Fish, Dry Beans,
Eggs, & Nuts Group**
2 - 3 Servings

Fruit Group
2 - 4 Servings

**Bread, Cereal, Rice,
& Pasta Group**
6 - 11 Servings

foods we eat are of poor nutritional value and contain only calories from sugar. They are a poor source of nutrition, hence the term *empty calories*. Foods like these are prime candidates for elimination or reduction for individuals trying to lose or maintain weight.

In order for the diet to provide an adequate balance of nutrients, an adult should have approximately 165–180 grams of carbohydrate per day (based on a diet of 1200 calories). This would total from 660–720 calories (140–150 grams at 4 calories per gram). Adults are advised to have 55–60 percent of their total calories in carbohydrates.

What does all this jargon mean? Carbohydrates are essential in the diet and are not necessarily bad. In fact, most people should *increase* their intake of *complex* carbohydrates. Starches should not have the bad rap they receive. People consider potatoes fattening because they are high in starch, yet potatoes are reasonable to eat because of their nutrition. The *amount* eaten is usually the problem, along with the goodies that adorn some of these foods. For example, sour cream and

butter, which are mainly fat, rapidly increase the caloric intake involved in eating an innocent potato.

It is unwise to follow a low-carbohydrate diet except under medical supervision. Some popular diets which restrict carbohydrate to less than 100 grams per day make it very difficult to maintain adequate nutrition. A sensible plan with 55–60 percent of your calories from carbohydrate is best.

Try to be on the lookout for simple sugars in your diet. These tend to come from foods with many calories and little nutrition. Examples are crackers, doughnuts, pastries, soft drinks, candy, and so forth.

These simple sugars stimulate insulin release. Since insulin is related to hunger, you will feel hungry in less time with simple sugars than with complex sugars. Moving away from candy and other sweet foods, toward vegetables and other complex carbohydrates, is a wise decision.

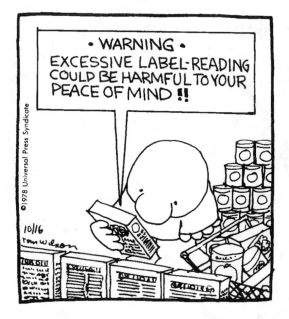

Carbohydrates and extra calorie burning

For many years, a simple statement has ruled in the minds of most experts—"A calorie is a calorie." The feeling was that calories were handled in the same way by the body no matter where they came from. If you ate 3500 calories of oat bran and tofu, you would gain the same weight as you would by eating the same calories from a triple cheeseburger and onion rings. No longer.

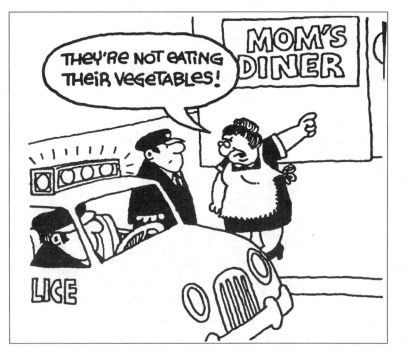

The body has an easier time converting fat calories to body fat than it does converting carbohydrate calories. Between 20–25 percent more energy is required for the body to handle carbohydrate than to handle fat. As an example, let's say you eat 100 calories of a high-fat food like butter. On another day, you eat 100 calories of a food high in complex carbohydrates, like a whole grain cereal. Your body will use 20–25 percent more calories to metabolize the carbohydrate. Therefore, the calories from fat and carbohydrate are not equal once they enter your body.

This is good news. Foods high in complex carbohydrates are good to eat for health reasons, and you will burn more calories when you eat them. Many people report that it is much easier to lose weight when they cut back on fat and eat more fruits, vegetables, and grains. With this in mind, let's look at the Vegetable Group of the Food Guide Pyramid.

Vegetables in your diet

Do you remember your mother saying to you, "Eat your vegetables, they're good for you"? Mom was right, vegetables are good for you. In fact, both fruits and vegetables are so important in the diet that the Food Guide Pyramid breaks them into separate groups.

Vegetables are an excellent source of Vitamins A and C, and folate. In addition, they provide minerals, including iron and magnesium, and as I mentioned earlier, they are an excellent source of carbohydrates. Vegetables are also naturally low in dietary fat. This is good news for people losing weight.

Most Americans fall short in their consumption of vegetables, perhaps because adding produce to their diet is inconvenient, time-consuming, or boring. Vegetables may not appeal to everyone's palate, especially in the ways they are usually prepared, but they are an important ingredient to a healthy and low-fat diet.

How many servings?

The suggested number of daily servings is three to five. This may sound like a lot, but it is actually less than you may think. For in-

Vegetables

Description	Calories	Protein (g)	Carb. (g)	Fat (g)
Asparagus, boiled (½ cup)	22	2.3	4.0	.3
Beets, boiled (½ cup)	26	.9	5.7	.0
Broccoli, boiled (½ cup)	23	2.3	4.3	.2
Brussels Sprouts (½ cup)	30	2.0	6.8	.4
Cabbage, raw (1 cup)	16	.8	1.6	.2
Carrots, boiled (½ cup)	35	.9	8.2	.1
Cauliflower, boiled (½ cup)	15	1.2	2.9	.1
Celery, raw (½ cup diced)	11	.4	2.6	.1
Corn—yellow, boiled (½ cup)	89	2.7	20.6	1.1
Cucumber, raw (½ cup diced)	7	.3	1.5	.1
Eggplant, raw (½ cup pieces)	11	.5	2.6	.0
Green beans, boiled (½ cup)	22	1.2	4.9	.2
Lettuce, raw (1 cup)	10	.8	2.0	.2
Lima beans, boiled (½ cup)	109	7.4	21.2	.3
Mixed vegetables, canned (½ cup)	39	2.1	7.6	.2
Mushrooms, boiled (½ cup pieces)	21	1.7	4.0	.4
Okra, boiled (½ cup slices)	25	1.5	5.8	.1
Onion rings, frozen (7 rings)	285	3.7	26.7	18.7
Peas, green, boiled (½ cup)	67	4.6	12.5	.2
Potato, canned w/o skin (½ cup)	54	1.3	12.3	.2
Potato, French fried (10 pieces)	158	2.0	20.0	8.3
Potato, hash brown (½ cup)	163	1.9	16.6	10.9
Potato, mashed (½ cup)	111	2.0	17.5	4.4
Potato, scalloped (½ cup)	105	3.5	13.2	4.5
Squash—zucchini, boiled (½ cup)	14	.6	3.5	.1
Sweet potato, boiled (½ cup)	172	2.7	39.8	.5

Note: Each of the food items listed above counts as one serving. This table should be used as a guide for the foods listed. Since food values vary by brand name it is important to read the food labels for these foods.

stance, just one-half a cup of boiled green beans, one medium carrot, two stalks of celery, or half of a broccoli spear make one serving.

How much is a serving?

As a general rule, the following will serve as a simple guide to help you include the right amount of vegetables in your daily diet:

- ☑ 1 cup of raw leafy vegetables
- ☑ ½ cup of other vegetables, cooked or chopped raw
- ☑ ¾ cup of vegetable juice

The chart on this page may help you to better understand the portion size of a serving. The foods listed count as a single serving.

Serving tips

There are a large variety of vegetables for you to choose from in our food supply. With a little creativity and planning, vegetables can become a fun and enjoyable part of your everyday diet. Here are some serving tips that you may find helpful:

Fresh vegetables make excellent snacks that you can easily take with you to work, school, or simply enjoy around the house. Celery, carrots, cauliflower, green peppers, cucumbers, and broccoli are good choices.

Steaming vegetables can also be fun and can add variety to your meals. Best of all, it is easy to do and does not leave a big mess. While steaming the vegetables, you can add herbs or other seasonings to add flavor or serve the steamed vegetables with a splash of lemon.

Think of creative ways to add vegetables to the foods you already eat and enjoy. Adding a slice of tomato, two large leaves of lettuce or spinach, and a pickle on the side turns a sandwich into a meal that includes one serving of vegetables.

When you eat fast-food, be creative. Most fast-food establishments now offer vegetable alternatives to french fries. Try a garden salad or baked potato next time. But be careful with dressings and toppings - make sure they are low-fat. Remember to watch those *hidden calories*.

Assignment for this lesson

This lesson began with behaviors to help you serve and dispense food in a reasonable way. These are the behaviors to practice: Remove serving dishes from the table; Leave the table after eating; Serve one portion of food; Follow the Five-Minute Rule; and Avoid dispensing food. Watch for Impossible Dream Thinking, and banish the thoughts that are holding you back. Add up the daily grams of carbohydrates in your diet to see if they make up about 55–60 percent of your daily diet, and try to eat the recommended number of servings from the Vegetable Group.

T F 47. It is best to take all of what you will eat in one serving so you will not need additional helpings.

T F 48. No exercise can help you lose fat in specific parts of the body.

T F 49. Impossible Dream Thinking is having fantasies and images about weight loss, life as a thin person, etc.

T F 50. Carbohydrates are not as important as other nutrients, and they should make up only about 30 percent of your daily diet.

T F 51. The Food Guide Pyramid suggests three to five servings each day from the Vegetable Group.

T F 52. Fat soluble vitamins give you energy, but water soluble vitamins do not.

(Answers in Appendix C)

Monitoring Form—Lesson Nine

Today's Date:

Time	Food and Amount	Calories
	Total Daily Calories	

Assignment this week	Always	Sometimes	Never
1. Remove serving dishes from table			
2. Leave table after eating			
3. Serve one portion			
4. Follow the five-minute rule			
5. Avoid dispensing food			
6. Watch out for Impossible Dream Thinking			
7. Daily servings from the Vegetable Group			
8. Less than _____ calories each day			
9. My diet has _____ grams of carbohydrate			

Food Groups for Today	Physical Activity	Minutes
Milk, yogurt, and cheese ❑ ❑ ❑		
Meat, poultry, etc. ❑ ❑ ❑		
Fruits ❑ ❑ ❑ ❑		
Vegetables ❑ ❑ ❑ ❑ ❑		
Breads, cereals, etc. ❑ ❑ ❑ ❑ ❑ ❑ ❑ ❑ ❑ ❑ ❑		

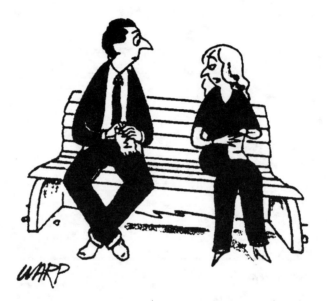

"When your mother told you to eat something green every
day, I don't think she had M & M's in mind."

Here we are, Lesson Ten already! I would now like to raise the potentially touchy, but important issue of family relationships. We will also cover pressures to eat from other people. This is another place where the "R" (Relationships) part of the LEARN program can be helpful, because offers and even demands to eat from others can be hard to resist. We will then move to a new category of Attitudes, the Imperatives, and I will discuss stress and eating. I will also discuss the benefits of jogging and cycling as physical activities. Finally, under Nutrition, I will point out the role of vitamin C and the B complex vitamins (the water soluble vitamins) in healthy eating and the role of fruit in your diet.

For you and your family to read

Some time ago, I traveled to Argentina and was invited to speak before a large meeting of a group called FAMALCO in Buenos Aires. Loosely translated, FAMALCO stands for "Families Anonymous of Relatives Fighting Against Obesity." This group was an outgrowth of ALCO, a large, nationwide, self-help group for obesity patterned after Alcoholics Anonymous (AA), much the way Overeaters Anonymous in North America is patterned after AA. FAMALCO is similar in nature to AL-ANON, which is for families of alcoholics. I was inspired by the innovative nature of FAMALCO. It is unfortunate that no such group exists in our country. I would like to share what I learned with you and your family, so *please ask your family to read this.*

The FAMALCO meeting began with moving testimonials from husbands, wives, children, and parents of people struggling with their weight. Some of the family members expressed sorrow about the weight problem, while others related dismay, sympathy, anger, and hostility. One thing common to all was the pain, suffering, and frustration experienced by both the overweight person and the family. FAMALCO allowed the family members to discuss these issues with others in the same situation and provided many opportunities for the families to learn new ways to help the overweight family member and to help themselves.

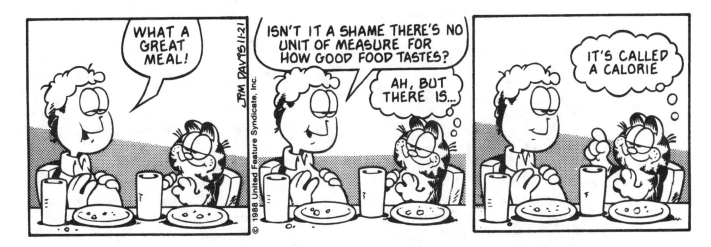

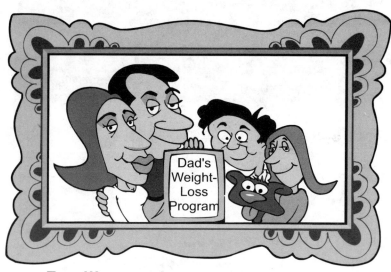

Families can be a great resource for a person losing weight.

This meeting reinforced my belief that families can be a great resource for a person losing weight, but that harmony between the individual and the family requires a special effort from both parties. Communication is the first step. The burden falls to the family member losing weight to express how he or she feels and how the family can help. This is difficult sometimes when the person resents the family's response to his or her weight. However, you must talk, express, and communicate.

The same responsibility applies to the family. The overweight person may have only a superficial knowledge of how the family feels. When the family finally expresses its feelings, the individual is likely to be relieved because the cards are on the table. This permits open discussion, positive communication, and suggestions from the person losing weight and the family about how they might help each other. I now recommend that the family and you read the section in Lesson Six on "Communicating With Your Partner." The guidelines presented there can be used to begin and sustain the communication.

When I completed my lecture before FAMALCO, the audience responded with a warm, loud ovation. I assured the audience that I had learned at least as much from them as they had learned from me. I was even more certain of this when I listened to the speaker following me, Dr. Alberto Cormillot.

Dr. Alberto Cormillot is a prominent physician and public official in Buenos Aires, known all over Argentina for his work on weight loss. He developed a comprehensive approach to overweight that would rival any in the world. In his talk, Dr. Cormillot listed a number of things the family should or should not do. They are as relevant in our country as they are in his.

Things the family should avoid

- **Do not hide food from the person losing weight.** He or she will find it and feel resentful.

- **Do not threaten.** Behavior is best changed with a soft touch, not coercion, so be nice.

- **Do not avoid social situations because of the person's weight.** This will batter the self-esteem of the family member losing weight and will breed resentment in the family.

- **Do not expect perfection or 100 percent recovery.** Weight problems are something a person learns to control, not cure. There will be periods of misery, weight gain, and overeating. The individual's achievements should be appreciated and the setbacks ignored.

- **Do not lecture, criticize, or reprimand.** These rarely help. The person needs to feel better, not worse.

- **Do not play the role of victim or martyr.** Overweight has many causes, both psychological and physiological. It is unfair for the family to blame the overweight family member and to feel victimized. Support and encouragement will do more than guilt and shame.

Things the family can do

- **Keep a positive attitude.** This sounds trite, but can be very important. It is not easy to be upbeat and encouraging when a program grinds on for months and months. Extra effort from the family can make life much easier for the person losing weight.

- **Talk with others in your situation.** Being in a family where a weight problem exists generates strong feelings in

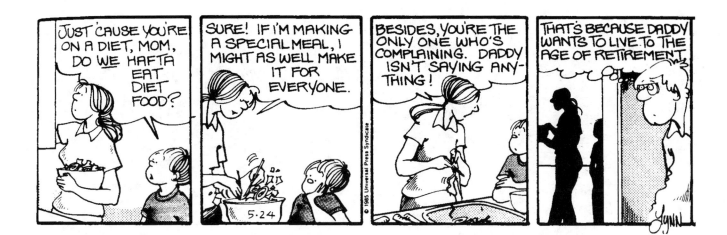

the family members. It can help to talk about these with others who deal with the same issues. Many good ideas can be generated from this process.

- **Keep the home and family relaxed.** This will permit the person on a program to pay attention to the task at hand, changing eating and exercise habits.

- **Learn to ignore and forgive lapses.** The family can react many ways to mistakes, bouts of weight gain, and binges. The person losing weight feels bad when these occur, so it is best for the family to adopt a *hands off* policy and to forgive and forget.

- **Ask the person losing weight how you can help.** The best way to learn how to help is to ask. Family members are sometimes surprised by what the individual wants.

- **Exercise with the person on a program.** This is a wonderful and healthy way to spend time together. If only a daily walk, this provides time to talk and can help the person with the program.

- **Develop new interests with the family member losing weight.** There are so many things in life to enjoy, and developing new interests can be good for everybody. Individuals losing weight sometimes feel they are embarking on a new life. New activities can involve the family in this process.

To summarize this section for the family, there are many ways the family can help the person losing weight. It begins with communication and proceeds to the things listed above. Both the family and the overweight person are responsible for making these happen.

Dealing with pressures to eat

A major challenge for individuals on weight loss programs is to cope with pressure to eat. Friends, relatives, and strangers, some well-meaning and some not, can make it difficult to lose weight by encouraging you to eat. There are a number of reasons for this.

They may be uncomfortable eating in front of you. People agonize about eating when another person is not. They offer food to be polite, even though they know the offer won't be accepted. You can tell them that you do not feel uncomfortable and that they should eat if they wish.

They may be jealous of your success. Others with weight problems may be jealous of your success. Thin people may also be jealous that you are accomplishing something and are proud of your achievement. This is their problem, so don't let it become yours by agreeing to eat.

They may not want you to succeed. This is rare, but it spells trouble for the person on a program. You can spot it in acts of sabotage. The person may develop a sudden craving for your favorite food or may say demoralizing things like, "You have always failed before and will fail again." There are several reasons why another person would act this way, but I do

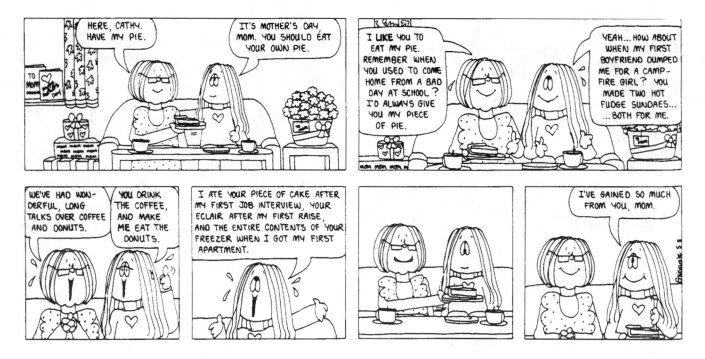

not want to launch into a lengthy psychological analysis. You are best off ignoring these comments. Confronting the person rarely helps and can make the situation worse. Again, this is their problem, so don't let it influence you. If they offer you food or encourage you to eat, refuse in a polite way, but be sure to refuse. The person will get the message and will quit trying.

They think you are starving. These people can imagine themselves in your shoes and are certain they would be ravenous. Since so many people associate food with love, encouraging you to eat is one way to show concern. Assure them that you are fine and that they can help by ignoring your diet and by not offering you food.

They want to test your determination. They may want to tease you or to see how serious you are about your program. It seems cruel, but it happens. Show them just how serious you can be.

Be polite, but be firm

When you get pressures to eat, stand up for yourself and refuse. Avoid being aggressive or insulting, even if you suspect evil motives. The polite approach works best. After a few polite refusals, most people will learn that their pressures will not work and will quit pestering you.

If Aunt Irma offers you fudge, you might say, "Gee Irma, I love your fudge, but I'm not very hungry." If your husband stops to get ice cream with you in the car, say "I hope you enjoy it, but I really don't want the calories." If a co-worker says, "Let's go out and get something fattening for lunch," you can reply with, "I'm struggling to avoid those foods, so I'd better not go. If we can go to a place with a salad bar, I'll be glad to join you."

If you have trouble being assertive, try to predict the situations in which you might be pressured to eat. Plan a response, and practice it so you arrive prepared to be polite and firm.

Another attitude trap: Imperatives

Imperatives are words that imply urgency and no room for error. Examples of imperative words are *always*, *must*, and *never*. If you are like most people who have tried to lose weight before, your vocabulary is peppered with imperatives. Using these words can pave the path to trouble. Here are some examples from my clients.

◆ "I will *never* eat more than 1200 calories."

◆ "I *must never* eat cookie dough ice cream again."

◆ "I will eat a salad for lunch *every* day."

- "I will *always* say no when Vicki offers me coffee cake."

- "I must *always* control my cravings for sweets."

- "Chocolate is my downfall, so I will avoid it *always*."

- "I will exercise *every* day."

- "I *must* have *perfect* control of my eating."

- "I will *always* control the moods that make me eat."

These thoughts can float around in your mind waiting to take pot shots at your control. If you exceed your calorie level some day, you can recover from the extra calories if your control stays intact. However, the imperatives can get a clean shot at you if your mind cranks out thoughts like, "I should never eat more than I'm told." When this happens, you may be a goner. Disappointment occurs, and one can lose sight of positive accomplishments because of a few mistakes.

Individuals who feel they should avoid certain foods are especially likely to fall prey to the imperatives. If you forbid yourself peanuts, you will be fine for a week or two. You may then start to crave peanuts, wonder how they would taste, and fantasize about a peanut feast when the program ends. You might then eat some peanuts, either because you are offered some or you break down and buy them. Feeling like a failure might then weaken control even further and dichotomous thinking can lead to *falling off* your program.

Watch out for those ATTITUDE traps

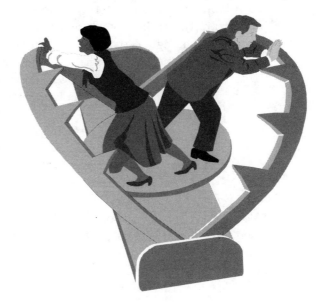

Try to find imperatives in your vocabulary. What do you expect of yourself, and how can you banish words like *never* and *always* from your internal conversations? Replace the imperatives with language that allows some room for error and flexibility. Remember, there is no such thing as a perfect person.

Here are some examples of common imperative statements and some methods to counter them. These may apply to you in one way or another, but if they do not, you can use them as examples to form your own methods of dealing with the imperatives. Once again, being prepared can make you ready to deal with most difficult situations.

Imperative and Counter Statements (examples)	
Imperative Statement	**Counter Statement**
I will never eat candy bars.	I will do my best to eat fewer candy bars, but if I have one, it is a sign to increase my control, not to let down.
I will never get depressed because it makes me eat.	Everybody feels down at times. If I get depressed I must think of reacting with something other than eating—walking may be a good choice.
I will exercise every day.	This is my goal, and I will do my best to reach it. When I can't, I will try harder the next day.

The imperatives are habits just like other behaviors and attitudes. To develop a new habit, practice is the key. It seems funny to practice thinking a certain way, but it really works. Once you know what attitudes give you trouble, you can gradually weaken their ability to influence you by replacing them with positive approaches.

Stress and eating

A very interesting (and unexplained) paradox is that stress makes some people eat more and some people eat less. Scientists are working to understand this, but one thing is clear—stress is often cited as a major issue for people who wish to lose weight.

When I discuss the complexity of weight loss with clients in our clinic, the issue of stress arises repeatedly. Some people point to a specific stressful event to explain why they gained weight in the first place. Others say that stress makes them want to eat all the time, so they nibble. Still others feel that stress threatens their ability to maintain weight loss and puts them at risk for relapse.

It is no surprise that stress exerts such an important effect on eating. There are clear links between stress and health. Health problems ranging from the common cold to chronic diseases like heart disease, diabetes, and asthma are thought to be affected by stress. It is reasonable to believe that reducing stress would make many people happier and healthier, and that control over eating and weight would be facilitated in the process.

Do you feel that stress influences your eating? Here are some questions to ask yourself:

❶ When you feel pressure to accomplish something, do you feel pulled toward food or pushed away from it?

❷ If you were sitting at a desk working on a project that had to be done quickly, would you want to be eating something?

❸ Do you believe food is something you use to feel better when you are stressed?

❹ Does stress make you eat more?

If you answered "yes" to any of these questions, stress and eating might be linked in important ways. The question then, is what to do about it?

There are two solutions. One is to respond to stress with activities other than eating. Lesson Thirteen discusses means for developing alternative activities. With a list of such alternatives, you can use the urge to eat as a signal to engage in another activity. Hence, the same stimulus (stress) might exist, but you would not react by eating.

A second solution is to reduce stress. This is an appealing possibility, because stress reduction might affect not only your eating but other areas of your life as well. It may be helpful, therefore, to learn stress management techniques. It would take another book the size of this to provide a complete stress management program, but I can provide a few details about stress and then refer you to materials or programs for more detailed information.

Stress is a fascinating interplay between body, mind, and environment. We each respond to situations in our environment in a unique way. Events that disturb one person mean nothing to another. Some people respond to stress with a racing heart and anger, while others respond with nausea and fear. What is certain is that the ways we think and

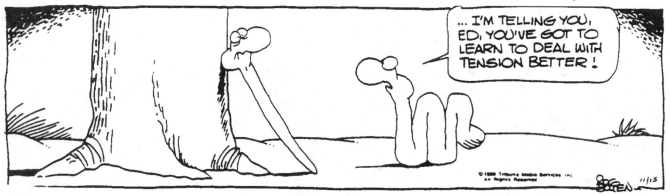

... I'M TELLING YOU, ED, YOU'VE GOT TO LEARN TO DEAL WITH TENSION BETTER!

act are key factors in how we handle stress. Therefore, there are a number of things a person can do to better manage stress. These are skills that you can learn, much as you are learning weight management skills in this program.

I will provide two examples here. The first is the use of relaxation training. Good stress management programs teach specific relaxation skills, so that when stress begins, a person has the ability to halt the process by countering a stress response with relaxation responses. Learning relaxation skills can be very helpful, and can help an individual calm down before an undesirable action occurs (like overeating).

The second example deals with what scientists have called *appraisal*. When an event occurs in our lives, we appraise the situation and then respond. The appraisal determines the response. One person who receives a negative evaluation from a boss might have a negative appraisal, suffer a blow to self-esteem, and feel depressed. Another might blame the boss, get angry, and strike back in some self-defeating way, while yet another might make a more positive appraisal and think of ways to improve work performance. The way we perceive and interpret events is crucial.

Both relaxation training and modifying the appraisal process are part of most stress management programs. So, how do you find one? The first possibility is to seek out stress management seminars or training programs. Local hospitals, YMCA's and YWCA's, colleges, and some corporate settings offer stress management programs. Some individuals find they need a formal program in a professional setting, so asking for leads from health professionals you know should be helpful.

Other people do not need a formal program and can use written materials in a very positive way. An excellent guide is a step-by-step manual by Drs. David Barlow and Ronald Rapee entitled *Mastering Stress: A Lifestyle Approach*. The book is published by the American Health Publishing Company (the company that publishes *The LEARN Program For Weight Control*). Information can be obtained by calling 1-800-736-7323 or by contacting The LEARN Education Center at the address provided toward the end of this manual.

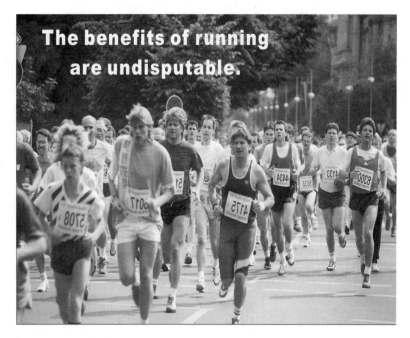

The benefits of running are undisputable.

Let's consider jogging and cycling

What a change there has been in society's attitude about exercise, particularly running. As recently as the early 1970s, the longest race in most track meets was two miles, and most people had trouble believing that kooks actually raced for six miles in cross country meets.

Jogging and running

Now it seems routine for people to brag about doing their three, five, ten, or even more miles. The number of people who proclaim themselves runners is staggering. There are running magazines, running clubs, and even running software packages for computers. It is tempting to poke fun at this hysteria and to pass it off as a fad. That would, in my opinion, be a mistake.

Before I discuss running in more detail, let me emphasize again the virtues of brisk walking. Running is fine, but for people who still have many pounds to lose, brisk walking is easier and brings nearly all the benefits. This section is designed to show that running can be helpful to some people, but walking is a fine alternative.

The benefits of running are indisputable. Many positive physical changes occur, as discussed in Lesson Two. What is often overlooked are the psychological advantages. I am not talking about the widely touted *runner's high*, but about a general sense of accomplishment, self-confidence, well-being, and good feelings.

This psychological advantage may come from running itself, or may simply result from the mastery of something new. At a sports medicine conference I attended in The Netherlands, where I lectured on the psychological benefits of exercise, Dr. John Garrow, an outstanding researcher from England, asked me a telling question. He asked if people would get the same positive effects from something unrelated to exercise, such as learning to play the cello.

Dr. Garrow was questioning whether something inherent to the exercise would be beneficial or whether the effects were due to the excitement of improving at any activity. This is a difficult question to answer. From a practical standpoint, exercise is a good means for producing this mastery because it carries physical benefits as well. After all, it burns more calories than playing the cello!

Cycling

Cycling has the advantages of running, and for some people is more enjoyable. Riding a stationary bicycle indoors or a traditional bike outdoors is good exercise. It spares the knees, ankles, and feet from the pounding they take when running, and is nice for heavy people be-

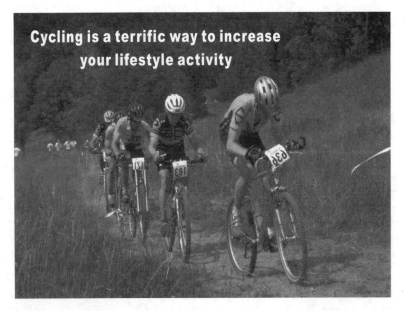

Cycling is a terrific way to increase your lifestyle activity

cause weight is supported by the bike. It is an excellent method for burning calories.

If cycling outdoors is feasible for you, give it a try. Cycling to work is terrific when possible. If not, consider buying a stationary bicycle for your home. I have one and like to alternate between running, cycling, and playing tennis. The cycling is nice in bad weather, and I can do it while watching the news or listening to music.

Running and cycling are not the only exercises, but they are good ones. These activities (along with walking and swimming) are top choices among my clients, so please give them a try. If you are doing something else regularly, stick with it. If you are sporadic in your habits or have not tried anything seriously, consider lacing up the shoes to hit the road or hopping on a bike to sail down the street.

More about water soluble vitamins

In Lesson Seven, I introduced the topic of vitamins and discussed the difference between water soluble and fat soluble vitamins. Let's look closer at the water soluble vitamins.

Vitamin C: good or bad?

No matter what we hear, people continue to think that vitamin C helps to cure and prevent colds. It has been ascribed other wondrous qualities as well. I recently read reports of a study where vitamin C had been used with cancer patients, as the vitamin advocates recommend. It did no better than a placebo. The advocates claim that the dosage was faulty. It is difficult for the public to make wise decisions when the scientists cannot agree. So, what do we do about vitamin C?

The Recommended Daily Allowance (RDA) for vitamin C is 60 mg, which is relatively easy to consume just by eating a balanced diet. This much vitamin C is contained in one serving of citrus fruit. Why then, do people take much larger doses than suggested? The vitamin pushers recommend that we take not two or three times the RDA, but 100 or 1000 times the amount. Does it help?

Vitamin C (ascorbic acid) is used by the body for teeth, bones, cells, and blood vessels.

It is absolutely essential for health. Vitamin C can be obtained from citrus fruits, berries, fruit juices, green vegetables, tomatoes, cabbage, and potatoes.

Studies have been done on the use of large amounts of vitamin C in hopes it will cure various illnesses. As with the cancer study I mentioned above, these studies typically show no advantage for taking more than recommended. This has been shown most convincingly with the common cold. Still, people cling to the hope it will help and send the nearest family member scurrying to the store for orange juice when they get the sniffles.

Since so many people take so much vitamin C, we must be concerned about possible dangers. Fortunately, vitamin C is water soluble. Excessive amounts, for the most part, are excreted through the urine, so your body only uses what it needs. However, there is some evidence that vitamin C can build up in body tissue when large doses are taken.

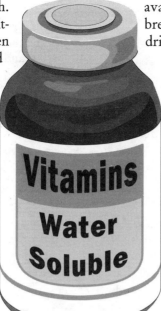

B complex vitamins

The B complex vitamins are also water soluble. This complex includes vitamin B_1 (thiamine), vitamin B_2 (riboflavin), niacin, vitamin B_6, and vitamin B_{12}. Each serves a different purpose and has different recommended amounts for healthy functioning.

Vitamin B_1 is necessary for the heart and nervous system because of its role in carbohydrate metabolism. It is available in enriched cereals, bread and other flour products, fish, meat, liver, milk, poultry, and whole grain cereals. Vitamin B_2 is important in carbohydrate metabolism and tissue repair. It is necessary for the skin and prevents light sensitivity in the eyes. It is available in leafy green vegetables, lean meat, liver, milk, eggs, and dried yeast.

Niacin is important for the metabolism and absorption of carbohydrate, so it plays a key role in converting food to usable energy. It is

available in enriched cereals and bread, eggs, lean meats, liver, and dried yeast.

Vitamins B_6 and B_{12} are becoming more popular in health food stores. Vitamin B_6 is used for metabolism of protein, carbohydrate, and fat, and is available in many foods, including chicken, fish, liver, whole grain cereals, and egg yolks. Vitamin B_{12} helps prevent anemia and aids in the work of the nervous system. It is found in lean meat, liver, kidney, milk, salt water fish, and oysters.

As with vitamin C, the B complex vitamins are being hawked in health food stores and nutrition centers for all sorts of ills. Most people get enough of the B vitamins from normal eating. There are some conditions for which additional B vitamins are needed, but these should be diagnosed by a physician, not a store clerk. Since these vitamins are water soluble, extra amounts will be excreted, but your money goes just where the extra vitamins end up.

What about multiple vitamins?

It is reasonable to take a well-formulated multiple vitamin if you are concerned about getting enough vitamins and minerals in your diet. Check the label to see what percentage of the RDA's they provide, and do not exceed 100 percent. Remember though, chances are that you need no supplements if you eat a balanced diet.

Don't be confused by the fancy sounding vitamins at your store. There is no advantage to natural vitamins (another health food ploy). The store brand generic vitamins are as good as the more expensive brand names.

Buy a multiple vitamin, which should contain the basic vitamins and minerals you need. Also, be leery of vitamins that are supposed to help with things like stress. If you think you have some special vitamin deficiency, consult a dietitian or physician.

Facts, fantasies, and fiber

Over the years, many parents have implored their children to eat more roughage. This basically good advice was about the only attention fiber received until the 1970s, when there was an explosion of interest in the topic. Books and magazines carried fiber diets, and sales of bran cereals increased dramatically. Other high fiber foods also appeared in the stores. Is this a positive development or is the fiber craze destined to pass with other food fads?

Dietary fiber comes primarily from the tough cell walls of plants. These materials include cellulose, hemicellulose, lignin, and pectin (which is used by home canners to turn fruit juice to jelly). Fiber is not broken down by digestion like other foods and basically retains its structure during its transit through the digestive system. The strand-like quality of fiber maintains its rigid structure.

Fiber absorbs water during the digestive process. This moisture helps with movement of waste products through the bowel. A brief lesson of digestion should clarify this process.

When you chew and swallow food, both the chewing and saliva begin to break food down into smaller nutrients. Stomach acid continues the process as food moves along, then more digestion continues in the small intestine. Toward the end of the line, waste products combine with water in the large intestine and are eliminated as stools. A stool with much water is larger and softer and moves through the colon more easily. A stool with little moisture is small and hard and creates the discomfort of constipation.

Much of the desirable moisture that facilitates movement of the stools comes from fiber. This is why increased fiber is prescribed for people with problems in the gastrointestinal tract such as diverticulitis, irritable bowel syndrome, and constipation. Some experts claim that fiber also reduces the risk of serious diseases like atherosclerosis and cancer of the colon.

The study of fiber and health gained momentum with the discovery that Africans living in rural settings rarely get diverticulitis. This occurs when a bubble or mucous membrane pushes out from inside the intestine. Their diet averages 25 grams of fiber per day, compared to 6 grams per day for the typical American. Cancer of the colon follows a similar pattern—it occurs rarely in rural Africa and often in industrialized countries. Furthermore, rates for these diseases have increased in the U.S. during this century, during which time fiber intake has decreased dramatically (due to the fiber being refined out of foods and to less reliance on fruits and vegetables).

Of course, fiber in the diet is only one of many factors which distinguish the rural Africans from us. One such factor is fat in the diet, which has also been linked to disease. There are dozens of non-dietary factors (stress, etc.) that might be involved. What does this mean for our diet?

With the current state of science, it is not possible to say that increased fiber in the diet protects against disease, but there are strong hints in this direction. The comparisons between rural and industrialized cultures have now been joined by laboratory studies, so that government agencies like the National Cancer Institute advocate increased fiber in the diet.

The average American should increase the fiber in his or her diet. Fiber comes from fruits, vegetables, and cereals. The chart below shows high fiber foods. The government has

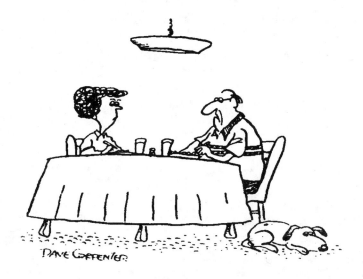

"High fiber, no salt, low cholesterol. No wonder the dog doesn't beg anymore."

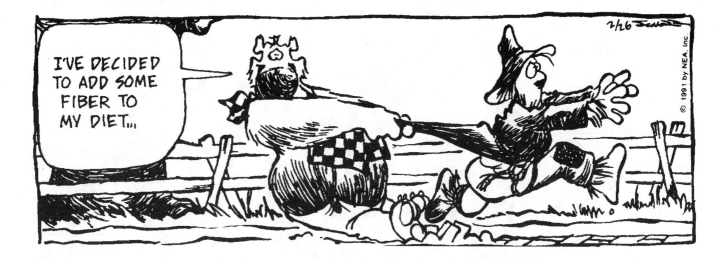

not yet established strict guidelines for daily intake of fiber. Most nutritionists suggest that a healthy goal is to aim for an average intake of 25 to 35 grams of fiber each day. Try to increase the number of these foods in your diet. They may help control your appetite, because they do add bulk. They may also have health benefits.

Fruit in your diet

Fruit and fruit juices are an important ingredient of a well balanced diet. Fruits are naturally low in sodium and dietary fat, and they are an excellent source of fiber. They provide generous amounts of Vitamins A and C and potassium. Vitamin A is essential for the growth of teeth, skin, and bones, and it is important for good vision.

Most Americans fall short in their daily consumption of fruits. This is particularly true of children and adolescents. When this happens, the body suffers from a lack of important vitamins, minerals, and fiber. Here are some tips that may help you add fruit to your diet.

Breakfast

Breakfast is an important meal—one that should not be skipped. This is a good opportunity to have a serving of fruit. Six ounces of fruit juice is a good way to start the day. But be careful to make sure you are drinking 100 percent fruit juice. Many of the fruit drinks, ades, and punches on the market contain only a small percentage of actual fruit juice and have a lot of added sugar.

If you have cereal for breakfast, top it off with fresh fruit instead of sugar. Strawberries, blueberries, bananas, and grapes are smart choices and take little time to prepare. If you are in a rush, take the fruit with you. Keep fresh oranges, bananas, kiwifruit, apples, peaches, or pears available to take with you.

Snacks

Fruit makes a good snack—whether in the morning, afternoon, or evening snack.

High Fiber Fruits, Vegetables, and Cereals

Fruits

Apples*	Cherries	Oranges	Pineapple
Apricots*	Dried fruit	Peaches*	Plums*
Bananas	Figs	Pears*	Prunes
Berries	Grapefruit		

*with peel

Vegetables

Asparagus	Corn	Mushrooms	Rhubarb
Beans	Eggplant	Okra	Sauerkraut
Broccoli	Endive	Onions	Spinach
Brussel sprouts	Green beans	Parsnips	Squash
Cabbage	Greens, all	Peas	Tomatoes
Carrots	Lettuce	Potatoes	Turnips
Cauliflower	Lima beans	Radishes	Watercress
Celery			

Cereals

Brans	Oatmeal	Shredded wheat
Whole wheat cereal		

The Food Guide Pyramid

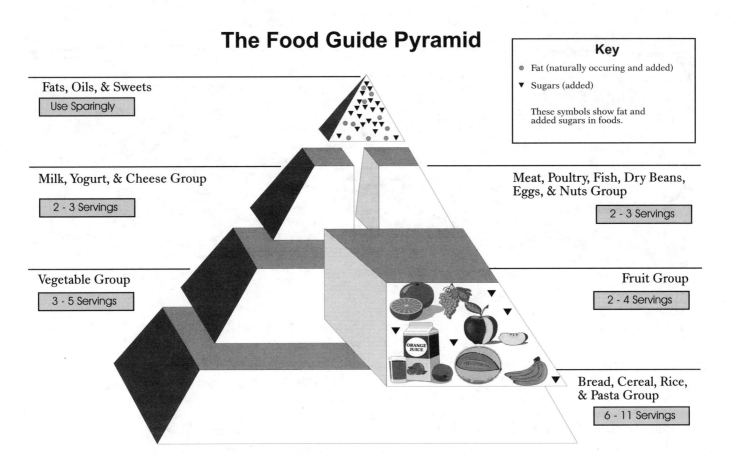

Fats, Oils, & Sweets
Use Sparingly

Key
- Fat (naturally occuring and added)
- ▼ Sugars (added)

These symbols show fat and added sugars in foods.

Milk, Yogurt, & Cheese Group
2 - 3 Servings

Meat, Poultry, Fish, Dry Beans, Eggs, & Nuts Group
2 - 3 Servings

Vegetable Group
3 - 5 Servings

Fruit Group
2 - 4 Servings

ORANGE JUICE

Bread, Cereal, Rice, & Pasta Group
6 - 11 Servings

Canned juices are also convenient and easy to take with you when you are on the go. Instead of a soda or cup of coffee, drink fruit juice. If you don't have fresh fruit available for a snack, canned fruit will do fine, but watch out for the heavy syrup and added sugars.

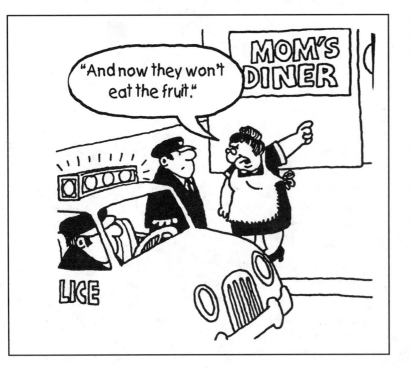

Lunch

If you take your lunch to work or school, include some fresh or canned fruit. Fruit is a healthy substitute for dessert. If you eat out, it is still possible to have some fruit. Many restaurants now offer fresh fruit as an appetizer or for dessert, but there are still some that do not offer fruit on the menu. If fruit is not available, ask for fruit juice.

Dinner

Dinner time is a good opportunity to review your fruit intake for the day. If you missed a serving or two during the day, add a glass of fruit juice to your evening menu. Fresh fruit can also be included with your meal (e.g., a fruit salad) or as a dessert.

How many servings?

The Food Guide Pyramid suggests two to four servings per day from the Fruit Group. This is less than you may think and should not be difficult to include in your daily diet.

Fruits

Description	Calories	Protein (g)	Carb. (g)	Fat (g)
Apple, w/skin (1 med)	81	.3	21.1	.5
Apple juice (6 oz)	87	.15	21.8	.2
Applesauce, sweetened (½ cup)	97	.2	25.5	.2
Apricots (4 med)	68	2.0	15.7	.5
Apricot nectar, canned (6 oz)	106	.7	27.1	.2
Banana (1 med)	105	1.2	26.7	.6
Blackberries, raw (1 cup)	74	1.0	18.4	.6
Blueberries, raw (1 cup)	82	1.0	20.5	.6
Cantaloupe, raw (1 cup)	57	1.4	13.4	.4
Casaba melon, raw (1 cup)	45	1.5	10.5	.2
Cherries, raw (10 med)	49	.8	11.3	.7
Dates, dried (10 med)	228	1.6	61.0	.4
Figs, raw (3 med)	111	1.2	28.8	.6
Fruit cocktail, in water (½ cup)	40	.5	10.4	.1
Grapefruit, raw, pink (½ med)	37	.7	9.5	.1
Grapefruit juice, fresh (6 oz)	72	.9	17.0	.2
Grapes, raw (½ cup)	29	.3	7.9	.2
Grape juice (6 oz)	116	.8	28.4	.2
Honeydew melon, raw (½ cup)	66	1.6	15.4	.6
Kiwifruit, raw (1 med)	46	.8	11.3	.3
Mandarin oranges (½ cup)	46	.8	11.9	.0
Mango, raw (1 med)	135	1.1	35.2	.6
Nectarine, raw (1 med)	67	1.3	16.0	.6
Orange, raw (1 med)	65	1.4	16.3	.1
Orange juice, fresh (6 oz)	8.	1.3	19.4	.4
Papaya, raw (1 med)	117	1.9	29.8	.4
Peach, raw (1 med)	37	.6	9.7	.1
Peach, in light syrup (½ cup)	68	.6	18.3	.1
Peach nectar (6 oz)	101	.5	26.0	.1
Pear, raw (1 med)	98	.7	25.1	.7
Pear, canned in light syrup (½ cup)	72	.3	19.1	.1
Pear nectar (6 oz)	112	.2	29.6	.0
Pineapple, raw (½ cup pieces)	38	.3	9.6	.4
Pineapple juice (6 oz)	103	.8	25.4	.2
Raspberries, raw (1 cup)	61	1.1	14.2	.7
Strawberries, raw (1 cup)	45	.9	10.5	.6
Watermelon, raw (1 cup)	50	1.0	11.5	.7

Note: Each of the food items listed above counts as one serving. This table should be used as a guide for the foods listed. Since food values vary by size and brand name it is important to read the food labels for these foods.

How much is a serving?

Servings from the Fruit Group are relatively easy to remember. The chart above includes food items that count as a single serving. As a general rule, the following count as one serving:

- ☑ 1 medium apple, orange, banana, peach, or pear
- ☑ ½ cup of chopped, cooked, or canned fruit
- ☑ 1 cup of small berries
- ☑ ¾ cup or 6 oz of fruit juice

Selection hints

In most parts of the country, certain fruits are seasonal which makes it necessary to choose from a variety of different fruits. Variety is important because different fruits provide different amounts of important nutrients. The following tips may be helpful in your selection:

Choose citrus fruits, melons, and berries regularly—these are rich in Vitamin C.

Choose fresh fruits as often as you can—they do not have added sugars and other preservatives. Try to avoid fruits that are canned or frozen in heavy syrups and sweetened fruit juices—you'll save many unwanted calories this way.

Choose fruit juices that are pure fruit juice and that do not contain large amounts of added water and sugars.

Assignment for this lesson

Keep a lookout for pressures to eat. Be polite but firm when you encounter people who want you to eat. Look also for Imperatives in your thoughts and banish them to Never-Never Land. Consider jogging and cycling, and consider the vitamins you take in light of the information discussed above. Keep track of your daily intake of fiber and try to average 25 to 35 grams per day. And finally, try to eat the recommended number of servings from the Fruit Group.

Self-assessment questionnaire

Lesson Ten

T F 53. When someone offers you food, it is best to accept it as a sign of their friendship.

T F 54. Imperatives are words like *always* and *never*. They leave no room for error.

T F 55. There are many benefits to jogging and cycling. They are good forms of exercise for people trying to lose weight.

T F 56. Vitamin B$_{12}$ is the only vitamin for which mega-doses are recommended.

T F 57. Fruits, vegetables, and cereals tend to be high in fiber.

T F 58. Most Americans eat plenty of fruits and should not worry about increasing their daily intake.

(Answers in Appendix C)

Monitoring Form—Lesson Ten

Today's Date:

Time	Food and Amount	Calories
	Total Daily Calories	

Assignment this week	*Always*	*Sometimes*	*Never*
1. Refuse offers to eat			
2. Banish imperatives			
3. Try jogging or cycling			
4. Watch vitamins			
5. Daily servings from the Fruit Group			
6. Less than _____ calories each day			
7. My diet has _____ grams of fiber			

Food Groups for Today	*Physical Activity*	*Minutes*
Milk, yogurt, and cheese ❏ ❏ ❏		
Meat, poultry, etc. ❏ ❏ ❏		
Fruits ❏ ❏ ❏ ❏		
Vegetables ❏ ❏ ❏ ❏ ❏		
Breads, cereals, etc. ❏ ❏ ❏ ❏ ❏ ❏ ❏ ❏ ❏ ❏ ❏		

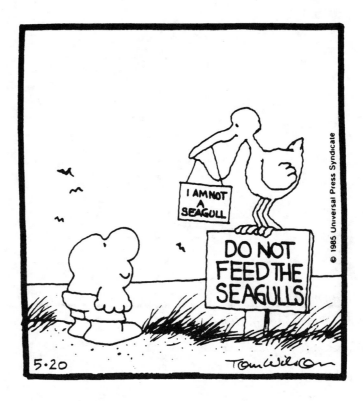

With ten lessons behind us, it is hard to believe that there is still so much to learn. In this lesson, we will begin with a discussion of lifestyle tips to help you with eating away from home. I will discuss aerobics and calisthenics in the Exercise section. We then move to activities that can bring more pleasure to a program partnership, and I will discuss the fat soluble vitamins. Finally, the Bread, Cereal, Rice, and Pasta Group of the Food Guide Pyramid will be discussed.

Eating away from home

Trips to restaurants can be a mine field of temptation. The best intentions can crumble when you are enjoying yourself with people who feast on delicious foods. Two aspects of this concern us. The first is how much we eat, but there are methods for keeping eating under control. The second is to control our *response* to the event.

One trip to a restaurant never torpedoed any program with its calories alone. An extraordinary meal of 5000 calories could bring only a pound and a half of weight. The *response* to those calories, however, could lead to trouble. Your attitudes during and after these events are as important as what you eat.

Eating at restaurants

It is hard to be virtuous at restaurants. This is a real problem for people in business or those whose lifestyle includes eating away from home. What should you do when dessert comes with the meal? What about a waitress who pours 14 gallons of dressing on your salad? How do you deal with a hot loaf of bread the waiter delivers before the meal even begins? How can you refuse when the dessert cart rolls up like a Brink's truck ready to unload its treasures?

Order a la carte meals. You may be inclined to order full meals because the cost is less than for the sum of its parts. This group plan is a booby trap because you order more than you need simply because the price seems attractive. However, the logic is faulty.

The regular price for a roast beef sandwich might be $5, but for $6 you could get French fries and cole slaw which would normally cost $1 each. The package deal makes sense only if you wanted the other two items anyway. If not, you are saving money you never would have spent. Most of these extras are high-calorie foods like French fries. Order just what you want.

Watch the salad dressing. Since salad dressing is high in fat (oil), eating more than you need really boosts the calories. Ask for salad dressing on the side so you are not at the mercy of a heavy handed server. Better yet, leave the salad dressing off completely.

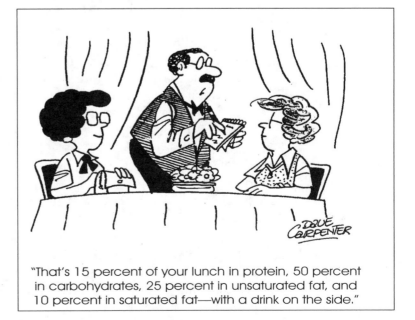

"That's 15 percent of your lunch in protein, 50 percent in carbohydrates, 25 percent in unsaturated fat, and 10 percent in saturated fat—with a drink on the side."

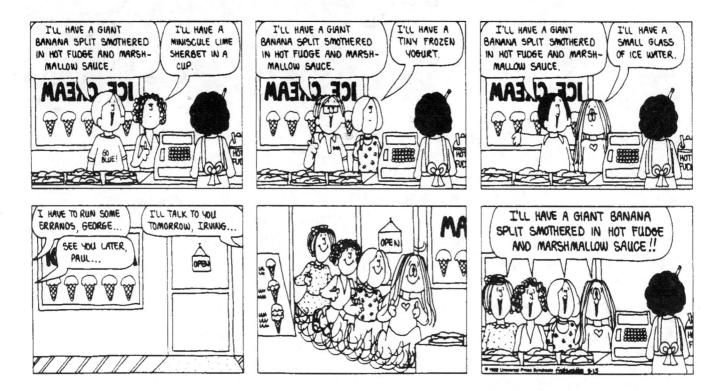

If you need dressing, consider bringing your own bottle of low-fat dressing. Many people do this, and unless you're at the White House for an awards banquet, you shouldn't be embarrassed.

Watch for hidden calories. Many foods contain calories that are added in subtle ways. These *hidden* calories are important to consider. Think about rich sauces added to meats and vegetables in French restaurants, oils added in Italian restaurants, and things breaded and fried in any restaurant. If you cannot guess what is in a dish, ask the waiter or waitress.

Watch alcohol. Alcohol is loaded with calories, and it is easy to consume more than you want in the spirit of being social. This is a real temptation when you sit in the bar area waiting for a table in the restaurant.

When you order alcohol, avoid the hard liquor and sweetened drinks. A jigger of whiskey has 110 calories and a Tom Collins has 180 calories. White wine is a better choice, and better yet is a white wine spritzer. You could also order club soda or tomato juice.

Alcohol generally has *empty* calories. Its sugar brings calories with little or no nutrition. You can estimate the calories in alcohol by remembering that the following drinks have about 100 calories: 12 oz of light beer, 8 oz of regular beer, 3½ oz of wine, and 1 shot of liquor. You may want to refer to the chart on page 83 as a reminder of calories in alcohol.

Beware of the breadbasket. Keep an eye out for that wondrous basket. It comes when you are hungry and excited about being at the restaurant. You can refuse the breadbasket, but if one arrives against your will, let it rest across the table. If you are still tempted, imagine there is a mousetrap under the napkin that covers the bread!

There are some people who actually benefit from the breadbasket. They are the ones who use a piece of bread (without butter) to take the edge off their hunger, so that they will eat less of higher-calorie foods later in the meal. You might try this approach, but don't use it as an excuse to eat lots of bread and then eat what you would anyway.

Bread does *not* have empty calories. It is an important part of your diet: Breads and Cereals comprise the largest of the five food groups of the Food Guide Pyramid. The purpose of watching the breadbasket is not to cut down on bread, but to avoid eating lots of bread just because it's there.

Be wise with dessert. Do you deserve dessert when you eat out? After all, you don't get special desserts often, so why not enjoy yourself? Ignore this rationalization and get dessert under two conditions: 1) you are still hungry; 2) you have planned it in your day's calories. Think about fresh fruit or gelatin. Both taste good and have far fewer calories than traditional choices.

Engage your partner. Restaurants are a place where your partner can help. This can begin before you arrive for the meal. Some individuals decide with their partners what to order in advance, before their restraint is weakened by the smells and atmosphere of a nice restaurant. Some even have their partner order for them. At the restaurant, the partner can keep the breadbasket in a safe place and can help by not pushing drinks or desserts.

Watch your emotional response. If you eat more than you plan, be careful not to consider it a catastrophe. We have been working to avoid the attitude traps, such as considering some foods *illegal* and setting unrealistic goals of never overeating. If you feel guilty, reread the earlier material, and be prepared to rebound from a bout of overeating by eating less, not more. Do *not* use this as a rationalization to overdo it, but keep these events in perspective and use them as a sign that you should do better the next meal or the next day.

These are techniques used by individuals to control their eating in restaurants. You may think of others yourself. For example, you might drink extra water to help fill up before the meal comes. Have fun, but keep control!

Are aerobics for you?

The answer is probably "No!"—or so you think. I used to feel the same way. I remember when coaches and teachers used calisthenics as punishment or as a way to *build character*. Push-ups, sit-ups, squat thrusts, and leg lifts ranked somewhere below staying after school on my list of favorite activities.

The situation is much different today. Calisthenics have been replaced with aerobics, slimnastics, Jazzercise®, and the like. This signals not only a change in terminology but a change in the way exercise is viewed. In my opinion, the changes are positive.

When aerobic training became popular, using exercise to build strength took a back seat

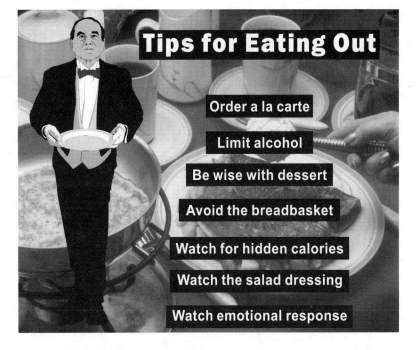

Tips for Eating Out

Order a la carte

Limit alcohol

Be wise with dessert

Avoid the breadbasket

Watch for hidden calories

Watch the salad dressing

Watch emotional response

to improving the condition of the heart. This involves getting the heart rate up and keeping it there. Many different movements can accomplish this, hence the use of dance and other types of movement in aerobics classes. This makes exercise more interesting and more healthy than the calisthenics of old.

Aerobic activities require a large increase in the body's use of oxygen. This is best accomplished by use of large muscle groups, and it involves some form of vigorous and rhythmic movement. Running, cycling, swimming, and rope jumping are examples, but so are dancing to fast music and the other movements you associate with aerobics classes. As I mentioned before, these are the *only* type of exercises that will improve cardiovascular conditioning. They are *not* the only exercises that will help you lose weight, but they are certainly among the best.

Aerobics can be done in so many ways that they are suitable for almost everybody. If you want to do it alone, there are books, TV shows, videotapes, and records. Most of these workout approaches are aerobic in nature. If you would like company, aerobics classes are held at the YMCA, YWCA, exercise centers, and in many companies, churches, and community centers. You can do aerobics at your own pace, even if you are with a group, so don't worry about the shape you're in. There are many excellent books available on aerobic

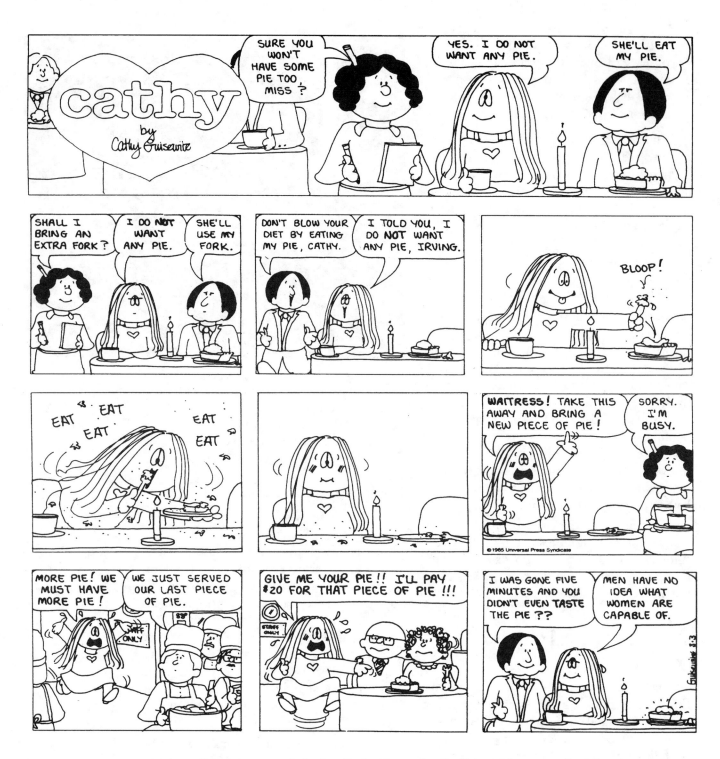

exercises. I suggest any of the books by Dr. Kenneth Cooper, which are available in most bookstores. These discuss what to do, how much to do, and how to have fun.

Many people losing weight use more than one form of exercise. This breaks monotony and gives you a chance to do whatever your mood dictates. You might run some days, bicycle other days, and do aerobics on days when a class is scheduled. This allows you to be flexible with your schedule, the weather, and your moods.

Pleasurable partner activities

There are many nice things you can do with your partner. These can be used as rewards from you to your partner, from your partner to you, or as a joint bit of pleasure to

Pleasurable Partner Activities

Take a romantic walk

Take a bath together

Plan a day at the park

Buy fancy underwear

Send flowers

Pick fresh fruit

Go bowling

Buy a nice wine

Play a new sport

See the city

Send a singing telegram

Plan a mystery weekend

See a movie

Buy cologne or perfume

Get gift certificates

Get a nice plant

Buy a tape or CD

Make Sunday breakfast

Ride bicycles

Go window shopping

Go on a picnic

Get a puppy or a kitten

Send a card

Go to a museum

Get a board game

Buy a new book

Buy a pedometer

Buy exotic lovemaking book

Find a lover's lane

Do your partner's laundry

Write a thank you note

Plan a surprise party

Fix something broken

Balance the checkbook

Watch the sunset

Do an erotic massage

_____ _____

_____ _____

_____ _____

_____ _____

_____ _____

_____ _____

_____ _____

_____ _____

_____ _____

_____ _____

_____ _____

acknowledge efforts from both of you. The list shown here gives many possible activities. Some are appropriate for partners in romantic relationships while others are for any partnership.

Share these ideas with your partner and use them for special times. If you are working together as a team, it will be nice to have some fun in addition to the work. Remember that there are many nice partner activities not on the list, so be creative. Add as many ideas to the list as you can.

More about fat soluble vitamins

In Lesson Ten I discussed the water soluble vitamins. In this lesson we will focus on the vitamins that are fat soluble. Vitamins A, D, E, and K are fat soluble. They are stored in fat tissue in the body if consumed in excess. This is why toxic doses are a more important issue with fat soluble than water soluble vitamins. You should be especially wary of people who promote large doses of these four vitamins. As with all vitamins, no more than the Recommended Daily Allowance (RDA) is suggested. Review the chart in Lesson Seven for the RDA of all vitamins.

Vitamin A is used for growth of the skin, bones, and teeth and is important in vision. It is found in leafy green vegetables, yellow vegetables, milk, eggs, fortified margarine, liver, and kidney. Vitamin D is crucial for development of bones and teeth, and helps the body use calcium and phosphorus. It is abundant in cod liver oil, and is found in egg yolk, milk, tuna, and salmon.

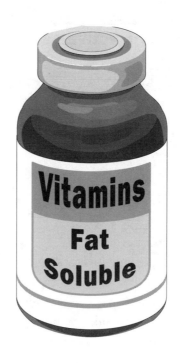

Vitamin E is useful for the functioning of red blood cells, and helps the body use essential fatty acids. Vitamin E is present in wheat germ, egg yolks, vegetable oils, cereals, and lettuce. Vitamin K is used by the liver in the production of prothrombin. It is found in liver, cabbage, spinach, and kale. The RDA has not yet been established for vitamin K.

Above all, watch out for bold claims. Taking extra amounts won't do a thing for weight loss and may damage your health.

Breads, cereals, rice, and pasta in your diet

Foods from this group of the pyramid are good sources of complex carbohydrates. These foods are good sources of *low-fat* energy and provide essential vitamins, minerals, and fiber. Foods from this group should make up the largest part of your daily diet. It is important, however, to watch out for the *hidden fats* and *calories* in some of these foods. Bread, cookies, and pastries, for example, typically include sugar and butter, oil, or margarine. Remember, it is easy to eat too many calories

Bread, Cereal, Rice, and Pasta

Description	Calories	Protein (g)	Carb. (g)	Fat (g)
Bread, wheat (1 slice)	61	2.3	11.3	1.0
Bread, white (1 slice)	64	2.0	11.7	.9
Bagel (½)	82	3.0	15.5	.7
Cereal, cheerios (1 oz)	111	1.4	19.6	1.8
Cereal, corn flakes (1 oz)	110	2.0	25.0	1.0
Cookies, chocolate chip (2 med)	99	1.1	14.6	4.4
Cookies, oatmeal (2 med)	124	1.6	17.8	5.2
Danish, 1 small (1 oz)	125	2.0	13.5	7.5
English muffin, plain (½)	68	2.3	13.1	.6
Pancakes, 4 in. diameter (1)	62	1.9	9.2	1.9
Pasta, enriched cooked (½ cup)	100	3.3	18.7	1.2
Pie, fruit, 2—crust, 8 in. (1/12 piece)	116	.9	18.3	4.6
Rice, enriched cooked (½ cup)	141	1.2	21.5	6.0

The Food Guide Pyramid

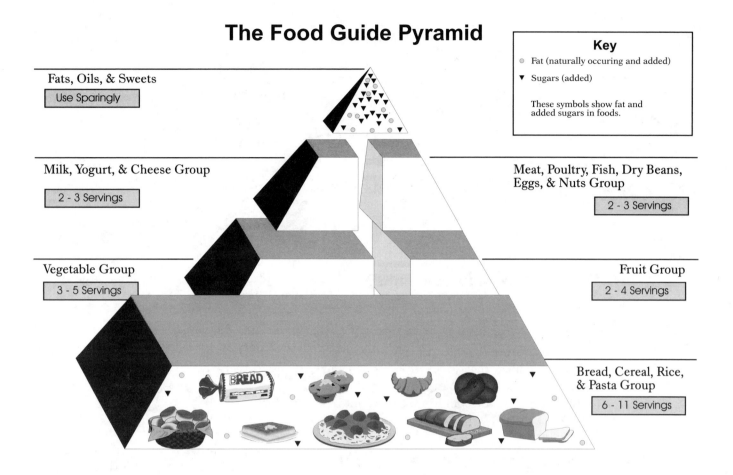

from this food group that do not provide good nutrition. Making wise food choices from this group is important.

Selection hints

The following guidelines will help you to make good choices from the Bread, Cereal, Rice, and Pasta Group:

Dietary fiber is important for good health, and foods from this food group are good sources of fiber. Choose several servings a day from whole grains, which are found in whole-wheat breads and whole-grain cereals.

Foods that contain low amounts of fat and simple sugars are the best choices for a healthy diet. Choose foods made with small amounts of sugars and fats. These food items include bread, English muffins, rice, and pasta.

Some foods from this group that are made from flour are typically high in fat and sugars. These include cookies, pastries, croissants, doughnuts, and cakes. Keep these foods to a minimum and use low-fat and sugar substitutes when possible.

Spreads and toppings can add many unwanted calories to the foods in this group while providing very little nutritional value. The best advice is to leave these items off or to at least use low-calorie or low-fat toppings, spreads, and sauces.

Most pasta stuffings and sauces use butter or margarine. Use only half of the recipe amount. If milk or cream is called for, use low-fat milk.

If pasta sauces or stuffings call for meat, use lean meat. Trim away any visible fat before cooking, and drain all oil before including in your sauce or stuffing.

How much is a serving?

Servings from this group are simple to remember. As a general rule, the following count as a single serving:

- ☑ 1 slice of bread
- ☑ 1 oz of ready-to-eat cereal
- ☑ ½ cup of cooked cereal, rice, or pasta

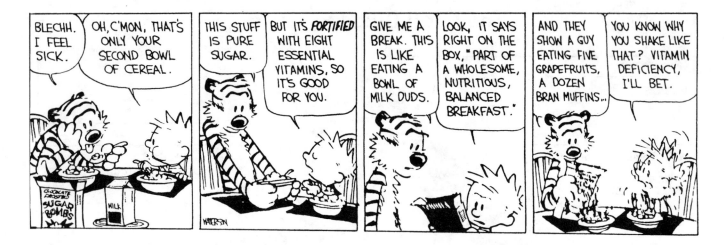

How many servings?

The Food Guide Pyramid suggests 6 to 11 servings each day from the Bread, Cereal, Rice, and Pasta Group. While this may sound like a lot, remember that foods from this group should be the largest part of your daily diet. The chart here includes foods that count as a single serving.

Breakfast cereal: the good, the bad, the sugar coated

Most of us grew up eating cereals for breakfast. The experience included not only the cereal, but reading the box, twisting and tilting the box in all directions to beat our brothers and sisters to the free prize, and saving box tops and proofs of purchase for the wonderful toys we could buy.

Today's marketing of breakfast cereals is clever indeed. Cereals are associated with cartoon characters and sports figures. The manufacturers are sensitive to our nutrition conscious culture and to the bad rap given to sugar coated cereals. Witness, for example, how some old favorites have changed names. *Sugar Smacks* are now *Honey Smacks*, *Super Sugar Crisp* is now *Super Golden Crisp*, and *Sugar Frosted Flakes* are now simply *Frosted Flakes*. Some cereals of questionable nutritional value are advertised on television as "part of a nutritious breakfast." The nutritious breakfast they show includes foods like juice, milk, muffins, fruit, and the like, so I suppose one could replace the cereal with a rock and make the same claim.

Breakfast plays an important role in our daily diet. One characteristic common to overweight persons is that they seldom eat breakfast. As they lose weight, many resume eating breakfast. Since cereal is part of the usual breakfast picture, the listing in the cereal table on the following page may be helpful in choosing a cereal with both calories and healthy eating in mind. The ratings have been adapted from an article in *Consumer Reports* magazine published in October, 1996. If you are interested in even more information, I urge you to read the article itself.

Cereals can be good sources of fiber and other nutrients, because the basic grains from which cereals are made (oats, wheat, corn, etc.) contain many nutrients for the calories. However, cereals differ greatly in nutritional value. Some have as much as 16 grams (three teaspoons) of sugar in every serving, so more than half the weight of the cereal is sugar.

The article in *Consumer Reports* points to cereals as "best choices" if each serving has 5 grams or more of fiber, five grams or less of sugar, and three grams or less of fat. The authors point out that some cereals that sound healthy may have fat and sugar in surprisingly high amounts. Raisin Nut Bran, Quaker 100 percent Natural Oats, and Blueberry Morning cereals have more than three grams of fat per serving, and Cracklin' Oat Bran has a whopping eight grams of fat per serving, including three grams of saturated fat. Some cereals have less than one gram of fiber per serving and 10 grams or more of sugar (e.g., Cocoa Puffs, Cocoa Pebbles, Trix, Frosted Flakes, Fruity Pebbles). It pays to look at the labels, not the name of the cereal.

A Nutrition Scorecard for Cereals

The cereals below represent nutritious and not-as-nutritious choices based on the *Consumer Report* comparison of more than 100 top-sellers. All are national brands; similar store brands should have similar nutrition. Note that cereal ingredients change fairly often. If you're concerned about nutrition, check a cereal's label before buying.

Best Choices
High fiber, very low sugar, low fat

(A serving from this list has 5 grams or more of fiber, 5 grams or less of sugar, and 3 grams or less of fat.)

General Mills Fiber One

Kellogg's All-Bran Extra Fiber

Kellogg's All-Bran Original

Nabisco Shredded Wheat (regular, spoon-size, and wheat 'n bran)

Ralston Wheat Chex

Other Choices
Very low sugar, low fat

(A serving from this list has 5 grams or less of sugar, 3 grams or less of fat, and 0 to 4 grams of fiber.)

General Mills Kix

General Mills Cheerios

General Mills Total Corn Flakes

General Mills Total Whole Grain

General Mills Wheaties

Health Valley Honey Clusters & Flakes with Apples & Cinnamon

Kellogg's Corn Flakes

Kellogg's Crispix

Kellogg's Rice Krispies

Kellogg's Product 19

Kellogg's Special K

Ralston Rice Chex

Ralston Corn Chex

Other Choices
High fiber, low fat

(A serving from this list has 5 grams or more of fiber, 3 grams or less of fat, and 6 to 20 grams of sugar.)

Familia Original Recipe Swiss Muesli

Kellogg's Bran Buds

Kellogg's Complete Bran Flakes

Kellogg's Frosted Mini-Wheats

Healthy Choice Multi-Grain Squares

Healthy Choice Raisin Squares

Nabisco Frosted Wheat Bites and 100% Bran

Post Fruit & Fibre Dates, Raisins, Walnuts

Post Grape-Nuts

Post Premium Bran Flakes

Ralston Multi Bran Chex

Raisin Brans (from various manufacturers)

Plenty of fat

(A serving has more than 3 grams of fat.)

General Mills Cinnamon Toast Crunch

General Mills Raisin Nut Bran

Kellogg's Cracklin Oat Bran

Post Banana Nut Crunch

Kellogg's Blueberry Morning

Kellogg's Great Grains Raisin, Date, Pecan

Quaker 100% Natural Oats, Honey & Raisins

Little Fiber, Plenty of Sugar

(A serving has less than a gram of fiber and at least 10 grams (2 teaspoons) of sugar.)

General Mills Cocoa Puffs

General Mills Reese's Peanut Butter Puffs

General Mills Trix

Kellogg's Cocoa Krispies

Kellogg's Frosted Flakes

Kellogg's Pop-Tarts

Post Cocoa Pebbles

Post Fruity Pebbles

Post Honey-Comb

Post Waffle Crisp

Ralston Cookie-Crisp Chocolate Chip

Assignment for this lesson

We began this lesson with a discussion of techniques for eating away from home. Use these to keep your eating under control. Try aerobic activities as part of your physical fitness routine, and remember all the ways to do aerobic activities: on your own, at the YMCA or YWCA, and at spas, community centers, and places of work. Use the suggestions for partner activities if you are using the partnership approach. Watch to see that you get the vitamins you need, but avoid falling victim to the vitamin hawkers who promise that large doses will cure nearly any ill. And finally, try to eat the recommended number of servings from the Bread, Cereal, Rice, and Pasta Group.

Self-assessment questionnaire

Lesson Eleven

T F 59. Alcohol is dangerous for people losing weight because it contains many calories and weakens dietary restraint.

T F 60. Ordering a la carte meals at restaurants helps avoid unwanted calories that come in *package* meals.

T F 61. Aerobic activities are designed to build strength in the shortest possible time.

T F 62. Vitamin E is associated with virility and may help in the remedy of alcoholism.

T F 63. Foods from the Bread, Cereal, Rice, and Pasta Group are a good source of complex carbohydrates, however, they may contain hidden fat.

T F 64. One characteristic common to overweight persons is that they seldom eat breakfast.

(Answers in Appendix C)

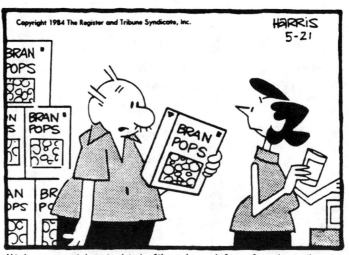

"It's a new idea in high-fiber breakfast foods. When the cereal is gone, you eat the box!"

Monitoring Form—Lesson Eleven

Today's Date:

Time	Food and Amount	Calories
	Total Daily Calories	

Assignment this week	Always	Sometimes	Never
1. Techniques for eating out			
2. Try aerobic activities			
3. Daily servings from the Bread & Cereal Group			
4. Less than _____ calories each day			

Food Groups for Today	Physical Activity	Minutes
Milk, yogurt, and cheese ❑ ❑ ❑		
Meat, poultry, etc. ❑ ❑ ❑		
Fruits ❑ ❑ ❑ ❑		
Vegetables ❑ ❑ ❑ ❑ ❑		
Breads, cereals, etc. ❑ ❑ ❑ ❑ ❑ ❑ ❑ ❑ ❑ ❑		

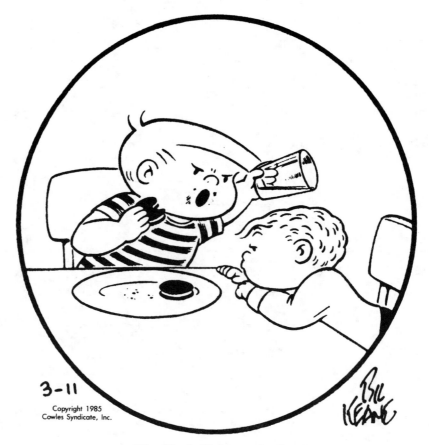

"Go ahead. Make my day."

Here we are, Lesson Twelve —three-quarters of the way through the program. We have poured through mountains of information and have done plenty of homework. It is time to integrate this into a practical approach you can use permanently. To do this, we will learn about the Behavior Chain. This gives you a system for deciding which of many techniques to use in a given situation. I consider this extremely important.

Bringing it all together: the behavior chain

We need to organize the information in this program into a logical picture. We have covered ways to identify problem situations, along with techniques (more than 70 by now) to help you control eating and increase exercise. We are still left with an important challenge.

What each person needs is a mental card file or computer data base to summon the right technique at the right time in a given situation. For example, if playing a card game (let's say bridge) with your friends is a high-risk situation, you could look in your file under "Playing Bridge" for a list of techniques. The card in your file would list different aspects of this situation that would determine its degree of risk. These aspects might be who the friends are, whether they serve food, how hungry you are, how well your program has been going, and so forth. Then when a situation arises, perhaps the arrival of potato chips and dip, your card would list several responses.

The Behavior Chain is the path to this process. It is a method for breaking eating episodes into discreet parts. When you examine each part, ideas emerge for stopping eating in its tracks. The ideas that follow can truly increase your understanding of eating.

A chain and its links

We can view eating as a chain of events which contains many links. The links string together like an ordinary chain. We can use a familiar phrase: *A chain is only as strong as its weakest link*. The good news is that you *want* to break this chain, so attacking at the weakest link is ideal.

If we return to the example of playing bridge with friends, eating the potato chips resides at the end of a long chain. Preceding it were links like having the chips available, going to the card game hungry, having friends offer the food, and so forth. The chain could be broken at any of these points.

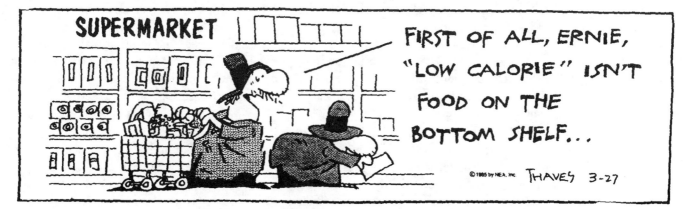

SUPERMARKET

FIRST OF ALL, ERNIE, "LOW CALORIE" ISN'T FOOD ON THE BOTTOM SHELF...

© 1985 by NEA, Inc   THAVES 3-27

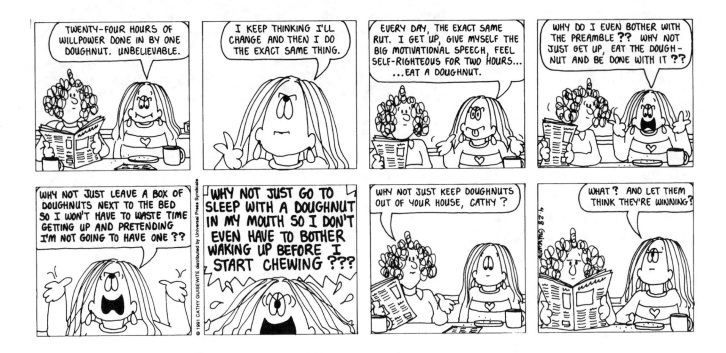

Each act of eating can be viewed with the chain in mind. Once you identify the links in your chain, you can spot the best link to break and how to break it. The more links you break, and the earlier in the chain you break them, the easier it will be to control eating.

A sample behavior chain

Let's illustrate the chain concept with the example of Laura. In her chain, Laura ate 10 cookies, felt guilty, and then ate even more. Laura's eating occurred in a chain which included many links before the eating and several links after the eating. We could help Laura control her cookie intake by analyzing this chain. Remember that this is an example to illustrate the *principle* of a chain. Think about how this concept applies to your situation.

Laura's chain began when she bought the cookies. She was home on Saturday afternoon and was tired and bored. She got the urge to eat and then ate the 10 cookies while watching TV. She felt guilty and ate more cookies later. We can find 12 links in Laura's chain. These are shown in the figure displayed on page 164 .

These are the twelve steps to Laura's dilemma. It started when (1) Laura bought the cookies. She then (2) left the cookies on the counter where they were plainly visible. She was (3) home on Saturday afternoon, which

she knows from experience is a high-risk time and place for overeating.

She was (4) tired and bored. She (5) felt an urge to eat and (6) went to the kitchen. She (7) took the cookies to the den and (8) ate them while watching TV. She (9) ate rapidly until she felt full, then (10) felt guilty and like a failure. This (11) weakened her restraint further until (12) she ate even more cookies.

Is Laura an innocent victim of an inevitable chain, or can she do something to interrupt it at a critical point? As you probably guessed, Laura has many options of interrupting the chain. Before we discuss these, think of your own lifestyle and the eating habits you have. How do they exist as chains, and what are the links in the chains?

Take some time now to draw a picture of an eating chain that applies to you. Use the blank chain provided on page 166 to fill in the details. You can use Laura's chain as an example, but make the situation specific to you. Pick a high-risk situation that really gives you trouble. Examples might be arriving home from work, watching television in the evening, feeling depressed or lonely, etc.

Your chain can contain fewer links or more than the blank chain permits, but try to include each important detail. You will see how the links are inextricably tied together to form a sequence of events that is hard to stop once it gets started. If you come armed with techniques for dismantling the chain, you will increase your control.

Interrupting the chain

Your mind was probably buzzing with ideas as we were discussing Laura's eating chain and as you were writing your own chain. We can use Laura's chain for an example of how a chain might be broken. Some of the possible ways Laura might interrupt her chain are shown below.

Analyzing your eating chain

This chain concept could be a key part of your program. If you can analyze your eating according to the chain notion, you can devise

Link	Link Breaking Techniques
Buy cookies	Shop from a list Shop on a full stomach Shop with a partner Have a partner do your shopping Buy cookie mix (needs baking)
Cookies on counter	Store in opaque container Freeze cookies Store in inaccessible place
Home during high-risk	Go shopping Schedule programmed activity Plan an enjoyable activity
Tired and bored	Exercise Get more sleep
Urge to eat	List of alternatives to eating Wait five minutes; urge may pass Separate hunger from cravings
Go to kitchen	Use alternative activities Get some exercise Leave house Low-calorie foods available
Take cookies to den	Eat in one place
Eat while watching TV	Do nothing else while eating
Eat rapidly until full	Put food down between bites Pause during eating Serve one cookie at a time Stop automatic eating
Feel guilty, like a failure	Watch dichotomous thinking Banish imperatives Set realistic goals Plan adaptive response
Restraint weakens	Resolve to increase control Read LEARN Manual for ideas
More eating	Examine chain, use techniques Watch attitude traps

Sample Behavior Chain

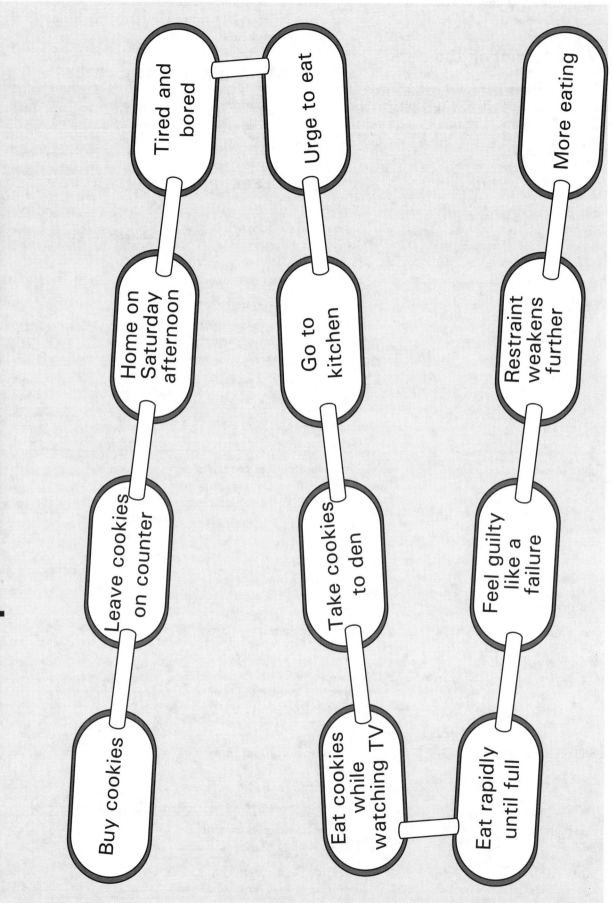

Buy cookies → Leave cookies on counter → Home on Saturday afternoon → Tired and bored → Urge to eat → Go to kitchen → Take cookies to den → Eat cookies while watching TV → Eat rapidly until full → Feel guilty like a failure → Restraint weakens further → More eating

many ways to get control. Contrast this with the common approach which relies solely on willpower once the chain is advanced and food beckons.

Now we can go to work on *your* chain. Look at each of the links in the chain and write down at least two ways the chain could be broken at each link. With Laura's chain, we listed 34 ways to break at least one link. Use the information you have learned in the program to think of *link-breaking techniques*. You might refresh your memory on techniques by referring back to the Monitoring Forms from previous weeks.

There are several things to remember when listing these techniques. The first is to concentrate on the weakest links. For instance, if eating ice cream is the final link in your chain, it might be easier to avoid buying the ice cream initially than to count on willpower when confronted by the food. This leads to the second point, which is to interrupt the chain as early as possible. This does not diminish the importance of interrupting the steps late in the chain, but starting early in the chain gives you more links to work with.

I know what happens when I read things where the author asks me to fill something out. I usually think it's not worth the effort and I read ahead. You may feel that you need not go through this exercise, and you might be correct. Remember, however, that the act of writing these things down will make you think and analyze your high-risk situations like never before.

Using the stairs

Climbing stairs is a handy way to increase your exercise. It is an ideal way to work extra activity into your lifestyle. It is an efficient way of burning calories. As you may know, climbing stairs burns more calories per minute than almost any activity. Its major virtue, however, is its ready availability. Most of us have several opportunities each day to use stairs. Stairs may be in our home, at work, and in stores. Let's see if we can exploit this opportunity.

People are willing to increase their use of stairs, but rarely think of it. This was shown in a study I did with several colleagues when I

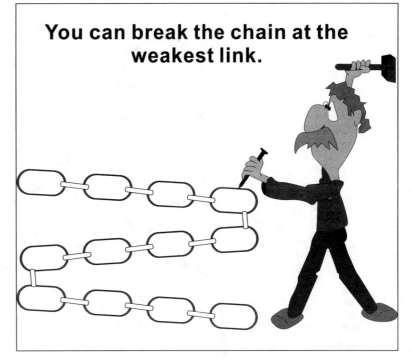

You can break the chain at the weakest link.

was at the University of Pennsylvania. We had observers measure the use of stairs in three public places where stairs and escalators were adjacent: a shopping mall in Philadelphia called the Gallery, a commuter train station, and a bus terminal. Our observers patiently recorded whether 40,000 people used the stairs or escalators.

The results were quite informative. Only 5 percent of people used the stairs. For every five normal weight people who used the stairs, only one heavy person did, which meant that only one percent of heavy people used the stairs. People would avoid the stairs even when they had to wait in a crowd to go up the escalator.

We then stationed a sign encouraging people to use the stairs at the base of the stairs and escalators. The sign carried the figure shown on page 167 and was designed for us by Tony Auth, the Pulitzer Prize winning political cartoonist of the *Philadelphia Inquirer*. The sign made a big impact. It nearly tripled the number of people using the stairs, and increased the number of overweight people using the stairs by seven-fold. It appeared that people were willing to use the stairs if reminded to do so.

Here is a bit more encouragement. Studies in England and the U.S. were done to investigate the link between exercise and life span

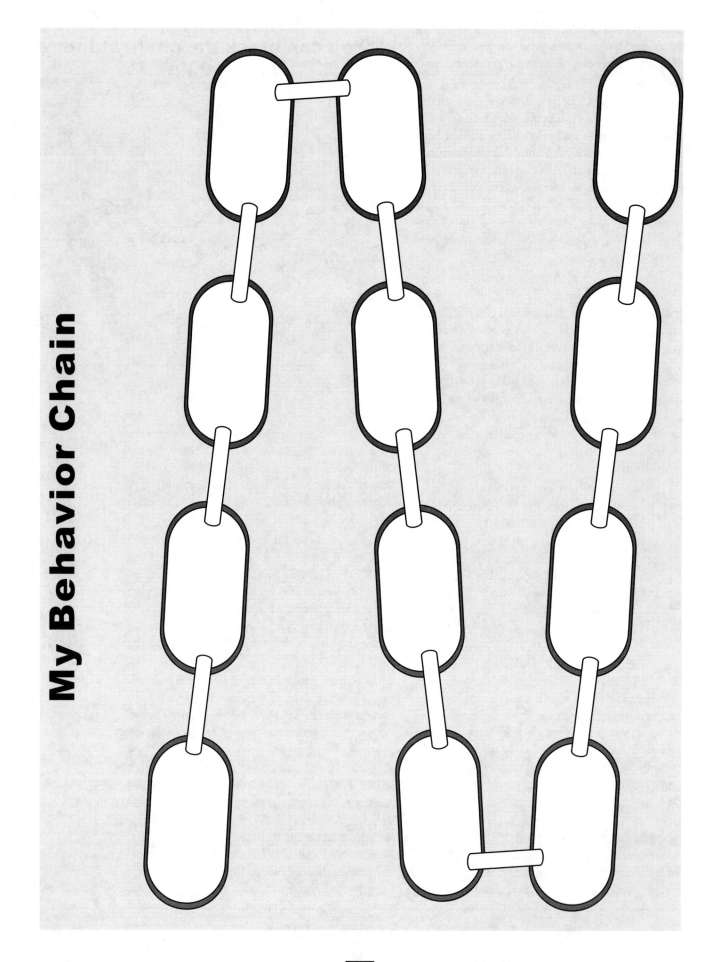

My Behavior Chain

(longevity). People who exercised regularly lived longer than those who were sedentary. The U.S. study, done by Dr. Ralph Paffenbarger from Stanford University, found that people who climbed only 50 stairs (not flights) or more each day had reduced risk of heart attack.

The value of using the stairs is not well known, but some people are regular stair climbers and are proud of it. Our study with the stairs and escalators was reported in many newspapers because of a wire service article. I received letters from all over the country from people who had been climbing the stairs for years for their exercise program. Some even reported running in a race, which is up the stairs of the Empire State Building! This is way beyond what I have in mind for people losing weight, so let's examine ways to use the stairs sensibly.

There are many clever ways to use stairs. At work, try the bathroom and water cooler on another floor. This will add several trips. Use the stairs at a mall in lieu of an escalator. If you work on the 9th floor of a building, take the elevator part way up and walk the remaining flights. Walk down all the flights. Use the stairs whenever possible at home. Walk to a different floor to make a phone call or to use the bathroom. Whatever you can do will add up.

Poultry: better than red meat?

An article by Bonnie Liebman in the *Nutrition Action Healthletter* provided some interesting facts about poultry. In only 20 years, the intake of chicken in the U.S. has doubled and of turkey has risen by two-thirds. This is a positive development because poultry can be helpful in reducing the intake of saturated fat.

The fact that poultry consumption is increasing is not lost on the beef and pork industries, and difficult though it is to believe, both are attempting to convince the public that their product is like chicken. You may hear ads stating that beef has no more cholesterol than chicken. This is not novel news, because beef is not particularly high in cholesterol. It does, however, have much more saturated fat

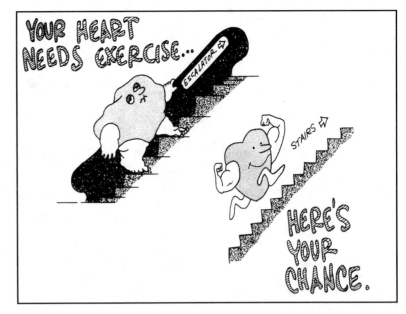

than chicken, and saturated fat is a worse culprit than dietary cholesterol in raising blood cholesterol. The YGSN (You've Got Some Nerve) award has to go to the campaign by the pork industry to characterize pork as the *other white meat*. This seems a direct attempt to make pork seem like chicken (pork has at least twice the saturated fat of chicken and turkey), and to distance pork from *red meat* (pork has at least as much fat as beef).

Birds differ in the amount of fat they provide. The leanest poultry is turkey. After poultry is cooked and skinned, chicken has double or triple the fat of turkey, and duck and goose have 50 percent more fat than chicken. The calories and amount of fat in various forms of poultry are in the table on the next page. As Liebman points out in her article, averages can be deceiving, because some cuts of red meat and some parts of poultry can have more or less fat than the average. In general, however, turkey breast without the skin has almost no fat, and chicken has about half the fat of lean red meats.

When preparing poultry, several factors should be considered. First, removing the skin reduces fat by about 50 percent. Second, fat intake is increased greatly when chicken is battered and fried, because the batter soaks up fat. A fried chicken breast from Kentucky Fried Chicken can have two or three times the fat of a roasted breast (even with the skin on). Finally, think of creative ways to use turkey and chicken in salads with fruits, pasta, and other

Calories and Fat in Poultry

(per 4 oz roasted portion)

Type of Poultry	Calories	Fat (g)
Duck, with skin	384	36.5
Duck, without skin	229	14.5
Goose, with skin	348	28.5
Goose, without skin	271	16.5
Turkey, light, with skin	187	6.0
Turkey, light, without skin	160	1.5
Chicken, light, with skin	253	14.0
Chicken, light, without skin	197	6.0
Chicken, dark, with skin	288	20.5
Chicken, dark, without skin	234	12.5
Ground turkey (3 oz)	191	12.5
Chicken hot dog	116	10.0
Turkey bologna (2 oz)	114	9.0

Note: Figures in table abstracted from Liebman, B. CSPI's Poultry Primer. Nutrition Action Healthletter, November 1986. Their source for calorie and fat information was USDA Handbook #8-5, #8-10, #8-13.

Fast food

Fast food restaurants are part of the American landscape. In 1970, there were 30,000 fast food outlets, rising to 140,000 by 1980. In 1995 there were 11,400 McDonald's alone, with three new McDonald's opening every day. Within a 15-minute drive of where I live in Connecticut, I bet I could find 25 fast food restaurants, and ocean occupies half of the available space! In addition to McDonald's, I would find Burger Kings, Kentucky Fried Chickens, Wendy's, Popeye's, and heaven knows what else. And with 24-hour service, breakfast, and drive-in windows, convenience has reached new levels. If you can believe it, 7 percent of the American population eats at McDonald's each day.

The world of fast food has undergone many interesting, and in a few cases, positive changes. Chicken has found its way onto the menu, but in some cases in better form than others (broiled chicken vs. chicken nuggets). Healthier oils are being used to cook French fries in some places, yet people are consuming fries (and therefore fat and calories) in record amounts. Some developments, such as drive-in windows and package deals (value meals), very likely increase the number of customers and amount eaten per customer.

The table shown in Appendix E lists foods from a number of the major fast food chains and shows the values for calories, fat, carbohydrate, and protein. The foods vary widely in their nutritional value. Foods from these restaurants can be high in saturated fat, sodium,

foods. This can make for some innovative dishes. The cookbooks listed in Lesson Six provide many ideas for making interesting dishes from these foods.

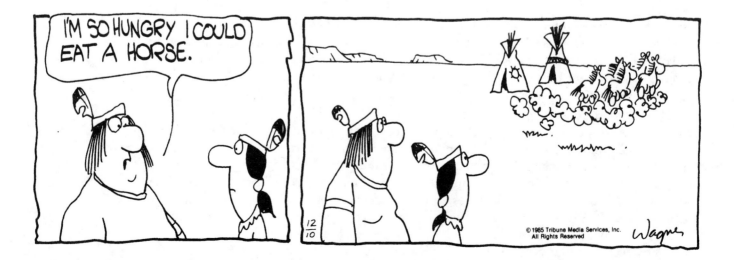

cholesterol, and calories, and low in calcium, vitamins A and D, and fiber. Soft drinks such as Coca Cola and Pepsi are not listed in the table. Calorie values for soft drinks are listed in the Calorie Guide in Appendix F.

The news is not all bad, however. One can walk into some fast food chains and escape with a reasonable meal. I hope the figures shown in the fast food table will be helpful in accomplishing this.

Assignment for this lesson

Much of this lesson focused on the Behavior Chain. Be sure to fill out the blank chain in this lesson and devise plans to break as many links as possible. Use this idea of the Behavior Chain in analyzing your high-risk situations and in planning in advance for countering pressures to eat. It may be useful to draw out more than one chain to help with your most difficult situations. For your exercise, see if there are ways to work extra stair climbing into your lifestyle. Continue monitoring your intake of the recommended number of servings from the five food groups of the Food Guide Pyramid.

Self-assessment questionnaire

Lesson Twelve

T F 65. Once the eating chain begins, it is not possible to stop because the links are so strong.

T F 66. A Behavior Chain, like any chain, is only as strong as its weakest links.

T F 67. It is best to interrupt an eating chain at one of its last links when you know what foods confront you.

T F 68. Using stairs is a convenient and accessible way for many people to increase activity.

(Answers in Appendix C)

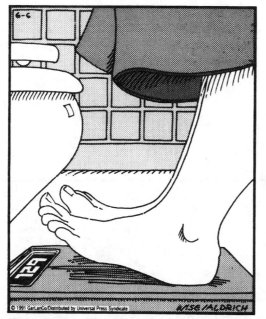

If you stand on the scale just so, you weigh less.

Monitoring Form—Lesson Twelve

Today's Date:

Time	Food and Amount	Calories
	Total Daily Calories	

Assignment this week	Always	Sometimes	Never
1. Sketch behavior chains			
2. Break links in chain			
3 Increase use of stairs			
4. Daily servings from the five food groups			
5. Less than _____ calories each day			

Food Groups for Today	Physical Activity	Minutes
Milk, yogurt, and cheese ❑ ❑ ❑		
Meat, poultry, etc. ❑ ❑ ❑		
Fruits ❑ ❑ ❑ ❑		
Vegetables ❑ ❑ ❑ ❑ ❑		
Breads, cereals, etc. ❑ ❑ ❑ ❑ ❑ ❑ ❑ ❑ ❑ ❑		

This lesson begins the last four of the program. In many ways, these may be our most important lessons because we turn our attention to permanent maintenance of weight loss. Central to this are three terms: *lapse*, *relapse*, and *collapse*. These will be discussed, as will methods to handle urges to eat, and I will discuss our toxic food environment.

Preventing lapse, relapse, and collapse

Far too often, a minor slip propels a person to misery. The guilt from a slip makes a person susceptible to more slips and can ultimately lead to loss of all control. This is a gloomy picture, but good news is around the corner! There *are* ways to turn the tables.

Maintenance of weight loss may be the greatest challenge facing overweight persons. Losing weight is difficult enough, but keeping it off ranks up there in difficulty with winning the lottery and finding a compassionate auditor from the Internal Revenue Service. Most overweight people have lost and regained weight many times, so something must be done to interrupt these cycles. The trick is to prevent slips from occurring and to respond constructively when they do occur.

Everyone makes mistakes. Some bounce back and use the slip as a signal to increase control. It is common, however, for the slip to

cause a negative emotional reaction (guilt and despair) which builds until all control is lost.

There are two paths to success. The first is to avoid or prevent slips and mistakes and the second is to respond to slips with coping techniques that put *you* in control. I will cover each path separately. In this lesson, we will work on preventing slips and in Lesson Fourteen I will emphasize recovery from slips.

Much of my discussion on this topic is drawn from the excellent work of Dr. G. Alan Marlatt and Dr. Judith Gordon, both psychologists from the University of Washington. They have studied the situations associated with relapse in overweight persons, alcoholics, smokers, drug addicts, and compulsive gamblers. They have also proposed methods for preventing relapse. Their work is described in a classic book entitled *Relapse Prevention* (Guilford Press, New York, 1985—call 1-800-736-7323 for ordering).

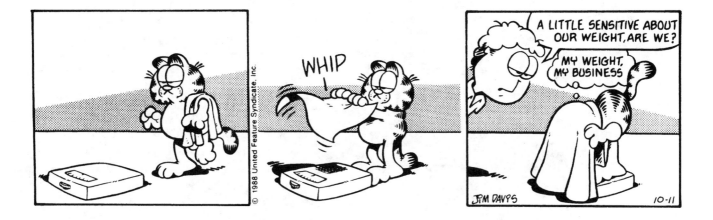

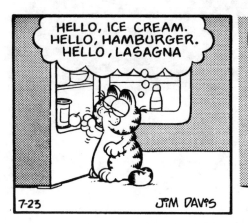
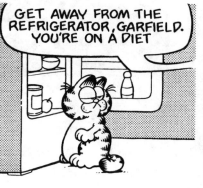
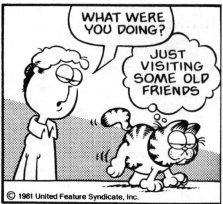

Distinguishing lapse, relapse, and collapse

I have used several terms to describe deviating from your weight control plan: mistake, lapse, slip, error, etc. Relapse implies something different and collapse is yet another matter. We fuss with these words because the terms we use can be important.

In recovering alcoholics, one slip or lapse is considered by many to be a relapse (i.e., "one drink a drunk"). The same is thought by some to be true for people who stop smoking. Having a single cigarette begins an inevitable path to relapse. However, there is abundant evidence that this is not true.

Many recovering alcoholics have had at least one drink since their reformation, and it is a rare ex-smoker who has not had a cigarette. Yet, they recover from their lapses and prevent a relapse. The same is unquestionably true with overweight individuals.

A *lapse* is a slight error or slip, the first instance of backsliding. It is a discreet event like eating a *forbidden* food, exceeding a calorie level, or gaining weight. *Relapse* occurs when lapses string together and the person returns to his or her former state. When relapse is complete and there is little hope of reversing the negative trend, *collapse* has occurred.

The most important message is that

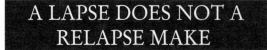

A LAPSE DOES NOT A RELAPSE MAKE

The person who can view a lapse for what it is, an unfortunate but temporary problem, is prepared to respond positively to life's inevitable setbacks.

Identifying urges and high-risk situations

The concepts of *urge* and *high-risk situations* were introduced earlier in the program. Distinguishing cravings (urges) from hunger was discussed in Lesson Three, conquering cravings was covered in Lesson Four, and the Behavior Chain was introduced in Lesson Twelve. These were all leading to the point we face now, the need to spot trouble before it occurs. Urges can now become a signal for corrective action.

Let's look back over what you have learned. You know much more about your eating than before, so let's take advantage of that information. Think carefully about when you are most likely to find your eating threatened. Is it when you have certain feelings, like loneliness or frustration? Is it when you have to deal with some person? Is it when you feel bad about your life and your weight? Is it when someone offers you food? Look back over your Monitoring Forms and your weight loss experience to identify these situations.

Now that you are a pro at identifying urges and high-risk situations, let's plan ahead. We will learn a technique called *outlasting the urges* and will learn to use alternatives to eating when the high-risk situations arise. These become our armor when we are barraged with temptation.

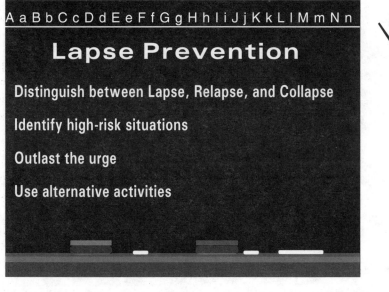

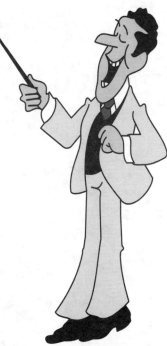

Outlasting the urges

It is possible to prevent a lapse by dealing with urges. I title this section *Outlasting the Urges* because an urge will usually go away if you just wait it out. This is easier said than done sometimes, but the rewards are high when you succeed.

Dr. G. Alan Marlatt, the psychologist mentioned previously, feels that an urge can be compared to a wave building in the ocean and then breaking on the beach. Conquering the urges is like surfing. A wave begins small, builds to a crest, breaks, and then subsides. Urges follow a similar course. They usually build gently to their strongest point and then weaken and gradually fade away.

The wave analogy is much different than the way people usually think about urges. Some people feel that an urge builds and builds and will create havoc unless it is gratified by eating. Actually, gratifying an urge by eating makes urges stronger and more frequent. In contrast, letting the urge pass, like the wave rolling in, will weaken it. If you can outlast enough of the urges, they will fade to obscurity.

The image of *urge surfing* is a good one. Pretend you are learning to surf. As the wave rolls in, you can battle it and be wiped out, or you can maintain your balance and *ride* the wave until it subsides.

Being a good urge surfer involves identifying the urges early in their development and then readying your skills to ride the wave. If the wave is upon you at full strength before you recognize it, you may wipe out no matter how well you surf. If you recognize the wave early, but cannot surf, you will also wipe out. Therefore, both parts are important—early recognition and skills to cope with the urges.

Simply waiting for the urge to pass can be all you'll need, but not always. Some urges and high-risk situations are stronger than others, so techniques other than waiting are necessary. One such technique is the use of alternative activities.

Using alternative activities

The principle of using alternative activities is simple. When you get the urge, do something else. If you use urges as a signal for positive activity, eating will become less rewarding and the old associations between urges and eating will diminish. When you see food, think about food, or feel hungry because you are lonely, eating is simply a habit created by an association. We can make new associations.

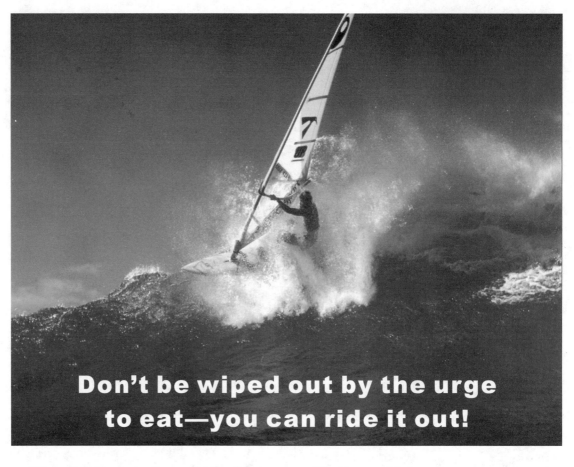

Don't be wiped out by the urge to eat—you can ride it out!

When you recognize urges, think of an activity that is incompatible with eating. For instance, typing a letter and jumping rope are incompatible—both cannot be done at once, unless you are Rubber Man. If you were addicted to typing and agreed to jump rope each time you got urge to type, the strength of your addiction would fade.

This same approach can work with eating. One cannot play the tuba and eat, so tuba practice would be a good alternative to eating. You might think of more practical methods that would involve activities you enjoy.

Making a list, checking it twice

Make a list of activities you could use when you are tempted to eat. The list should contain more than one activity so you have several choices. If you vow to consult the list when you want to eat, your control can improve. Make certain the list contains enjoyable activities so you will actually do them in lieu of eating.

The list provided on the next page contains ideas for incompatible activities. Some can be done at home, others take you out of the house. Some take little time while others are more involved. Many are examples from my clients. Do they give you more ideas?

Now that you have ideas from the list, it is time to establish your own list. Write out the activities that would make good alternatives for you. Add as many activities as you can. They should be both enjoyable and feasible. Some may require planning and the right timing, like going to a movie. Others should be available at a moment's notice so you can spring into action when an urge hits.

Try consulting the list when you get the urge to eat. If you can distract yourself for even a few minutes, the urge to eat can fade and your control can increase. Studies have shown that hunger comes and goes during the day, so not succumbing the instant an urge hits can give you precious time to think. Do your best to ride the wave!

Incompatible Activities to Eating

Walk the Dog	Play a Board Game
File Coupons	Ride a Bike
Go to a Movie	Brush Your Teeth
Call a Friend	Read This Manual!
Shop for Plants	Frame Some Pictures
Take a Shower	Refinish Furniture
Listen to Music	Play Music
Take a Drive	Knit a Sweater
Read a Romantic Book	Work in a Garden
Read a Sexy Book	Visit a Museum
Go to the Zoo	Buy a Gift
Buy a New Magazine	Plan a Vacation
Kiss Somebody	Paint a Picture
Wash the Car	Buy Tickets
Kiss Somebody Again	Work on a Hobby
Write a Letter	Visit a Neighbor
Get Some Exercise	Donate to Charity
Look at Photo Album	Imagine Being More Fit

My Alternatives to Eating

1. _____
2. _____
3. _____
4. _____
5. _____
6. _____
7. _____
8. _____
9. _____

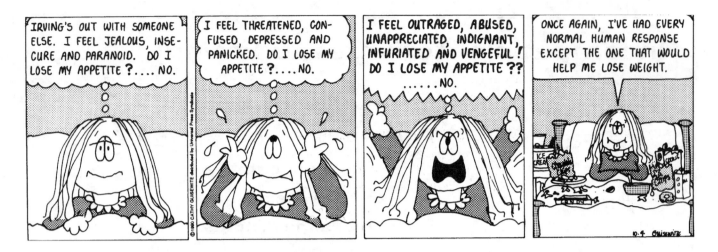

Bracing yourself against a toxic environment

People with weight problems face a difficult, even toxic environment. The temptations to eat are constant, powerful, and compelling. If you pause for a moment to think, you might be surprised by how we accept this without the slightest protest.

Think of the number of fast food restaurants you find within a 15-minute drive of your home. In addition to the national chains like McDonald's, Burger King's, Wendy's, and Kentucky Fried Chicken's, there are local and regional restaurants. Most now have drive-thru windows, which make it easier and faster to get loads of calories and fat. Most now serve breakfast and some are open 24 hours. Nearly every service station has been or is being closed and remodeled to contain a mini-market and almost every mall has a food court. There are vending machines everywhere and fast food chains like McDonald's are showing up in airports, airplanes, and even hospital lobbies!

Let's take another example. Many of the fast food restaurants offer package meals called value meals. More bad food for less money— some value, eh? They also offer, at a seemingly good price, the opportunity to get extra large drinks and fries, when you "supersize it." This is so much a part of our landscape that the word "supersize" has become a verb in our vocabulary.

The value meals and the supersize portions are a powerful and effective means the companies have of marketing their foods.

Food advertising is also a problem. Madison Avenue's brightest minds set to work to convince us that we should eat foods that can often be very high in calories, fat, and sugar. The average American child sees 10,000 food commercials each year, 95 percent of which are for fast foods, sugared cereals, candy, and soft drinks.

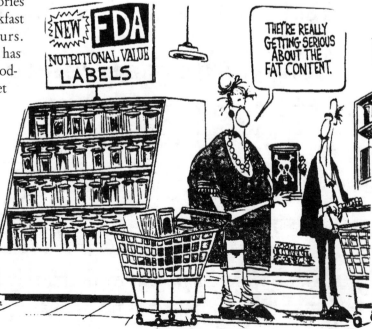

It is not stretching the language to say that we are exposed to a toxic food environment. We are exposed to and are encouraged to consume things that can cause deadly diseases such as heart disease and cancer. We rail against the tobacco companies for exposing us to temptations to smoke (especially when the inducements are aimed at children), but we remain remarkably quiet when the same thing happens with unhealthy food. I expect that over time a more militant attitude will begin to occur with the public.

What does this mean for you? It means that you must find creative ways to resist the environmental pressures to buy bad foods. Part of this lies in developing an attitude, in some cases an angry one. When you see the drive-thru sign, remember that it is designed to make it easier for you to spend your money on products that can harm you. When you see the junk food stores in the food court, remember that they are in business to feed their bad food to as many people as possible. When you fill your car with gas, remember that there is an industry that sells chips, pastries, ice cream, and soft drinks that wants you to succumb. Get mad, and resist!

The other way to deal with this pressure is be aware of it and avoid exposure as much as possible. When you can, avoid going around these places. If at the mall, stay away from the food court. Use a credit card to pay for gas at the pump rather than go inside where the food is. Try not to drive by the fast food places when you are hungry. Most of all, keep alert to these inducements to eat and see that you, and not a multi-billion dollar food industry, is in charge of your eating and your health.

Hard work at the office

Most people think that working in an office is the perfect setting for getting flabby. Wrong! Certain office activities require great effort. The table below shows just how strenuous life in the office can be.

Office Calories

Activity	Calories
Throwing in the towel	0
Beating around the bush	35
Bending over backwards	75
Hitting the nail on the head	75
Dragging your heels	90
Tooting your own horn	100
Flirting at the water cooler	150
Avoiding the boss	175
Jumping to conclusions	200
Climbing the walls	250
Passing the buck	300
Making mountains out of molehills	400
Running around in circles	450
Throwing your weight around	500

Assignment for this lesson

There are several activities for your assignment. The first is to distinguish lapse from relapse, and the second is to identify high-risk situations. This information forms the basis for the next two parts of the assignment—to outlast the urges and to use alternative activities to eating. Finally, recheck your diet to make sure you are eating enough fiber. Review the information on fiber in Lesson Seven if you need to.

Self-assessment questionnaire

Lesson Thirteen

T F 69. When a person lapses, relapse is close behind because nothing can interrupt the negative cycle of lapses and binging.

T F 70. It helps to have a list of alternatives to eating for use when urges strike.

T F 71. The emphasis on fiber may be dangerous because fiber is indigestible material that can harm the intestinal system.

(Answers in Appendix C)

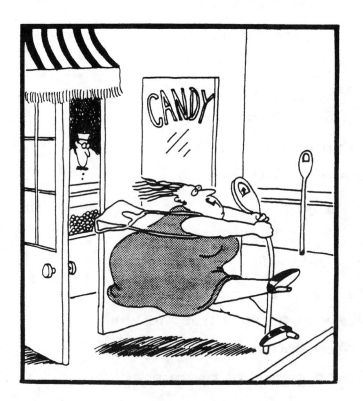

Monitoring Form—Lesson Thirteen

Today's Date:

Time	Food and Amount	Calories
Total Daily Calories		

Assignment this week	*Always*	*Sometimes*	*Never*
1. Identify high risks			
2. Outlast urges			
3. Alternative activities			
4. Daily servings from the five food groups			
5. My diet has _____ grams of fiber			
6. Less than _____ calories each day			

Food Groups for Today	*Physical Activity*	*Minutes*
Milk, yogurt, and cheese ❑ ❑ ❑		
Meat, poultry, etc. ❑ ❑ ❑		
Fruits ❑ ❑ ❑ ❑		
Vegetables ❑ ❑ ❑ ❑ ❑		
Breads, cereals, etc. ❑ ❑ ❑ ❑ ❑ ❑ ❑ ❑ ❑ ❑		

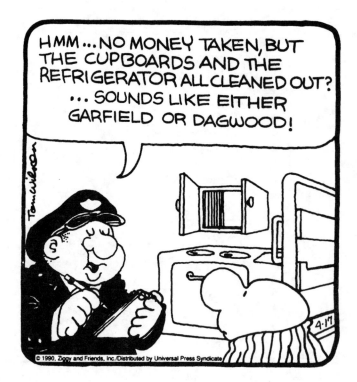

In Lesson Thirteen, we noted two ways to keep the reins on urges and to prevent the common journey from lapse to relapse to collapse. One path, preventing lapses, can be attained by avoiding high risk situations and by using alternative activities to short-circuit the urges. This lesson will focus on the second path—to cope with lapses once they occur. We will also cover the role of cholesterol in the diet.

Coping with lapse and preventing relapse

Lapses are inevitable. By this point in the program, most people losing weight have experienced peaks of joy and valleys of distress. It is the rare person who has not eaten some high-calorie foods, overeaten at a special event or holiday gathering, or resorted to favorite foods when times got tough. The issue is not so much *whether* the lapses occur, but the person's *reaction* after they occur.

An example might elucidate this. Two friends, Judy and Joan, were both on a weight loss program and attended a wedding. Both overate at the buffet, to the tune of 2000 calories. Judy did it on shrimp and steak, whereas Joan fixed her attention on bread and desserts. The extra 2000 calories should not sink their weight loss efforts because the calories amount to less than a pound of weight. Judy and Joan, however, reacted quite differently to the 2000 calorie lapse.

Judy felt guilty about the wedding episode and told herself, "I blew my eating plan." She then thought, "What the heck, I blew it already, I might as well enjoy myself." She ate more when she got home, felt guilty the next day, and continued the overeating for five days. Joan, on the other hand, felt bad about the 2000 calorie lapse, but responded in a more constructive manner. She reflected on what happened and planned accordingly. She increased her walking an extra 15 minutes for the next four days and cut back on her calorie intake.

How can we learn from Joan and master our lapses? Following six specific steps can be a big help. These are adapted from the work of Dr. G. Alan Marlatt mentioned in Lesson Thirteen.

❶ **Step 1: Stop, look, and listen.** A lapse is a signal of impending danger, like a train signal and the crossing gates. Stop

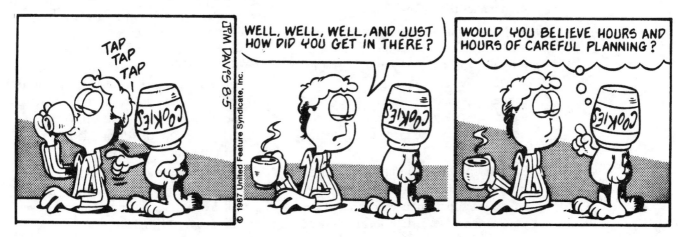

Mastering a Lapse

1. **Stop, look, and listen**
2. **Stay calm**
3. **Renew your program vows**
4. **Analyze the lapse situation**
5. **Take charge immediately**
6. **Ask for help**

what you are doing, especially if the lapse has started, and examine the situation. What is occurring? Why is a lapse in progress? Consider removing yourself to a safe location where you won't be tempted and where you can think in a rational manner.

❷ **Step 2: Stay calm**. If you get anxious or blame yourself for the lapse, the situation may get worse. You may conclude that you are a hopeless binge eater and that control is impossible. Coming to these conclusions is easy when you get all worked up. Try to separate yourself from the situation, and view it as an objective observer would—that one lapse does not prove failure. Keeping a cool head makes the following steps easier.

❸ **Step 3: Renew your weight-loss vows**. Take a minute to remind yourself of how far you have come, the progress you have made, and how sad it would be if one lapse canceled out all your hard work. Restate your program goals and renew the vows you made when dieting began.

❹ **Step 4: Analyze the lapse situation.** Instead of blaming yourself for letting go, use the situation to learn what places you at risk. Do certain feelings create

the risk? Is it the presence of food, other eating, other activities, etc.? Did you do anything to defend against the urge? Did it work? Why or why not? What thoughts did you have?

❺ **Step 5: Take charge immediately**. Leap into action with your planned techniques. Leave the house, feed the remaining food to the disposal, or do whatever works for you. The alternative activities you listed in Lesson Thirteen will be a good place to start. Don't wait, and be decisive. Waiting is an excuse for letting go even more. Jump on that lapse like a dog on a bone! Remember that it is usually easier to get control if you leave the situation.

❻ **Step 6: Ask for help.** Partners, friends, coworkers, and others can be a real source of support. You might review the material on Relationships from earlier lessons where we discussed who to ask for help, how to ask, and how to respond if help is given. If you could really use support during lapses, don't be shy about asking for help.

These six steps are easy to remember. You can even write them on a small card to keep in your wallet or purse. Using them, however, will require some effort.

182

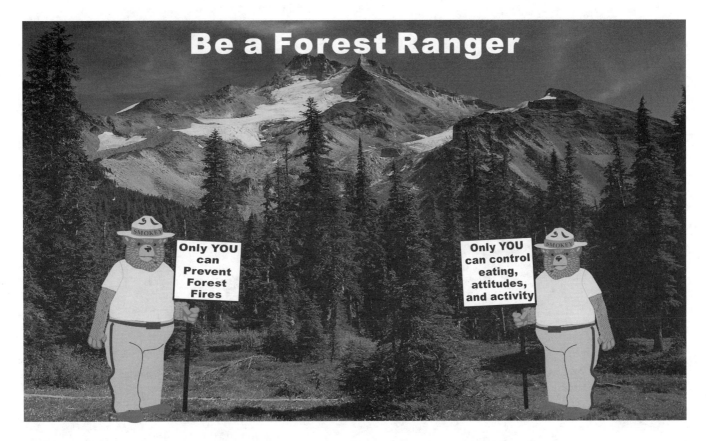

Becoming a forest ranger

Consider yourself a Forest Ranger on the lookout for fires. Your job is to prevent fires and to put them out quickly if they start. Your lapses are like the fires. You will try to prevent them, but when they do flare up, extinguish them immediately. Occasionally a fire may seem out of control, but don't lose the forest!!

Let's develop this idea of the Forest Ranger a bit further. Your job is to take control over your eating, exercise, and weight. The Ranger's job is to keep control over the forest. The Ranger must do everything possible to prevent fires from breaking out. Since fires may be difficult to control once they start, the Ranger believes in "an ounce of prevention..." Prevention is also important for you. You have learned dozens of ways to take control of your eating so that lapses will not occur. As you know, the key is to be prepared for high-risk situations, to plan in advance, and to keep the right attitude.

The Forest Ranger's second task is to stop the spread of fires once they do occur. The Ranger's ability to do this will determine whether the forest is spared or destroyed. A lapse in your eating is like the fire that breaks out. Whether you bounce back and spare your diet, or let the mistake destroy the progress you have made (lapse, relapse, then collapse) depends on your ability to use the techniques described here.

Please remember the dual tasks that confront both you and the Forest Ranger. You are concerned with both prevention and with crisis management. Identify the situations where you are most likely to confront problems. Then plan to use both your prevention techniques and the constructive methods you have learned to deal with lapses.

These are the ways to prevent lapses and to stop lapses dead in their tracks. The information here and in Lesson Thirteen is, in my opinion, crucial for long-term success. We will review it in the next lesson. Please refer back to these lessons if you find yourself in trouble. This dual approach of preventing problems and of coping with problems when they do arise allows you to hit temptations from two angles.

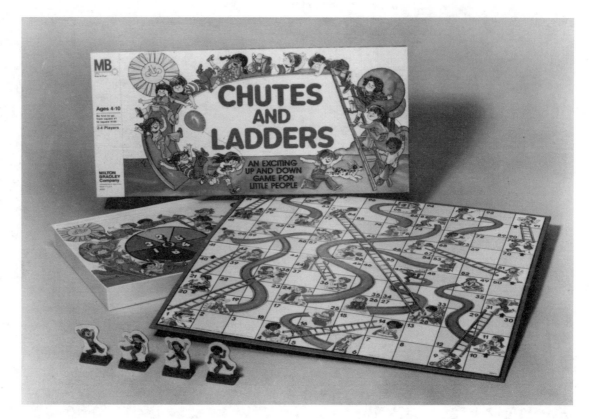

Life on chutes and ladders

There is a well-known children's board game called "Chutes and Ladders," known formerly as "Snakes and Ladders." Many adults remember the game from their own childhood or from playing with their children. The basic idea behind the game provides a good moral to remember as we discuss lapse, relapse, and collapse.

In Chutes and Ladders, players use a spinner to advance over the 100 spaces on the board. At some point there are ladders which advance a player by many spaces. At other points, there are chutes which can send the player back many spaces. For example, a player who lands on space nine is shown cutting the lawn for his parents. For his effort, he can advance to space 31, which shows the boy going to the circus. A player landing on space 95 is greeted by a picture of a boy who hits a baseball through a window. His transgression sends him back to space 75 where he is emptying his piggy bank.

Sometimes playing Chutes and Ladders goes without a hitch. You land on the ladders and avoid the chutes. Other times the chutes

seem to draw you like a magnet. However, even under the worst of circumstances, a player can reach the top of the board and win the game.

Let's say that the Milton Bradley Company made Chutes and Ladders relevant to the situations faced by individuals controlling their weight. One might advance up a ladder by eating under control at a buffet, but might slide down a chute by eating 400 peanuts at Happy Hour. Jogging would qualify one for a ladder and would speed the person toward the ultimate goal. Eating 15 of Cousin Clara's Cocoa Cremeballs would definitely hasten one's descent down a chute.

There are several points to remember from our hypothetical game of Chutes and Ladders. The first is that making progress up the ladders can always be interrupted by a chute. Even a program that goes smoothly for weeks can be stymied by setbacks. However, even the longest fall down a chute can be remedied by heading back up the board, hopefully with the aid of a few ladders. If you have the skills and the motivation to control eating and increase exercise, you will be poised to take advantage of the ladders and will advance more quickly.

Weight control, like life, has both chutes and ladders. Being prepared for this fact is half the battle. The other half is having the right attitude and behaviors to remain optimistic when trouble occurs, and to have skills in hand to rebound from lapses. Think now of the situations that can send you down a chute and plan some prevention strategies. Think also of the situations that can propel you up a ladder, then make them happen!

When children play Chutes and Ladders, landing on a chute can be discouraging. He or she may want to quit playing because the immediate setback overwhelms the knowledge that things might get better (there might be a ladder ahead). The immediate bad feelings created by a dietary mistake can make individuals want to quit. It is crucial to remember that life has its chutes, particularly when you're working hard to control your weight. Look ahead for the ladder, and by all means, **keep playing** the game.

Cholesterol

Cholesterol is a waxy substance necessary for the body's functioning. It can be manufactured by the body or can be eaten in food. High blood levels of cholesterol are related to risk for heart disease, and the blood level of cholesterol is determined in part by what you eat.

Cholesterol is carried in the bloodstream by something called lipoproteins. Some of the cholesterol is deposited on the walls of the arteries as fatty streaks. When these deposits build they form a fibrous plaque which makes the wall of the artery less able to adjust to blood flow. If the artery narrows enough to stop or seriously restrict the flow of blood, vital tissue can be deprived and die. The result is a heart attack if the coronary arteries are involved or a stroke if the blocked arteries supply the brain.

Knowing your own cholesterol level can be important. The National Cholesterol Education Program, a nationwide effort of the National Institutes of Health, suggests that the desirable level of blood cholesterol is below 200 mg/dl. The range from 200–239 mg/dl is considered borderline, and above 240 mg/dl is considered high. Where you fall in these cate-

Use skills and motivation to help propel you up the ladder of success.

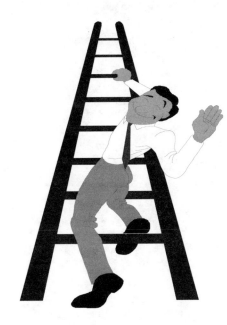

gories will indicate how often blood cholesterol should be checked, the degree to which diet should be changed, and whether special advice from a physician is necessary. It is advisable, therefore, to have your cholesterol level checked.

You may have heard talk about different types of cholesterol, particularly HDL (high density lipoprotein) cholesterol and LDL (low density lipoprotein) cholesterol. HDL is thought to protect against heart disease, so higher levels are better. LDL has the opposite effect, so lower levels are better. Scientists are learning more about how diet and exercise can be used to raise HDL and lower LDL but it appears that the same methods used to lower total cholesterol will have beneficial effects on HDL and LDL.

To help control blood cholesterol it is important to limit the amount of fat and cholesterol ingested, and to be sensitive to the type of fat you eat. Saturated fat from animal sources (fats from beef, lamb, pork, ham, butter, cream, whole milk, cheese) and saturated fat from vegetable sources (coconut oil, palm oil, cocoa butter) should be limited. It is desirable to limit saturated fats and to replace them with

Cholesterol Content of Common Foods

Food	Quantity	Cholesterol (mg)
Dairy Products		
Skim milk	1 cup (8.6 oz)	5
Buttermilk from skim	1 cup (8.6 oz)	5
Low-fat milk (1% fat)	1 cup (8.6 oz)	15
Whole milk (4%)	1 cup (8.7 oz)	34
Ice milk, soft serve	1 cup (6.2 oz)	35
Cream, half & half	1T (0.5 oz)	6
Whipping cream	1T (0.5 oz)	20
Butter	1T (0.5 oz)	29–35
Rich ice cream (16% fat)	1 cup (5.2 oz)	84
Low-fat cottage cheese	4 oz	6
Low-fat yogurt, vanilla/plain	8 oz	11–18
Swiss cheese	1 oz	28
Cheddar cheese	1 oz	28
Cream cheese	1 oz	31
American cheese	1 oz	41
Meats and Poultry		
Bacon, fried and drained	2 slices (0.8 oz)	12
Bologna	1 slice (1.3 oz)	14
Boiled ham	1 oz	15
Hog dog	1 (1.6 oz)	29
Pork chop, broiled, lean	4 oz	100
Roast turkey, light meat	4 oz	87
Fried chicken	4 oz fried in veg. oil	90–103
Ham roast, lean only	4 oz	100
Beef pot roast, lean only	4 oz	103
Sirloin steak, lean only	4 oz	103
Ground beef, broiled	4 oz	107
Roast turkey, dark meat	4 oz	115
Egg, large, poached	1 (1.7 oz)	242
Egg, scrambled in veg. oil	1 (2.3 oz)	263
Beef or calf liver, fried	4 oz	297
Chicken liver, simmered	4 oz	846
Fish and Seafood		
Canned salmon	4 oz	40
Clams, raw	4 (3 oz)	42
Cod	4 oz	57
Scallops, steamed	4 oz	60
Rainbow trout, fresh	4 oz	62
Canned tuna, oil pack	4 oz	63
Halibut steak, broiled	4 oz	68
Lobster	4 oz	96
Canned crab	4 oz	116
Shrimp	4 oz	170

Note: **Figures adapted from** *The Dictionary of Sodium, Fats, and Cholesterol* **by Barbara Kraus, New York: Putnam, 1974.**

polyunsaturated fats, which usually come from vegetable oils.

The table on the previous page may be helpful in guiding you in choosing foods low in cholesterol. It is important to remember that reducing saturated fat in the diet can have an even more powerful effect in lowering blood cholesterol than can reducing dietary cholesterol. Information on fat is provided in earlier lessons.

Assignment for this lesson

The main priority for this lesson is to use the six steps to deal with lapses. It is easy to remember the steps if you write them down on a card and keep them handy, perhaps in your wallet or purse. This way you will be prepared, so if trouble comes your way, you can whip out the card and put the brakes on any temptation.

Self-assessment questionnaire

Lesson Fourteen

T F 72. Getting nervous or anxious during a lapse is helpful because anxiety interferes with appetite and allows you to remove yourself from temptation.

T F 73. When dealing with a lapse, it is best to move quickly and decisively before control erodes even further.

T F 74. For controlling your blood cholesterol, it is important to limit intake of saturated fat.

(Answers in Appendix C)

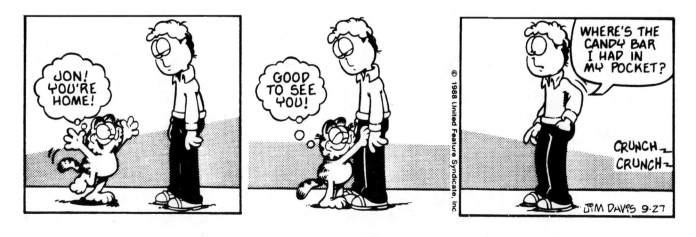

Time	Food and Amount	Calories

Monitoring Form—Lesson Fourteen

Today's Date:

Total Daily Calories		

Assignment this week		Always	Sometimes	Never
1.	Six steps for lapse			
2.	Be a Forest Ranger			
3	Alternative activities			
4.	Daily servings from the five food groups			
5.	Less than _____ calories each day			

Food Groups for Today		Physical Activity	Minutes
Milk, yogurt, and cheese ❑ ❑ ❑			
Meat, poultry, etc. ❑ ❑ ❑			
Fruits ❑ ❑ ❑ ❑			
Vegetables ❑ ❑ ❑ ❑ ❑			
Breads, cereals, etc. ❑ ❑ ❑ ❑ ❑ ❑ ❑ ❑ ❑ ❑			

Thre are now two lessons remaining in the LEARN program, and there are still important items to cover. In this lesson we will discuss material in the lifestyle and nutrition areas. We will deal with special events and holidays, and with the role of minerals in the diet. I will also introduce a lifestyle factor of major importance, the Master Monitoring Form. Let's forge ahead!

As described in the next lesson, I have written *The Weight Maintenance and Stabilization Guide*. It is a companion to *The LEARN Program* and is to be used as *The LEARN Program* ends. It is a step-by-step guide for losing more weight (if needed) or maintaining and stabilizing weight if you have lost to your goal. I wrote this guide in response to hundreds of requests for something dealing specifically with what to do after an initial program ends. This can be obtained by calling The LEARN Education Center (1–800–736–7323) or writing to the address provided at the end of this book.

The master monitoring form

There has been a Monitoring Form for each lesson in this program. You have recorded food intake, changes in the five LEARN areas (lifestyle, exercise, attitudes, relationships, and nutrition), and physical activity. This sets the stage for the Master Monitoring Form.

The Master Monitoring Form is similar to the forms you have seen throughout the program. It is unusual, in that it has blank spaces where techniques have been listed in other lessons. The aim is for you to list the techniques which best suit *your* needs. The new form appears toward the end of this lesson.

Keeping records is usually rated as one of the most important aspects of the program. Many clients continue to keep the records for years. Whether you do this or not depends on how long it takes for your new habits to become permanent. I recommend strongly that

you complete the records for at least eight more weeks.

The Master Monitoring Form contains the same standard sections for recording eating and exercise (on the left side and the bottom right side, respectively). The top right part, where the techniques have been listed, is blank. You can complete this part of the form with the techniques you consider most important.

I cannot predict what these techniques will be. For one person it will be to eat slowly, for another it will be to end dichotomous thinking, for another to do aerobic exercise at least

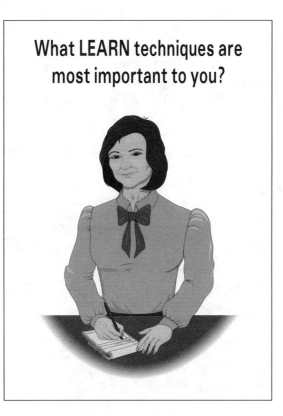

What LEARN techniques are most important to you?

four times a week, and for another to keep food out of sight.

These are only examples of the large list of techniques you have learned. Think back over your experiences and decide which techniques are necessary for you. The Master List of Techniques (Appendix A) described below will be helpful for this task.

When you have arrived at your list of key behaviors, enter them on your Master Monitoring Form. Make photocopies and use them as long as needed. Recording your food intake and your exercise is so important that I have not made these optional. When you add the behaviors I mentioned, your form will be complete.

We are beginning with the Master Monitoring Form in this lesson, so we have the opportunity to discuss your experience with it in the final lesson. Try to start right away, so you will have this experience under your belt for Lesson Sixteen.

Using the master list of techniques (Appendix A)

Appendix A contains a summary list of all the techniques I introduced in the program. Use this to review your progress and to determine which techniques were most important to you. Some techniques almost certainly did not apply. If you do no food shopping, the techniques in this area were not relevant. Focus on those most pertinent for you. They may be the techniques you struggled with

most, which is one sign that the habits they targeted are difficult to change.

Go through the list of techniques in Appendix A, and circle the ones that are most important in your attempts to lose weight. These are not necessarily the behaviors that are easiest for you. They should be the ones that are the keys to your future success. Circle any behavior you feel fits this bill. Think back carefully over your experience with earlier parts of the program, and consider programs you have been on in the past. Circle the behaviors that help you control your eating and increase your exercise.

Now that you have circled the important behaviors, it is time to narrow the list. You would like to end up with 5–10 behaviors that will be the final entries for your Master Monitoring Form. Having too few techniques can make you miss opportunities to change your habits, and having too many makes record keeping too complex. It is fine to modify the list as your habits change, but for now, this list should be your marching orders to yourself.

Holidays, parties, and special events

Do you get stuffed more than the turkey on Thanksgiving? Do you love the salted nuts people offer at parties? Do you feel obligated to eat when a host or hostess prepares an elegant meal? There are several ways to deal with these special occasions.

Holidays, parties, and special occasions can be a problem because eating is encouraged. Not only does temptation abound, but every-

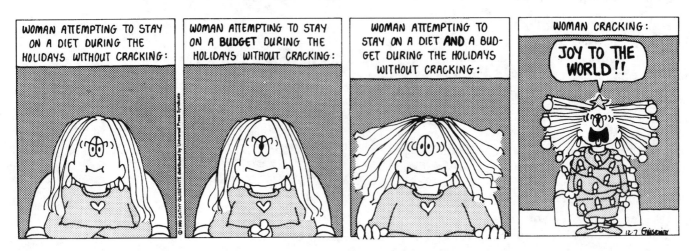

one else is eating, the food is good, there may be social pressure to "try some of this," and it is natural to *let go* when celebrating. The trick is to be prepared and to avoid the anxiety that comes from trying to diet and celebrate at the same time.

One common mistake is for individuals on weight-control programs to vow to eat nothing at the event. This is a real set-up, because they either feel guilty when they eat or feel deprived when they don't. You can enjoy yourself and still keep your virtue. Here are five methods for having fun and keeping the reins on uncontrolled eating.

❶ **Plan ahead.** Think about the event before you go. Try to anticipate both the food you will face and the actions of other people. Think about your own desires to eat and the external pressures from others. Have a general idea of what you will eat. You can call ahead and ask what will be served. You can make a tentative list of what you will eat and add up the calories. How does it fit with your day's calorie goal?

❷ **Eat something before you go.** Don't go starved to a special event. Everything will look good and you will forget that you only want to sample special foods. Have a salad, carrot sticks, cauliflower, or other low-calorie food before you go.

❸ **Eat only special foods.** Stay away from the potato chips, crackers, dip, nuts, bread and other foods that you can have any time. Use the chance to try new foods or foods you rarely have. Remember to make the best use of your calories.

❹ **Be the slowest eater.** Keep your eye on others and be the slowest eater at the event. Be the last to start and the last to finish. You will enjoy the food more and will feel satisfied with less. Pay attention to the texture, smell, and subtleties of taste. This will halt the rapid and automatic eating that brings so many calories.

❺ **Keep a proper perspective.** If you do eat more than you intend, keep a positive attitude. Don't turn an event into more than it really is: just another day with meals and calories. In the scheme of a month or year's worth of eating, what can one day mean? One day's indiscretion should not ruin any program. There are plenty of formerly heavy people who occasionally overdo it. Their trick is to bounce back. As I stated before, your reaction to the eating is more important than the eating itself. Your attitudes are central to your ability to control your eating both during and after the event.

The national walking movement

People are walking here, there, almost everywhere. The movement has been bolstered by the discovery that walking can be fun, can be done in the most interesting places, and can be done with a group of similarly minded people. There is also increasing knowledge about

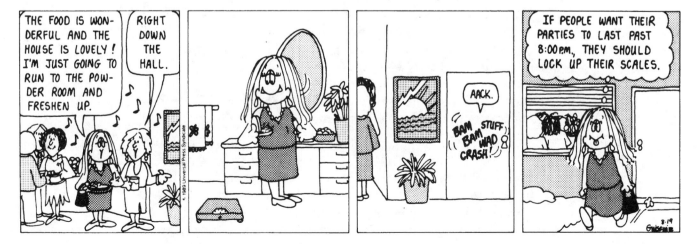

Resources for Walkers

American Volkssport Association

1001 Pat Booker Road, Suite 101
Universal City, Texas 78148
(210) 659–2112

Can send you a list of walking clubs in your area. An annual membership ($20 per individual and $25 for families) includes a subscription to *American Wanderer*.

Prevention Walking Club

Rodale Press
Box 6099
Emmaus, PA 18099
(800) 666-1216

Included as a separate section in *Prevention Magazine* dealing with all aspects of walking. Annual subscription $17.94.

Walkabout International

835 Fifth Avenue, Room 407
San Diego, CA 92101
(619) 231–7463

Club with chapters in various cities. Organizes & publishes information about walks.

Walking Magazine

9–11 Harcourt St.
Boston, MA 02116
(617) 266–3322

Bimonthly commercial magazine about walking. $14.95 per year for subscription.

Walking Handbook

The Cooper Institute for Aerobics Research
12330 Preston Road
Dallas, Texas 75230
(800) 635–7050

Forty-page handbook on all aspects of walking. $6.95 per copy (plus postage).

---

the health benefits of walking. Dr. Ralph Paffenbarger of Stanford University studied 17,000 college alumni who are now ages 53 to 90. Men who walked briskly nine or more miles each week had 21 percent lower risk of death from heart disease than men who walked less than three miles each week.

The popularity of walking has led Americans to do what they do best, organize. There are walking clubs, walking trails, walking magazines, special walking shoes, and even a clearinghouse for information on walking. Information on these aspects of walking can be a real resource for the person losing or controlling their weight. It can help insure that walking is done correctly and that the experience can turn from drudgery to an enriching experience, both socially and physically.

Walking clubs and informal groups have blossomed all over the country. An example is the American Volkssport Association. This group organizes walking events such as a volkswalk, a 6 or 12 mile nontimed walk where the object is to meet people while enjoying exercise. Another example is Walkabout International, a group that began as a small walking club in San Diego and now publishes a schedule listing more than 90 walks each month. Chapters have now formed in different cities. To find resources in your area, the information in the table here may be helpful. Also, check the weekend section of your newspaper for walking events, which may direct you to local clubs.

Minerals

The body contains some 60 different minerals, about 22 of which are essential for life. There are great differences in the amounts of various minerals in the body. An example from the book *Introductory Nutrition* by Dr. Helen Guthrie, from which much of this discussion on minerals is drawn, is that of cobalt and calcium. A deficiency in cobalt, which constitutes only two parts per trillion of body weight, can be mroe damaging than a deficiency of calcium, which accounts for fully 2 percent (two parts per hundred) of body weight. The essential minerals are listed in Lesson Seven.

Minerals serve to maintain the acid-base balance in the cells, to facilitate many biological reactions, to maintain water balance (sodium and potassium are the key minerals here), to form parts of essential body compounds, to regulate muscle contraction, to transmit nerve impulses, and to aid in growth of body tissue. It is important to consume sufficient amounts of minerals, but excessive amounts can be dangerous.

I will discuss three minerals of particular interest: calcium, sodium, and iron. These are the most frequently discussed minerals, and ones that have important implications for health. For a more detailed discussion of these and the other minerals, refer to the book by Dr. Helen Guthrie mentioned above.

Calcium

Most people think of calcium for its role in formation of bones and teeth. It does play this role, but so do other minerals. Also, this is not the only function of calcium. Approximately two percent of the body is calcium, almost all of which is in teeth or bones.

An infant's bones are soft and incapable of sustaining much weight. Calcium helps the bones harden, a process called calcification or ossification. Calcium is necessary throughout life to sustain bone strength, but the amount actually needed by the body is often misunder-

stood. Inadequate calcium early in life makes one more susceptible to osteoporosis (a serious bone disease) in later years. However, there is dispute about how much calcium is needed. Different amounts are necessary during infancy, childhood, pregnancy, adult life, and the later years. The figures range from 540 mg/day for infants to 1200 mg/day for adults. The general RDA for calcium is one gram (1000 mg) per day.

Milk and milk products form the greatest supply of calcium in our diet. People who drink milk and eat milk products usually receive adequate calcium; males are more likely to do this than females. For people who avoid milk products, it is almost impossible to consume enough calcium from other foods to meet dietary standards. In addition to milk products, calcium is available in cereals, beans, some meats, poultry, fish, eggs, fruits, and vegetables.

The two conditions most commonly associated with calcium problems are kidney stones and osteoporosis. The issue of kidney stones is an easy one; there is no evidence that calcium intake is associated with the formation of stones. Osteoporosis is a different matter.

Osteoporosis is the condition of diminished bone mass. It occurs mainly in middle-aged and elderly women and can cause shortened stature, susceptibility to bone fractures, and pain in the lower back. There are multiple causes, but in many cases, calcium and sometimes fluoride supplementation can arrest this destructive process. This is a condition for a physician to monitor, so if you suspect this is an issue for you, speak with a doctor.

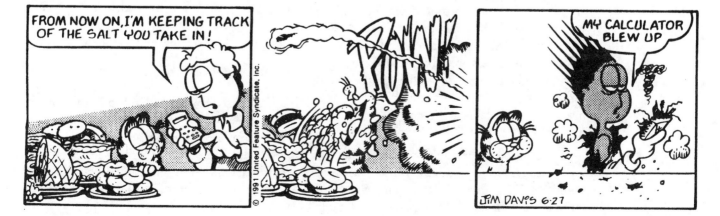

Sodium Content of Foods

Description	mg	Description	mg
Milk, Yogurt, and Cheese		**Fruits**	
Milk, 1 cup	120	Fruit, fresh, frozen, canned, ½ cup	Trace
Yogurt, 8 oz	160		
Natural cheeses, 1½ oz	110–450	**Bread, Cereal, Rice, and Pasta**	
Process cheeses, 2 oz	800	Cooked cereal, rice, pasta, unsalted, ½ cup	Trace
		Ready-to-eat cereal, 1 oz	100–360
Meat, Poultry, Fish, etc.		Bread, 1 slice	110–175
Fresh meat, poultry, fish, 3 oz	Less than 90		
Tuna, canned, water pack, 3 oz	300	**Miscellaneous**	
Bologna, 2 oz	580	Salad dressing, 1T	75–220
Ham, lean, roasted, 3 oz	1,020	Peanuts, roasted in oil, salted, 1 oz	120
		Potato chips, salted, 1 oz	130
Vegetables		Ketchup, mustard, steak sauce, 1T	130–230
Vegetables, fresh, or frozen (cooked), ½ cup	Less than 70	Corn chips, salted, 1 oz	235
Vegetables, canned or frozen with sauce, ½ cup	140–460	Dill pickle, 1 medium	930
Tomato juice, canned, ¾ cup	660	Soy sauce, 1T	1,030
Vegetable soup, canned, 1 cup	820	Salt, 1t	2,000

Sodium

Sodium is an important mineral which is present mainly in body fluids. It helps regulate fluid balance. Typical intake of sodium is between 3000 and 7000 mg per day, in the form of 7.5 to 18 grams per day of salt. A teaspoon of table salt provides 2000 mg of sodium, so to consume the three to seven grams of sodium daily means eating 1.5 to 4 teaspoons of salt. This seems like a lot, but the average person does it every day!

The suggested *safe and adequate* intake of sodium is 1100 to 3000 mg per day (½ to 1½ teaspoons per day). You can see that this is far below the average intake, so overconsumption of sodium is more a problem than underconsumption.

The sodium we consume comes from two sources: the salt naturally present in foods, and salt added during preparation and serving of food. Some foods, like bacon, are naturally high in sodium. Some foods have salt added in processing, as with some soups. Other foods usually have salt added after preparation (like french fries).

An example of having salt added is the case of potato chips. A potato has only 1 mg of sodium per 100 grams, while the same weight of potato chips has 340–1000 grams. The table above shows the salt content of foods. The table was adapted from the *Home and Garden Bulletin Number 252.*

Sodium has been implicated in hypertension. This is the reason that individuals with high blood pressure are often prescribed a low-sodium diet. It has been recognized recently that increased potassium can lower blood pressure, so a combination of sodium restriction and potassium supplementation may be beneficial for blood pressure control.

It is possible to reduce sodium intake to about 3500 mg per day by limiting the use of table salt and by avoiding foods high in salt. To reduce the level further, to the 2000 mg or so recommended for blood pressure control, a strict diet of foods naturally low in sodium is necessary. This means eating very little of foods like canned soups, broth, canned vegetables, olives, cured foods, pickles, and salted foods like potato chips and crackers.

Iron

Compared to calcium and sodium, iron exists in rather small amounts in the body. It is still essential. Iron is found mainly in the blood, but some iron is present in every cell. Its primary function is to facilitate the transfer of oxygen and carbon dioxide among body tissues.

The need for iron varies according to age and sex. For instance, an adult man needs 0.9 to 1.2 mg of iron per day. Adult women require almost twice as much (1.4–2.2 mg/day), and adolescent girls need even more (1.9–3.7 mg/day). Liver is the only food that provides appreciable iron, so adding iron to the diet is often necessary. Much of this is done with food products that are *fortified* or *enriched*. Some 30 states require that flour be enriched, so additional iron is available in bread products.

Iron deficiency is not common, but can be serious when it does occur. It can result in anemia, which is a deficiency in the number or quality of red blood cells. Iron supplementation can usually remedy this problem.

Most people receive adequate iron in the diet and do not need supplements to prevent pseudo-ailments like *iron poor blood*. People who suspect an iron problem should consult a physician or dietitian.

What does all this information on minerals mean? As with vitamins, most people receive adequate minerals if they eat a carefully chosen, balanced diet. However, there are special groups of people who require mineral supplements. Examples are needs for calcium in elderly women and iron in teenage girls. It is best to get specific advice from someone trained in nutrition.

Assignment for this lesson

Now is the time to begin keeping the Master Monitoring Form. Select the techniques important to you from the Master List of Techniques (Appendix A) and enter them on the form. We will discuss this in Lesson Sixteen, at which time you can develop a permanent version of the Master Monitoring Form.

Self-assessment questionnaire

Lesson Fifteen

T F 75. Certain techniques are essential for all individuals controlling their weight.

T F 76. Controlling your eating at a special event is easier if you eat something before you go.

T F 77. Iron deficiency is common and many people need to supplement their eating with additional iron.

T F 78. The average person consumes more than twice the safe and adequate intake of salt each day.

(Answers in Appendix C)

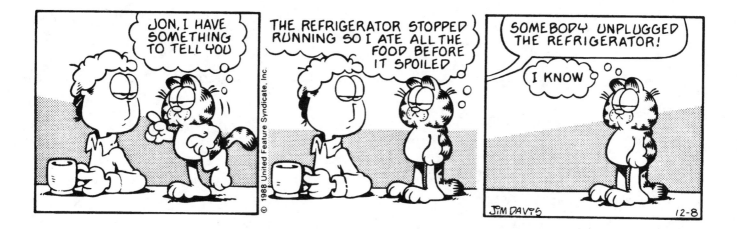

Master Monitoring Form—Lesson Fifteen   *Today's Date:*

Time	Food and Amount	Calories
Total Daily Calories		

Assignment this week	Always	Sometimes	Never
1.			
2.			
3			
4.			
5.			

Food Groups for Today	Physical Activity	Minutes
Milk, yogurt, and cheese ❑ ❑ ❑		
Meat, poultry, etc. ❑ ❑ ❑		
Fruits ❑ ❑ ❑ ❑		
Vegetables ❑ ❑ ❑ ❑ ❑		
Breads, cereals, etc. ❑ ❑ ❑ ❑ ❑ ❑ ❑ ❑ ❑ ❑ ❑		

Here we are, the final lesson in The LEARN Program. I hope you have enjoyed your voyage through the program and have acquired the skills you need for permanent weight control. We can now take the final few steps. Let's finish with a flurry of excitement!

Interpreting your progress

At this stage in the program, individuals have had different experiences and weight losses. Some have done well and attained their goal, and others still have weight to lose. There are those who struggled at times and succeeded at others, but are on their way to a positive outcome. Others struggled throughout and lost no weight at all. Let's reflect on *your* progress and use it to forge a picture of the future.

Making the transition from the structure of the program to *free living* can be tricky for some people. If you are fearful of this transition or have had difficulty in the past when ending a program, some work in the "A" (Attitudes) part of the LEARN model might help.

Some people who complete programs have an unfortunate way of not taking credit when credit is due. When they do well on a program they attribute their success to the program, but if they flounder, they blame themselves. I hear people say, "Weight Watchers really helped me lose weight" and later say, "The Weight Watchers program was good, I just couldn't stick with it." This attitude can eventually wear away a person's confidence.

I prefer a different attitude. If you do well on a program, the credit is yours. The program only provides ideas and techniques, but you have the responsibility for implementing them. It is similar to using tools to build a house. Having the right tools can help, but someone has to make the effort to put it all together. Giving the program credit for weight loss is like giving the hammer credit for building the house. When we hear a virtuoso perform a masterpiece on the piano, do we give the piano credit? Whatever you have achieved is yours to boast about. You deserve to feel good and to remember that *your* efforts were at work. What does this mean?

If you have been responsible for making progress, the progress can continue. If the program has been responsible, it would be natural for you to fall apart. This is not the case, obviously, but beware of the tendency to give the program credit when the credit is yours.

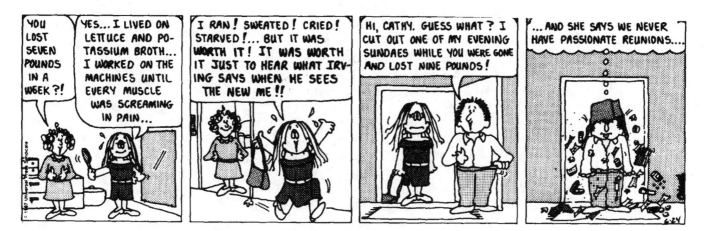

Like a batter on a baseball team, you don't have to hit a home run on every pitch!

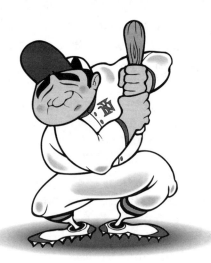

In the past several paragraphs, I have spoken about the program *ending*. Do you notice the contradiction in this idea and the basic concepts of The LEARN Program? A primary thrust of our effort has been to learn new behaviors and habits that can become permanent. In this sense, the program does not end. The key issue is whether you can take away changes that you will live with. If so, we have accomplished part of our mission. If not, try to identify the lessons in the manual that can best facilitate this notion, and then reread the material. The sections on Attitudes are a good place to start.

If you have done less well than expected, what can we conclude? Again, the natural tendency is to despair and blame yourself. I do not feel this is fair. Over the course of a lifetime, overweight individuals go through periods of being very motivated and having the strength to try a program, and periods where nothing seems to work and starting a program is a series of false starts.

There are peaks of strength and valleys of weakness, with lots of terrain in between. Individuals begin programs at many points in these stages. The ones who do best, of course, are those at the peaks. Those at the valleys have trouble. Others fall somewhere in the middle.

For a person who has not done well, I recommend two approaches. The first is to consider waiting until a peak comes along, and then try again. The right timing can be important. The second is to consider trying a different program. This program is not right for everyone, so if something else meets your needs, by all means try it.

Losing weight is like being a batter on a baseball team. You need not hit a home run on every pitch. Even if you strike out, you will have other chances at bat, and even if you go hitless in one game, there will be other games. You just want to avoid a prolonged slump! So, keep a positive attitude and keep trying.

Remember reasonable weight?

In the very beginning of this program, we discussed the concept of "reasonable weight." Because most people begin programs with expectations of what they will weigh that are based on arbitrary and unrealistic beauty ideals or even on landmarks in their lives (when they got married, finished school, etc.), what should be viewed as terrific progress gets dismissed.

Let me tell a story about Susan. She began a program at 185 pounds saying she wanted to be 125. Susan weighed 125 when she got married but began gaining weight after she had children and had been no less than 150 most of her adult life. In the 16 weeks on the program, Susan lost 25 pounds, and weighed 160. Instead of celebrating the 25 pounds she did lose, she was focused on the remaining weight. How reasonable is it for her to think that 125 is the only acceptable weight?

You may have lost as much weight as you set out to lose, but if not, which is the case with many people, it is important to view what you have done in a positive context. There is no reason to expect perfection—we do not expect the perfect job, the perfect hair, the perfect eyes, the perfect nose—the perfect life. Why, then, are we only satisfied with total weight loss? The answer is that society teaches us that weight is under total control of the in-

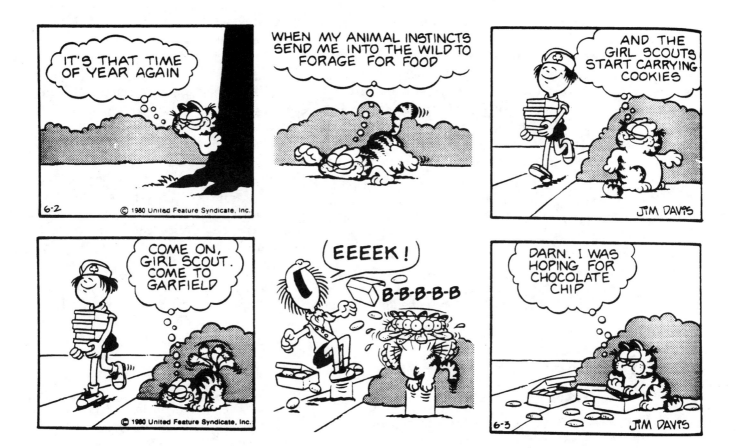

dividual and we have ideals that are highly unrealistic. It would be like saying there is only one acceptable eye color and that people with other colors were imperfect and weren't trying hard enough to change who they are.

You may be one of the many people who would like to weigh much less but will not or cannot. The choice, then, is whether to wage a wholesale assault on your self-esteem by feeling there is something wrong, or to accept what is reasonable and feel good about progress you are able to make. You know which path I favor.

A great deal of research has been done on goal setting. It won't surprise you to hear that people get frustrated, disappointed, and even depressed when they do not reach their goals. Goals, therefore, have to be challenging, but not impossible to reach. By setting realistic goals, and by rewarding yourself for reaching them, your self-esteem will increase and you will be in a much better position to sustain changes you make.

Examining your master monitoring form

I introduced the Master Monitoring Form in the last lesson to give you some experience with it. How did it work for you? This seemingly simple step of getting the form in good order can be quite important. It can help you define which techniques are important for you, and can provide feedback on how you are doing. Let's review the procedures for making the form work to your advantage.

As I mentioned in Lesson Fifteen, many clients generally list record keeping as one of the most important aspects of the program. You may remember from the early lessons that record keeping has several virtues. It reminds you of the techniques that can help you lose weight and can give you positive feedback about changes you make. It can also help control eating because there is always some accountability when the record is filled out every day.

You can add or delete techniques from the form you completed last week. The Master

List of Techniques (Appendix A) shows all the techniques used in the program. Pick the ones most likely to help. This is a good time to refer back to the Behavior Chain you completed in Lesson Twelve. This showed how trouble can be avoided by interrupting the eating chain at various places. This may give you clues for techniques to add to the Master Monitoring Form.

Don't hesitate to change the Master Monitoring Form in the weeks ahead. A blank form is provided in this lesson. Make as many copies as you need. I recommended in the last lesson that you continue to complete this form for at least eight more weeks. Do it well beyond this point if it will help. I know some people who have kept forms like this for more than 10 years.

Making your habits permanent

There are several keys to developing permanent habits. *Practice* is one such key. The 16 lessons in this program may not provide enough time for all your habits to change. Eating habits develop over years and years, so we must be patient for the changes to become permanent. By the time a person is 40, at least 40,000 meals have been consumed. This is lots of practice, so new habits may take time.

Another key is *awareness*. Try to remain a student of your eating and exercise habits. Be aware of what stimulates your eating and of methods for turning the tide. The Master Monitoring Form is designed with this in mind.

A note about breakfast

I mentioned in an earlier lesson that many overweight people skip breakfast. This happens because they may not feel hungry in the morning, they are in a hurry, or they feel that skipping breakfast is a good way to start off the day by saving calories. Most people who successfully lose weight resume eating breakfast as they lose weight. This prevents the situation where you find yourself famished later in the day. To eat breakfast is consistent with the

prevailing wisdom among health experts. There are some recent research findings that further support this view. Researchers at the University of Minnesota gave subjects one of five cereals ranging in fiber content, plus milk and orange juice, for breakfast at 7:30 a.m. At 11:00, the subjects were given a buffet lunch, and the amount eaten was carefully recorded. The subjects who had the high-fiber cereals ate fewer calories at lunch than did the people eating the low-fiber cereals. Especially important is that the people eating the high-fiber cereals ate fewer total calories (combining breakfast and lunch) than the subjects with the low-fiber cereals.

Starting the day with breakfast, especially a breakfast high in fiber, may help control calorie intake the rest of the day. In the research study I just described, subjects who ate the high-fiber cereals ate less at lunch even when they felt just as hungry as subjects having the other cereals. So, beginning the day with breakfast will probably help you control your weight. The guide to breakfast cereals in Lesson Seven will give you some guidance about the calorie and fiber content of various cereals. In addition to helping you eat less, the fiber may have positive health consequences.

Indeed, breakfast could be the foundation to developing overall healthy eating habits. This is especially true for children, since many habits learned as children carry over into adulthood. There are many creative ways to make breakfast fun, fast, and easy; it just takes a little planning and dedication. If you are a breakfast-skipper, the breakfast tips that follow may help you incorporate breakfast as an important part of your day. If you are still not convinced, try it for a couple of weeks. The benefits may surprise you.

- ◆ **No time?** Try getting up a few minutes earlier—10 minutes will do fine; once you are up and going you will not miss the time. This is plenty of time to have a glass of juice, a bowl of cereal, and some fruit.

- ◆ **Still no time?** Plan breakfast around foods that are ready to eat or take little time to prepare. Examples include canned or fresh fruit, juices, milk, instant breakfast mixes, ready-to-eat cold cereals, yogurt, cheese, bagels, and toast.

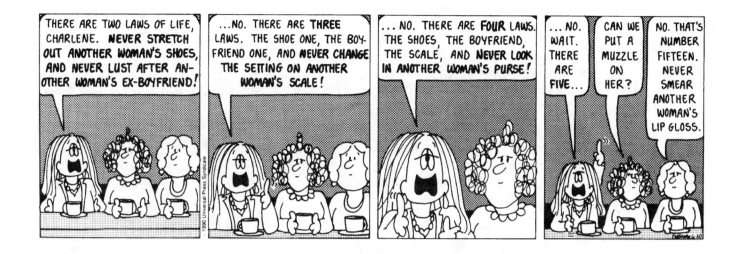

- **Take it to go.** If you still find yourself short on time, pack yourself a *breakfast-to-go* the night before, and eat the following morning when you have a few extra minutes. Try celery stuffed with cheese, fresh or dried fruits, canned juice or milk, breakfast bars, a bagel, or English muffin.

- **Be creative.** Top cereals with fresh fruit, add jelly or jam to toast, biscuits, or rolls, and add chopped nuts to hot cereals.

- **Not hungry?** Drink some juice, and take something with you for a snack later in the morning. Bread or crackers will do fine. You may wish to add some cheese or fruit. Then drink some milk or water.

- **Plan your breakfast the night before.** Make as much advanced preparation as possible. This way you are not confronted with the decision of what to prepare, and much of your meal can be ready and waiting for you when you wake up.

- **Start a breakfast partnership.** Enjoy the company of your spouse, a child, or a friend. Take turns making healthy breakfast choices. You can also take turns preparing breakfast with a breakfast partner.

Doing a master self-assessment

Appendix B and Appendix C contain the questions and answers for the Master Self-Assessment. These are taken from each lesson in the program. Try doing a Master Self-Assessment by answering the questions after the lessons and comparing your answers to those in Appendix C. You may want to study the manual until you get all the questions correct. Wrong answers can clue you to areas where you need to solidify your knowledge.

A special guide for weight maintenance

As I mentioned in the previous lesson, I received many requests from people using The LEARN Program to provide a follow-up guide. Some people wanted help with losing more weight while others wanted information on maintenance and stabilization. Now such a guide is available, *The Weight Maintenance and Stabilization Guide*. This detailed, step-by-step guide is designed to focus on approaches that are specific to long-term weight control.

The skills necessary to keep weight off are different from those needed to lose weight initially. One must settle into a routine that becomes stable. Long-term motivation and commitment are central to this endeavor, and one must solidify the thoughts, actions, and feelings necessary for permanent changes. The guide is written with just this in mind. It contains practical information drawn from the many suggestions I have received from people, from research done at our clinic at Yale and from many other research centers, and from many years of experience working with people on maintaining weight loss.

Information on obtaining *The LEARN Maintenance and Stabilization Program* is available by calling the LEARN Education Center at 1–800–736–7323 or by writing to the address listed at the back of this book.

Ending where we began

We can end where we began—with emphasizing the most important principles of all. You may recall that one of the first things I mentioned was a concept called self-efficacy. It tell us that the people most likely to make successful, long-term changes are those with the skills and confidence to do so. You have learned many skills — skills to help you confront difficult situations, to handle setbacks, to make changes you can live with, and to enjoy the whole process. You hold your weight control future in your hands. Use the skills and you'll do just fine.

You should be confident in your ability. You should not and could not be confident that you will be perfect, or that you will have an easy path to your goal. But, you can be confident that despite bumps in the road, occasional detours, and perhaps even getting lost on occasion, you can find your way back to the road and continue on your important journey.

Give yourself a pep talk when you need it. If you were your own coach, think about what you would need to hear to be most effective, and then inspire yourself in that way. Do whatever you can to be confident that you have the necessary skills, and then use the skills, use the skills, and use them some more. It can work.

Saying farewell

Let me offer my sincere hope that you enjoyed this program and that you are on your way to accomplishing your weight loss goals.

It can be a hard struggle, but with the right attitude and new habits, success can be yours. Keep up the spirit!

Finally, please contact me with your ideas and comments about this program. Success stories are welcome, as are suggestions for improving the program. I pay attention to what I hear and would like to hear from you. Send comments to me :

American Health Publishing Company
P.O. Box 35328, Dept. 10
Dallas, TX 75235-0328

You may also fax or e-mail your comments to me at the numbers listed in the very beginning of this book.

Good luck!!

Good Luck!

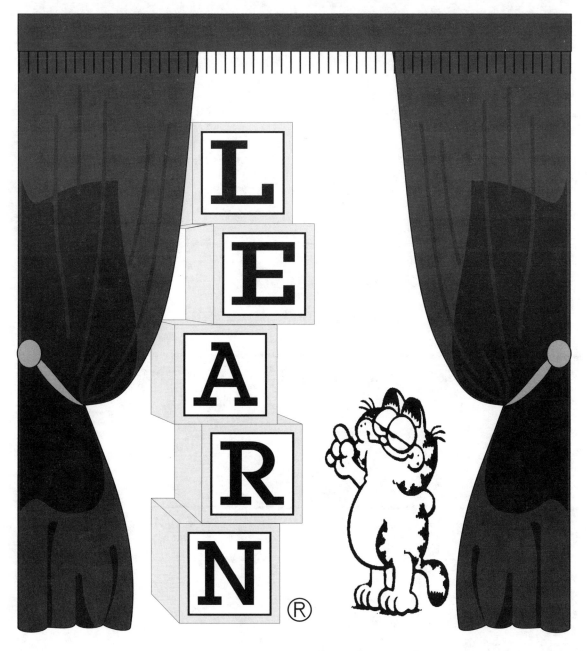

Master Monitoring Form—Lesson Sixteen   *Today's Date:*

Time	Food and Amount	Calories
	Total Daily Calories	

Assignment this week	Always	Sometimes	Never
1.			
2.			
3			
4.			
5.			

Food Groups for Today	Physical Activity	Minutes
Milk, yogurt, and cheese ❑ ❑ ❑		
Meat, poultry, etc. ❑ ❑ ❑		
Fruits ❑ ❑ ❑ ❑		
Vegetables ❑ ❑ ❑ ❑ ❑		
Breads, cereals, etc. ❑ ❑ ❑ ❑ ❑ ❑ ❑ ❑ ❑		

Master List of Techniques

Lifestyle Techniques

Exercise Techniques

Attitude Techniques

Relationship Techniques

Nutrition Techniques

Master Self-Assessment

		True	False
1.	Discovering the psychological roots of your weight problem is the most important factor in weight reduction.	____	____
2.	All overweight people have an excessive number of fat cells.	____	____
3.	There is no such thing as a slow or underactive metabolism.	____	____
4.	Very few people can accurately estimate the quantity and calories of foods.	____	____
5.	Record keeping may be the most important aspect of a weight loss program.	____	____
6.	Automatic eating is common in overweight people and distracts them from the taste of food.	____	____
7.	The Food Diary helps uncover patterns in your eating habits.	____	____
8.	Exercise isn't of much use for weight loss because it burns relatively few calories.	____	____
9.	Exercise can help prevent the loss of muscle tissue during weight loss.	____	____
10.	The calorie is the measure of the amount of fat in food.	____	____
11.	The calorie level necessary to lose weight is the same for all people.	____	____
12.	Walking one mile burns almost as many calories as running the mile.	____	____
13.	Expensive exercise suits are worth the money because the special materials help the body.	____	____
14.	Everyone should walk with a partner because the company increases pleasure.	____	____
15.	Overweight people do not experience hunger, only psychological cravings for food.	____	____
16.	Eating an extra 10 calories per day will add one pound of weight over a year.	____	____
17.	The ABC approach stands for Alternatives, Behavior, and Consciousness.	____	____

Master Self-Assessment *(continued)*

18. Shaping refers to encouraging others to help you lose weight. _____ _____

19. The five food groups are Milk and Yogurt Products, Vegetables, Fruits, Meats and Proteins, and Breads and Cereals. _____ _____

20. Ice cream and several other high-sugar desserts are not allowed on this program. _____ _____

21. Cleaning your plate is harmful because the server decides how much you will eat. _____ _____

22. Climbing stairs requires more energy per minute than many traditional exercises like swimming and jogging. _____ _____

23. If you,eat an equal number of servings from the five food groups of the Food Guide Pyramid, you will have a balanced diet. _____ _____

24. Eating on a schedule is not advisable because it is too regimented. _____ _____

25. Eating rapidly helps you enjoy food *more* because the taste buds get more stimulation. _____ _____

26. Pausing during a meal increases food intake because the body digests food and sends out signals to eat more. _____ _____

27. Your resting pulse will increase as you lose weight and get in better condition. _____ _____

28. You should tell your program partner in specific terms how he or she can help. _____ _____

29. Since too much dietary fat has been linked to heart disease and other health-related risks, it's best to eliminate all fat from your diet. _____ _____

30. The recommended daily intake of dietary fat is 30 percent or less of total calories. _____ _____

31. One gram of fat contains more than twice the calories of one gram of carbohydrate or protein. _____ _____

32. Saturated fat is usually solid at room temperature and is found only in animal foods, such as meats and dairy products made from whole milk or cream. _____ _____

33. Since all fruits and vegetables have only small amounts of fats, it is not as important to count the amount of fat in these foods as it is to count the dietary fat from meat and dairy products. _____ _____

34. It is wise to shop for food when you are hungry to test the new restraint you have learned. _____ _____

35. Buying foods that require preparation can increase your awareness of eating and help you eat less. _____ _____

36. Most people get enough exercise to realize the many health benefits of an active lifestyle.

37. Exercise must be done in specific amounts for it to aid you with weight loss.

38. Thirty minutes of moderate-intensity physical activity is now recommended for Americans.

39. All nutrients that we eat contain calories.

40. The recommended number of daily servings from the Milk, Yogurt, and Cheese Group is two to three.

41. Eating yogurt everyday can help you lose weight.

42. Keeping high-calorie foods stored out of sight can decrease impulsive eating.

43. Warming up and stretching before exercise is to strengthen your muscles.

44. To get a cardiovascular training effect, there must be the right combination of frequency, intensity, and time.

45. Fat thoughts can hinder a person's efforts to lose weight.

46. Light bulb or dichotomous thinking refers to your own *bright* ideas about weight loss.

47. It is best to take all of what you will eat in one serving so you will not need additional helpings.

48. No exercise can help you lose fat in specific parts of the body.

49. Impossible Dream Thinking is having fantasies and images about weight loss, life as a thin person, etc.

50. Carbohydrates are not as important as other nutrients, and they should make up only about 30 percent of your daily diet.

51. The Food Guide Pyramid suggests three to five servings each day from the Vegetable Group.

52. Fat soluble vitamins give you energy, but water soluble vitamins do not.

53. When someone offers you food, it is best to accept it as a sign of their friendship.

54. Imperatives are words like *always* and *never*. They leave no room for error.

55. There are many benefits to jogging and cycling. They are good forms of exercise for people trying to lose weight.

Master Self-Assessment (contented)

True   False

56. Vitamin B$_{12}$ is the only vitamin for which mega-doses are recommended.

_____ _____

57. Fruits, vegetables, and cereals tend to be high in fiber.

_____ _____

58. Most Americans eat plenty of fruits and should not worry about increasing their daily intake.

_____ _____

59. Alcohol is dangerous for people losing weight because it contains many calories and weakens dietary restraint.

_____ _____

60. Ordering a la carte meals at restaurants helps avoid unwanted calories that come in *package* meals.

_____ _____

61. Aerobic activities are designed to build strength in the shortest possible time.

_____ _____

62. Vitamin E is associated with virility and may help in the remedy of alcoholism.

_____ _____

63. Foods from the Bread, Cereal, Rice, and Pasta Group are a good source of complex carbohydrates, however, they may contain hidden fat.

_____ _____

64. One characteristic common to overweight persons is that they seldom eat breakfast.

_____ _____

65. Once the eating chain begins, it is not possible to stop because the links are so strong.

_____ _____

66. A Behavior Chain, like any chain, is only as strong as its weakest links.

_____ _____

67. It is best to interrupt an eating chain at one of its last links when you know what foods confront you.

_____ _____

68. Using stairs is a convenient and accessible way for many people to increase activity.

_____ _____

69. When a person lapses, relapse is close behind because nothing can interrupt the negative cycle of lapses and binging.

_____ _____

70. It helps to have a list of alternatives to eating for use when urges strike.

_____ _____

71. The emphasis on fiber may be dangerous because fiber is indigestible material that can harm the intestinal system.

_____ _____

72. Getting nervous or anxious during a lapse is helpful because anxiety interferes with appetite and allows you to remove yourself from temptation.

_____ _____

73. When dealing with a lapse, it is best to move quickly and decisively before control erodes even further. _____ _____

74. For controlling your blood cholesterol, it is important to limit intake of saturated fat. _____ _____

75. Certain techniques are essential for all individuals controlling their weight. _____ _____

76. Controlling your eating at a special event is easier if you eat something before you go. _____ _____

77. Iron deficiency is common and many people need to supplement their eating with additional iron. _____ _____

78. The average person consumes more than twice the safe and adequate intake of salt each day. _____ _____

Answers for Self-Assessment Questions

1. *False*   Psychological problems are not at the root of all cases of overweight. There is no evidence that uncovering these *causes* helps with weight loss.

2. *False*   People who have been overweight in childhood may have excessive fat cells, but other overweight persons may not. They have fat cells that are too large.

3. *False*   There are wide variations in metabolic rate among different people. Some are cursed with a *slow metabolism* and may be prone to easy weight gains in body weight.

4. *True*   One study found that persons losing weight who observed common foods and estimated quantity and calories averaged errors of 60 percent. Therefore, using a calorie guide and scale is important.

5. *True*   Persons who have lost weight and maintained their loss often report that record keeping was one key to their success.

6. *True*   Many overweight people eat without paying attention to all they consume. They miss the taste in much of what they eat.

7. *True*   The Food Diary helps you discover times, foods, feelings, and activities associated with eating.

8. *False*   Exercise has many benefits aside from the calories you burn. It is one of the *most* important aspects of weight control.

9. *True*   Exercise maximizes the loss of fat and can prevent the loss of muscle. Exercise combined with diet is preferable to diet alone for weight loss.

10. *False*   The calorie is a measure of the energy your body gets from a food. Fat supplies some of these calories in some foods, but so do carbohydrate and protein.

11. *False*   There are differences in how much weight people lose on the same caloric intake. Some people need to make a greater restriction in caloric intake than do others in order to lose weight.

12. *True*   How far you go is more important than how fast you go, so walking is an ideal exercise. Of course, running will get the job done faster!

13. *False*   Expensive exercise clothes contain no special materials and have no advantage over clothes most people have anyway. Their only advantage is cosmetic.

14. *False*   Many people do profit from exercising with a partner, but many enjoy doing their exercise alone. It is a matter of individual preference.

15. *False*   Overweight people experience physical hunger. However, they often confuse psychological cravings for this hunger and eat when there is no physical need.

16. *True*   As few as ten calories make a difference when added over a period like a year.

17. *False*   The ABC approach stands for Antecedents, Behavior, and Consequences. It shows the importance of what occurs before, during, and after eating.

18. *False*   Shaping refers to making gradual progress in a step-by-step fashion so that goals are attainable.

19. *True*   These are the five food groups of the Food Guide Pyramid. In order to have a balanced diet, a variety of foods should be eaten from these groups.

20. *False*   No foods are prohibited. You can learn to eat any foods in moderation. Making foods *illegal* only sets up a person for failure.

21. *True*   It is wise to break the habit of cleaning the plate so you, and not the server, determine how much you eat. By cleaning the plate, you admit that you have no control over eating, because you eat whatever is in front of you.

22. *True*   Climbing stairs is an excellent way to burn calories. However, most people cannot climb stairs for extended periods, so it is best considered a lifestyle activity in which exercise can be added to your daily routine.

23. *False*   Different numbers of servings are recommended for each of the five food groups. Refer to Lesson Five for specific information.

24. *False*   Eating on a schedule helps define the times you eat so that you minimize the times of the day associated with eating.

25. *False*   Taste buds catch nothing but a blur if the food shoots past like a rocket. Slowing down can help you enjoy food more.

26. *False*   Pausing gives the body a chance to signal that enough has been eaten. It can keep you satisfied with less food.

27. *False*   As your weight declines and you become more fit, your resting heart rate will probably decline, showing that your heart can accomplish its work with fewer beats.

28. *True*   Do not expect your partner to read your mind. Tell your partner exactly what he or she can do to help. Remember, be specific, ask for positive changes, and be nice to your partner in return.

29. *False*   Fat plays an important role in the body and should not be eliminated from your diet. It is important for good health, however, most people eat too much fat.

30. *True*   Fat, as a percentage of total calories eaten, should be 30 percent or less of your daily diet.

31. *True*   One gram of fat contains nine calories while one gram of carbohydrate or protein contain only four calories.

32. *False*   It is true that saturated fats are generally solid at room temperature, but is not true that saturated fats are found only in animal products. Coconut and palm oils also contain saturated fats.

33. *False*   It is important to be familiar with the fat content of *all* foods. Vegetables are usually low in fat, however, nuts are an example of vegetables that are very high in fat.

34. *False*   Shopping on an empty stomach is asking for trouble. You will do less impulse buying if you shop after eating.

35. *True*   Taking the time to prepare foods will give you a chance to make a determined decision to eat. Many times the food will not be worth the effort, so you can ask yourself how important the eating really is.

36. *False*   Only about 22 percent of the American adult population is active enough to realize health benefits. The rest are either totally sedentary or not active enough.

37. *False*   This concept of an exercise threshold is a barrier to exercise for many people. *Any* exercise can help, so do whatever you can.

38. *True*   Thirty minutes of incremental physical activity over most days (at least five) is now recommended for people to reach a moderate-level of physical fitness.

39. *False*   Vitamins, minerals, and water are considered nutrients essential to our bodies, yet, they contain no calories.

40. *True*   The Food Guide Pyramid recommends two to three servings daily from the Milk, Yogurt, and Cheese Group.

41. *False*   Yogurt may be used in many creative ways to *replace* other foods that have calories, however, there is no evidence that eating yogurt everyday helps people lose weight.

42. *True*   Remember the refrigerator battle cry, "Out of Sight, Out of Mouth!"

43. *False*   The two purposes of stretching and other warm up exercises are to loosen the muscles to avoid strain and to permit the heart and circulatory system to make a gradual transition from rest to hard work. You should warm up and cool down for at least five minutes each time you exercise.

44. *True*   These are the three parts of the formula, so if you wish to get a training or aerobic effect, you must do each part in specific amounts.

45. *True*   Each of us holds internal conversations, and many overweight individuals have *fat thoughts*. These thoughts and attitudes can greatly hinder weight loss efforts if they are not countered.

46. *False*   This refers to thinking that you are on or off a program, perfect or terrible with your behavior, and legal or illegal in your eating. This must be replaced with a more rational perspective.

47. *False*   It is best to take one portion at a time because it gives you time to decide whether you need more. It interrupts automatic eating.

48. *True*   Spot reducing is a myth. Your body adds and removes fat according to genetic and hormonal factors. You can reduce fat in general, but you cannot dictate where it will come from.

49. *True*   These images and fantasies can distract a person from the day-to-day behaviors needed to lose weight, and can lead to serious disappointment when the individual loses weight and significant life issues.

50. *False*   Carbohydrates should make up the largest portion of your daily diet (between 55 and 60 percent of total calories). It is important, however, to watch for *hidden* calories in these foods and to limit the *added* calories, such as toppings, butter, and dressings.

51. *True*   The Food Guide Pyramid suggests between three and five servings each day from the Vegetable Group.

52. *False*   Vitamins do not contain energy themselves, but aid in the breakdown of other nutrients into energy that the body can use.

53. *False*   It is nice to be friendly, but it is more important that *you* control what you eat. Be polite, but be firm in not yielding to pressure to eat.

54. *True*   These words are a setup for failure because they represent standards that no person can meet.

55. *True*   Jogging and cycling have both psychological and physical benefits. They are ideal for many people who are losing and maintaining weight.

56. *False*   There is no weight-loss advantage to taking mega-doses of any vitamin. Sticking with the Recommended Daily Allowances (RDA) is the best policy. This can usually be done by eating a balanced diet, and at most, can be accomplished with a multiple vitamin.

57. *True*   These foods are naturally high in fiber and are good additions to your diet if you wish to increase fiber intake.

58. *False*   Most American do not eat the recommended number of servings of fruit on a daily basis. Hence, most people should increase their intake of fruit.

59. *True*   Alcohol releases inhibitions and weakens dietary restraint. It contains little nutrition and many calories.

60. *True*   Package deals, like getting a hamburger, fries, and cole slaw together more cheaply than separately, deliver more food (and calories) than you may want or need. Only get the package if you are *sure* you want all its components.

61. *False*   Aerobic activities do little for strength. They increase the body's use of oxygen and improve the condition of your heart. They are valuable for both health and weight loss.

62. *False*   Unless you are vitamin deficient or have special dietary needs, you probably need no vitamin supplements. A balanced diet usually provides adequate vitamins.

63. *True*   Foods from this group are very high in complex carbohydrates and most people should increase their intake from this food group. Breads, cakes, cookies, etc., however, have *hidden* calories and it is important to watch out for these.

64. *True*   Many overweight people avoid eating breakfast because they may not be hungry first thing in the morning or because they hope to *save* calories by not eating. This typically leads to more calories being consumed during the day, however.

65. *False*   People losing weight sometimes feel the chain is out of control, but a chain *can* be broken by using the right techniques at the proper time in a given situation.

66. *True*   A behavior chain can be broken at any link. Concentrate on the weakest links, where the chain is easiest to break.

67. *False*   It can be difficult to interrupt a chain at one of the final links because the momentum created by the earlier links can be powerful. Consider breaking the early links before the process gets rolling.

68. *True*   Most people have access to stairs, so it is easy to add several flights to your routine.

69. *False*   Some people *think* that a lapse leads to relapse because they feel guilty at any mistake. By using special coping techniques, you can see that a lapse can be a signal to do better, not worse.

70. *True*   This can provide you with a list of enjoyable activities that can become associated with the signals that are used to stimulate eating.

71. *False*   Precisely because fiber is indigestible, it facilitates movement of food and waste products through the digestive system. Eating a high-fiber diet may also reduce risk for several chronic diseases.

72. *False*   Anxiety makes it hard to think and weakens restraint that might keep eating in check. It is best to stay calm during a lapse so you can make a rational plan for responding.

73. *True*   The longer you wait during a lapse, the more momentum builds for overeating. Acting swiftly and decisively is the best approach. Consider yourself a Forest Ranger. Your task is to prevent fires and to move quickly when a fire breaks out.

74. *True*   Saturated fat can raise your cholesterol level, so it is important to control the intake of foods high in cholesterol *and* foods high in saturated fat.

75. *False*   Different people respond to different techniques. It is best to select a small number of techniques that work for *you* and to focus on them.

76. *True*   Eating a low-calorie food before you go takes the edge off hunger. This can help you avoid high-calorie foods like chips and nuts, so you can use your calories for special foods you really want.

77. *False*   Iron deficiency is not common. Most people obtain adequate iron from normal eating and do not need the popular supplements.

78. *True*   Most experts recommend reductions in salt intake. Excess sodium comes from salt in foods naturally and from the salt we add to food.

Guidelines for Being a Good Group Member

Many programs deal with participants in groups. This is done for an important reason. Members of the group can provide tremendous help to one another. The help may come in the form of encouraging words, a pat on the back, ideas to solve a specific problem, or just the knowledge that others in similar circumstances care about you.

Importance of the group

From a problem-solving perspective, a group provides a shared experience that can help you develop an effective program. But beyond providing information, group members can provide support and encouragement. Most people losing weight encounter times when their motivation is high and other times when it is difficult to move in the right direction. When you take a detour from your program, the group can help the motivation return. When you are highly motivated yourself, you can encourage someone else in the group who may have trouble.

Good chemistry and teamwork

When a group has the right chemistry, it functions like a well-oiled machine. The meetings are enjoyable, informative, and motivational. Each group member receives as much as he or she gives, and all are better off for the effort.

The analogy of a sports team is especially appropriate. Let's take a basketball team, for example. We all know of teams with great individual players, but the team goes nowhere if the players do not work together. One player may have an opportunity to take a shot, but passing to a teammate who has a better shot will help the team. Teams with far less talent win championships by working together and helping one another. This intangible *team spirit* motivates everyone to work harder.

Each player receives and gives, and all benefit in the process.

Being a good group member is a **responsibility** of anyone entering a group. But more than duty, it is the best way to lose weight. Entering a group with a spirit of cooperation and the willingness to help others will insure that the help comes back to you. In the long run, you emerge the winner.

To be a good group member means following specific guidelines. There are things to do, things to say, and ways to act. The guidelines that follow can make this happen.

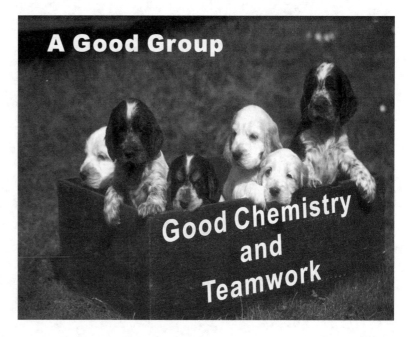

A Good Group

Good Chemistry and Teamwork

Guidelines and responsibilities

Attend meetings and be punctual

People in a group are responsible for attending meetings, not only for themselves but for others. When a group member misses a meeting, others in the group may worry about the person, may wonder if the absence is a sign of trouble, etc.

There will undoubtedly be times when you question whether you should attend a meeting. You might have overdone it on nacho chips, it may be rainy and miserable outside, or you may have had a difficult time with work or with the kids. These are the times when your program might be most in jeopardy, so it is important to attend the meeting. The group functions best when all attend, so remember that by joining a group you are agreeing to do your level best to make the meetings.

Being on time is another key factor. When you arrive late for a group, you draw attention to yourself, disrupt the proceedings, miss what has happened thus far, and force the group leader to either ignore what you have missed or cover it again. Showing up late, especially if it occurs chronically, is a sign of disrespect for other members of the group.

Sometimes, of course, being late is inevitable. You might have just arrived in town on the flight from Tokyo where you were thinking of acquiring SONY or Toyota. If you live in Arizona, you might have been attacked by the Abominable Cactus. Or you might have some more common reason like a traffic jam, late baby sitter, or deadlines at the office. These things are fine, but when you are late when you can help it, we start to worry.

Being late can be a sign of many things. Some people are always late because they fall into the Type A behavior pattern. They are always rushing and want to get in every last bit of activity before departing for the group. Such a person would cringe at sitting around for a few minutes with nothing to do. My advice is to go ahead and cringe, but be on time.

Sometimes group members are late because they have done poorly and want to avoid speaking with the group leader. Others might be angry at the group leader or dissatisfied with the program or their progress. These things are usually not done on a conscious level, but if you look closely at your reasons for being late, these things may be the driving factors. If you find yourself being late, or wanting to be late, think about the reasons.

Really listen

Sure, we all listen in a group, but do we **really** listen? Are you tuned in to what is happening? Do you hear the emotions behind the words that another group member might be using?

It is quite apparent when someone in the group is not listening. Yawning, rolling the eyes, looking out the window, or daydreaming are giveaways. It is easy to get distracted, especially if what is being discussed is not relevant to you, or if something else important is occupying your thoughts. It takes a real effort to listen carefully.

Being a good listener involves watching the person who is speaking. Do they look like they are expressing some strong emotions? Is the topic a sensitive one? Have you experienced a similar situation or feeling? Have you found some approach helpful with the problem? It is fine to ask questions if you don't un-

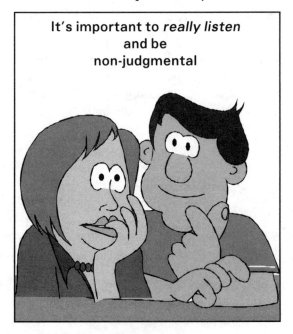

It's important to *really listen* and be non-judgmental

derstand what the person was saying, and it is certainly fine to respond with supportive statements or suggestions. It will be nice when others in the group do this for you, so start by really listening.

Be non-judgmental

This may sound like psychological jargon, but here is what it means to be non-judgmental. Sometimes you might feel that what another group member says or does is wrong, silly, or even stupid. There is a tendency to come down on these people or to point out the folly in their ways. The risk lies in being too negative, which can antagonize the person on the other end and make the remaining group members mad at you for being critical.

This does not mean that you are in a group where *everything is wonderful* and no negative emotions can be expressed. It is important to remember that there are different ways of saying things. What others say can be used as an opportunity for growth or an occasion to create bad feelings. The basic concept is for group members to accept one another. In such a climate, people in the group feel free to say things they might otherwise hide for fear of being criticized.

The chart provided below gives some examples of judgmental and non-judgmental statements. As you can see, the non-judgmental statements are supportive and understanding, and open the door for further discussion. They show others that you care about them and are willing to help.

Be an active participant

In any group, some people are more active than others. This is fine, and can reflect differences in personalities. Not everyone has to be chirping away like a magpie to benefit from the group. However, opening up to be an active participant can help both you and the other members of the group.

Being silent in a group sometimes reflects being shy or reserved. In other cases, it shows that a person is angry, resentful, or bored. Whatever the reason, try to speak up when you have something worth saying. If you would like to share some of your own experiences, would like to ask if anyone has a solution to a particular problem you face, or can provide ideas of your own about an issue, speak up. Many times what you have to say will be listened to with all the attention given to a group leader, and you might have ideas that the leader or others in the group do not have.

If you are more the silent type, don't feel pressured to be exceptionally talkative. Not everyone will participate equally or will speak the same amount. When you do have something to offer, please share it with the others.

Share the air space

Think of the air in the group room as the territory around an airport. If too many planes enter the air space, the situation becomes dangerously confusing. If one jet occupies more than its share of the air space, say by circling in an erratic pattern, it would be tough going for the others.

Being Non-judgmental

One person says	Judgmental Response	Non-judgmental Response
I just couldn't exercise this week.	You must be getting lazy.	It's hard to keep motivated to exercise.
I don't think this group is helping.	You are just making excuses.	Can we do something to help?
Others here don't understand me.	You talk too much.	I would like to. What can I do?

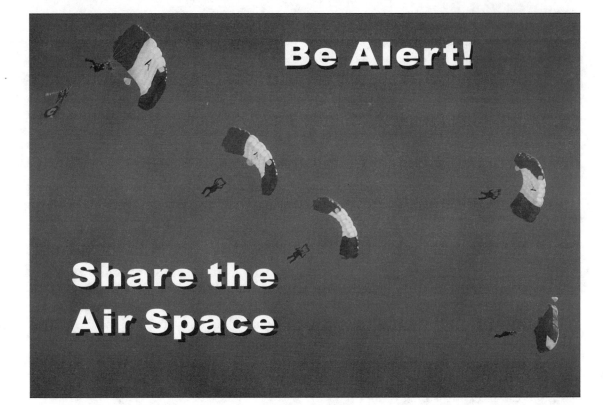

Be Alert!

Share the Air Space

In a group, there is only so much air space. Only so many voices can be heard and so many things said in the course of a group. For members of the group who are particularly verbal, there can be a tendency to monopolize the conversation and to crowd others from the air space.

Again, not everyone speaks the same amount, so if some people are naturally more active in the group, there is no need to pull in the reins. But if such a person interrupts or always speaks first, there may be a problem with sharing the air space. If the person takes a long time to make a point, or has to say something during every discussion, it may be time to open the air space to others. Look at the way you speak in the group, and see if any of these apply to you. If so, try to pull back and think before speaking. By all means speak up when you have something to say, and say what you feel, but try not to speak just because there is an opportunity.

Be supportive

One of the fundamental reasons there are groups is for group members to support each other. This can be motivating and encouraging. In fact, sometimes a kind word or a supportive gesture will mean more coming from a fellow group member than the exact same word or gesture coming from the group leader.

Group members should try to be nice, helpful, and understanding. When another group member is troubled by something, do what you can to show that you understand. You can offer moral support by showing that you understand that the person faces a difficult situation. Share similar experiences you might have had, and most of all, give some constructive suggestions if you can think of ways to help.

In summary

When you enter a group, you enter a situation in which you can reap impressive rewards. You have the opportunity to not only learn the facts and techniques of the program, but to support and be supported, learn and instruct, help and be helped. This does not happen automatically, so people must be serious about their responsibilities as group members. In so doing, they will benefit from you and you will benefit from them. All will be better off and the long-term result can be permanent weight loss.

Appendix E

Fast Food Guide

Description	Calories	Pro (g)	Carb (g)	Fat (g)
Arby's				
Roast Beef Sandwiches				
Arby's Melt w/ Cheddar	368	18	36	18
Arby Q	431	22	48	18
Bac 'N' Cheddar Deluxe	539	22	28	34
Beef 'n Cheddar	487	25	40	28
Giant Roast Beef	555	35	43	28
Junior Roast Beef	324	17	35	14
Regular Roast Beef	388	23	33	19
Super Roast Beef	523	25	50	27
Chicken				
Breaded Chicken Fillet	536	28	46	28
Chicken Cordon Bleu	623	38	46	33
Chicken Fingers (2 Pieces)	290	16	20	16
Grilled Chicken BBQ	388	23	47	13
Grilled Chicken Deluxe	430	23	41	20
Roast Chicken Club	546	31	37	31
Roast Chicken Deluxe	433	24	36	22
Roast Chicken Santa Fe	436	29	35	22
Sub Roll Sandwiches				
French Dip	475	30	40	22
Hot Ham 'N' Swiss	500	30	43	23
Italian Sub	675	30	46	36
Philly Beef 'N' Swiss	755	39	48	47
Roast Beef Sub	700	38	44	42
Triple Cheese Melt	720	37	46	45
Turkey Sub	550	31	47	27
Light Menu				
Roast Beef Deluxe	296	18	33	10
Roast Chicken Deluxe	276	20	33	6
Roast Turkey Deluxe	260	20	33	7
Garden Salad	61	3	12	.5
Roast Chicken Salad	149	20	12	2
Side Salad	23	1	4	.3
Other Sandwiches				
Fish Fillet	529	23	50	27
Ham 'n Cheese	359	24	34	14
Ham 'n Cheese Melt	329	20	34	13
Potatoes				
Cheddar Curly Fries	333	5	40	18
Curly Fries	300	4	38	15
French Fries	246	2	30	13
Potato Cakes	204	2	20	12
Baked Potato (Plain)	355	7	82	.3
Baked Potato w/ Margarine and Sour Cream	578	9	85	24
Broccoli 'N' Cheddar Bkd Potato	571	14	89	20
Deluxe Baked Potato	736	19	86	36

Description	Calories	Pro (g)	Carb (g)	Fat (g)
Soups				
Boston Clam Chowder	190	9	18	9
Cream of Broccoli	160	7	15	8
Lumberjack Mixed Vegetable	90	2	10	4
Old Fashion Chicken Noodle	80	6	11	2
Potato w/ Bacon	170	6	23	7
Timberline Chili	220	18	17	10
Wisconsin Cheese	280	10	20	18
Desserts				
Apple Turnover	330	4	48	14
Cherry Turnover	320	4	46	13
Cheesecake (Plain)	320	5	23	23
Chocolate Chip Cookie	125	2	16	6
Chocolate Shake	451	15	76	12
Jamocha Shake	384	15	62	10
Vanilla Shake	360	15	50	12
Butterfinger Polar Swirl	457	15	62	18
Health Polar Swirl	543	15	76	22
Oreo Polar Swirl	482	15	66	22
Peanut Butter Cup Polar Swirl	517	20	61	24
Snickers Polar Swirl	511	15	73	19
Burger King				
Burgers				
Whopper	640	27	45	39
Whopper w/ Cheese	730	33	46	46
Double Whopper	870	46	45	56
Double Whopper w/ Cheese	960	52	46	63
Whopper Jr. Sandwich	420	21	29	24
Whopper Jr. w/ Cheese	460	23	29	28
Hamburger	330	20	28	15
Cheeseburger	380	23	28	19
Double Cheeseburger	600	41	28	36
Double Cheeseburger w/ Bacon	640	44	28	39
Sandwiches/Side Orders				
Bk Big Fish Sandwich	700	26	56	41
Bk Broiler Chicken Sandwich	550	30	41	29
Chicken Sandwich	710	26	54	43
Chicken Tenders (8 Piece)	310	21	19	17
Broiled Chicken Salad	200	21	7	10
Garden Salad	100	6	7	5
Side Salad	60	3	4	3
French Fries (Med, Salted)	370	5	43	20
Coated French Fries (Med, Salted)	340	0	43	17
Onion Rings	310	4	41	14
Dutch Apple Pie	300	3	39	15

Fast Food Guide *(continted)*

Description	Calories	Pro (g)	Carb (g)	Fat (g)
Drinks				
Vanilla Shake (Medium)	300	9	53	6
Chocolate Shake (Medium)	320	9	54	7
Chocolate Shake (Medium)	440	10	84	7
Strawberry Shake (Medium)	420	9	83	6
Breakfast				
Croissan'wich w/ Sausage, Egg, and Cheese	600	22	25	46
Biscuit w/ Sausage	590	16	41	40
Biscuit w/ Bacon, Egg, Cheese	510	19	39	31
French Toast Sticks	500	4	60	27
Hash Browns	220	2	25	12

Dairy Queen

Description	Calories	Pro (g)	Carb (g)	Fat (g)
Burgers/Sandwiches/Side Orders				
Homestyle Hamburger	290	17	29	12
Homestyle Cheeseburger	340	20	29	17
Homestyle Double Cheeseburger	540	35	30	31
Homestyle DD Hamburger	440	30	29	22
Homestyle DD Cheeseburger	540	36	31	31
Homestyle Bacon Double Cheeseburger	610	41	31	36
Homestyle Ultimate Burger	670	40	29	43
Hot Dog	240	9	19	14
Cheese Dog	290	12	20	28
Chili Dog	280	12	21	16
Chili 'N' Cheese Dog	330	14	22	21
Fish Fillet Sandwich	370	16	39	16
Fish Fillet Sandwich w/ Cheese	420	19	40	21
Chicken Breast Fillet	430	24	37	20
Chicken Breast Fillet w/ Cheese	480	27	38	25
Chicken Strip Basket w/ Gravy	860	35	88	42
Chicken Strip Basket w/ BBQ Sauce	810	33	88	37
Grilled Chicken Breast Fillet	310	24	30	10
French Fries, Small	210	3	29	10
French Fries, Regular	300	4	40	14
French Fries, Large	390	5	52	18
Onion Rings	240	4	29	12
Ice Cream and Yogurt				
Vanilla Soft Serve, ½ Cup	140	3	22	4.5
Chocolate Soft Serve, ½ Cup	150	4	225	
Nonfat Frozen Yogurt, ½ Cup	100	3	21	0
Small Vanilla Cone	230	6	38	7
Regular Vanilla Cone	350	8	57	10
Large Vanilla Cone	410	10	65	12
Small Chocolate Cone	240	6	37	8
Regular Chocolate Cone	360	9	56	11
Regular Yogurt Cone	280	9	59	1
Small Chocolate Sundae	290	6	51	7
Regular Chocolate Sundae	410	8	73	10
Regular Cup of Yogurt	230	8	49	.5
Regular Yogurt Strawberry Sundae	300	9	66	.5
Small Misty Slush	220	0	56	0

Description	Calories	Pro (g)	Carb (g)	Fat (g)
Regular Misty Slush	290	0	74	0
Strawberry Misty Cooler	190	0	49	0
Small Chocolate Malt	650	15	111	16
Regular Chocolate Malt	880	19	153	22
Small Chocolate Shake	560	13	94	15
Regular Chocolate Shake	770	17	130	20
DQ Sandwich	150	3	24	5
Strawberry Shortcake	430	7	70	14
Banana Split	510	8	96	12
Chocolate Dilly Bar	210	3	21	13
Chocolate Mint Dilly Bar	190	3	20	12
Toffee Dilly Bar w/ Heath Pieces	210	3	24	12
Fudge Nut Bar™	410	8	40	25
Buster Bar	450	10	41	28
Peanut Buster Parfait	730	16	99	31
Small Dipped Cone	340	6	42	17
Regular Dipped Cone	510	9	63	25
Starkiss	80	0	21	0
Caramel & Nut Bar	260	5	32	13
Fudge Bar	50	4	13	0
Vanilla Orange Bar	60	2	17	0
Lemon Freez'r™ ½ Cup	80	0	20	0
Small Butterfinger Blizzard	520	11	80	18
Regular Butterfinger Blizzard	750	16	115	26
Small Chocolate Sandwich Cookie Blizzard	520	10	79	18
Regular Chocolate Sandwich Cookie Blizzard	640	12	97	23
Small Strawberry Blizzard	400	9	66	11
Regular Strawberry Blizzard	570	12	95	16
Small Heath Blizzard	560	10	82	21
Regular Heath Blizzard	820	14	119	33
Small Chocolate Chip Cookie Dough Blizzard	660	12	99	24
Regular Chocolate Chip Cookie Dough Blizzard	950	17	143	36
Small Reeses Peanut Butter Cup Blizzard	590	14	81	24
Regular Reeses Peanut Butter Cup Blizzard	790	19	105	33
Small Strawberry Breeze	320	10	68	.5
Regular Strawberry Breeze	460	13	99	1
Small Heath Breeze	470	11	85	10
Regular Heath Breeze	710	15	123	18
Choice Vanilla Big Scoop	250	4	27	14
Choice Chocolate Big Scoop	250	4	28	14
Strawberry-Banana Pizza, 1/8	180	3	29	6
Heath Treatzza Pizza 1/8 Pizza	180	3	28	7
M&M Treatzza Pizza 1/8 Pizza	190	3	29	7
Peanut Butter Fudge, 1/8 Pizza	220	4	28	10
Frozen Log Cake, 1/8 Cake	280	5	4	39
Frozen 8" Round Cake, 1/8 Cake	340	7	53	12
Frozen 10" Rd Cake, 1/12 Cake	360	7	55	12
Frozen Heart Cake, 1/10 Cake	270	5	41	9
Frozen Sheet Cake, 1/20 Cake	350	7	54	12

Description	Calories	Pro (g)	Carb (g)	Fat (g)

Hardee's

Breakfast

Description	Calories	Pro (g)	Carb (g)	Fat (g)
Rise 'N' Shine Biscuit	390	6	44	21
Jelly Biscuit	440	6	57	21
Apple Cinnamon 'N' Raisin Biscuit	200	2	30	8
Sausage Biscuit	510	14	44	31
Sausage & Egg Biscuit	630	23	45	40
Bacon & Egg Biscuit	570	22	45	33
Bacon, Egg, & Cheese Biscuit	610	24	45	37
Ham Biscuit	400	9	47	20
Ham, Egg & Cheese Biscuit	540	20	48	30
Country Ham Biscuit	430	15	45	22
Big Country Breakfast (Sausage)	1000	41	62	66
Big Country Breakfast (Bacon)	820	33	62	49
Frisco Breakfast Sandwich (Ham)	500	24	46	25
Regular Hash Rounds	230	3	24	14
Biscuit 'N' Gravy	510	10	55	28
Three Pancakes	280	8	56	2
Ultimate Omelet Biscuit	570	22	45	33

Sandwiches

Description	Calories	Pro (g)	Carb (g)	Fat (g)
Hamburger	270	14	29	11
Cheeseburger	310	16	30	14
The Boss	570	27	42	33
Cravin' Bacon Cheeseburger	690	30	38	46
The Works Burger	530	25	41	30
Mesquite Bacon Cheeseburger	370	19	32	18
Quarter Pound Dbl Cheeseburger	470	27	31	27
Chicken Fillet Sandwich	480	26	54	18
Regular Roast Beef	320	17	26	16
Big Roast Beef Sandwich	460	26	35	24
Grilled Chicken Sandwich	350	25	38	11
Mushroom 'N' Swiss Burger	490	28	39	25
Frisco Burger	720	33	43	46
Hot Ham 'N' Cheese	310	16	34	12
Fisherman's Fillet	560	26	54	27

Fried Chicken/Sides

Description	Calories	Pro (g)	Carb (g)	Fat (g)
Breast	370	29	29	15
Wing	200	10	23	8
Thigh	330	19	30	15
Leg	170	13	15	7
Cole Slaw (4 oz)	240	2	13	20
Mashed Potatoes (4 oz)	70	2	14	0
Gravy (1½ oz)	20	0	3	0
Baked Beans (5 oz)	170	8	32	1

Salads/Fries

Description	Calories	Pro (g)	Carb (g)	Fat (g)
Side Salad	25	1	4	0
Garden Salad	220	12	11	13
Grilled Chicken Salad	150	20	11	3
Fat Free French Dressing	70	0	17	0
Ranch Dressing	290	1	6	29
Thousand Island Dressing	250	1	9	23
French Fries (small)	240	4	33	10
French Fries (medium)	350	5	49	15
French Fries (large)	430	6	59	18

Shakes/Desserts

Description	Calories	Pro (g)	Carb (g)	Fat (g)
Shake (Vanilla)	350	12	65	5
Shake (Chocolate)	370	13	67	5
Shake (Strawberry)	420	11	83	4
Shake (Peach)	390	10	77	4
Vanilla Cone	170	4	34	2
Chocolate Cone	180	5	34	2
Cool Twist Cone	180	4	34	2
Hot Fudge Sundae	290	7	51	6
Strawberry Sundae	210	5	43	2
Peach Cobbler (6 oz)	310	2	60	7
Big Cookie	280	4	41	12

Jack In The Box

Breakfast

Description	Calories	Pro (g)	Carb (g)	Fat (g)
Breakfast Jack	300	18	30	12
Pancake Platter	400	13	59	12
Sausage Croissant	670	21	39	48
Scrambled Egg Pocket	430	29	31	21
Sourdough Breakfast Sandwich	380	21	31	20
Supreme Croissant	570	21	39	36
Ultimate Breakfast Sandwich	620	36	39	35
Hash Browns	160	1	14	11

Sandwiches

Description	Calories	Pro (g)	Carb (g)	Fat (g)
Chicken Caesar Sandwich	520	27	44	26
Chicken Fajita Pita	290	24	29	8
Chicken Sandwich	400	20	38	18
Chicken Supreme	620	25	48	36
Grilled Chicken Fillet	430	29	36	19
Spicy Crispy Chicken Sandwich	560	24	55	27

Burgers

Description	Calories	Pro (g)	Carb (g)	Fat (g)
Hamburger	280	13	31	11
Cheeseburger	320	16	32	15
Double Cheeseburger	450	24	35	24
Jumbo Jack	560	26	41	32
Jumbo Jack w/ Cheese	650	31	42	40
Grilled Sourdough Burger	670	32	39	43
Ultimate Cheeseburger	1030	50	30	79
¼ lb. Burger	510	26	39	27

Salads

Description	Calories	Pro (g)	Carb (g)	Fat (g)
Garden Chicken Salad	200	23	8	9
Side Salad	70	4	3	4

Mexican/Teriyaki

Description	Calories	Pro (g)	Carb (g)	Fat (g)
Taco	190	7	15	11
Monster Taco	283	12	22	17
Chicken Teriyaki Bowl	580	28	115	1.5

Sides/Desserts

Description	Calories	Pro (g)	Carb (g)	Fat (g)
Seasoned Curly Fries	360	5	39	20
Small French Fries	220	3	28	11
Regular French Fries	350	4	45	17
Jumbo French Fries	400	5	51	19
Super Scoop French Fries	590	8	76	29
Onion Rings	380	5	38	23
Egg Rolls–3 Piece	440	3	54	24
Egg Rolls–5 Piece	750	5	92	41
Chicken Strips (breaded) 4 Piece	290	25	18	13
Chicken Strips (breaded) 6 Piece	450	39	28	20
Stuffed Jalapenos–7 Piece	420	15	29	27

Fast Food Guide *(continted)*

Description	Calories	Pro (g)	Carb (g)	Fat (g)
Stuffed Jalapenos–10 Piece	600	22	41	39
Bacon & Cheddar Potato Wedges	800	20	49	58
Hot Apple Turnover	350	3	48	19
Cheesecake	310	8	29	18
Chocolate Chop Cookie Dough Cheesecake	360	7	44	18
Carrot Cake	370	3	58	15

Kentucky Fried Chicken

Chicken

Description	Calories	Pro (g)	Carb (g)	Fat (g)
Breast, extra crispy	353	27	15	21
Breast, original recipe	257	26	8	14
Drumstick, extra crispy	173	13	6	11
Drumstick, original recipe	147	14	4	9
Kentucky Nuggets (one)	46	3	3	3
Thigh, extra crispy	371	20	14	27
Thigh, original recipe	278	18	9	20
Wing, extra crispy	218	12	8	16
Wing, original recipe	181	12	6	13

Side Orders

Description	Calories	Pro (g)	Carb (g)	Fat (g)
Baked Beans	105	5	19	1
Buttermilk Biscuit	269	5	32	14
Corn on the Cob	176	5	32	3
Cole Slaw	103	1	12	6
Kentucky Fries	268	5	34	13
Mashed Potatoes & Gravy	62	2	10	2
Potato Salad	141	2	13	9

Long John Silver's

Fish/Seafood

Description	Calories	Pro (g)	Carb (g)	Fat (g)
Large South of the Border	1380	35	167	64
Regular South of the Border	690	18	84	32
Large Classic	1470	35	170	72
Regular Classic	730	18	85	36
Large Ceasar	1460	36	167	73
Regular Ceasar	730	18	83	37
Large Ranch	1460	35	170	72
Regular Ranch	730	18	85	36
Large Cajun	1450	36	170	70
Regular Cajun	730	18	85	35
Batter-Dipped Fish Sandwich	320	17	40	13
Ultimate Fish Sandwich	430	18	44	21
Flavorbaked™ Fish Sandwich	320	23	28	14
Popcorn Fish	290	13	27	14
Flavorbaked Fish (1 Piece)	90	14	1	2.5
Clams	300	11	31	17

Chicken

Description	Calories	Pro (g)	Carb (g)	Fat (g)
Large South of the Border	1370	36	162	64
Regular South of the Border	690	18	81	32
Large Classic	1450	36	165	72
Regular Classic	730	18	83	36
Large Ceasar	1450	37	162	73
Regular Ceasar	730	18	81	37
Large Ranch	1450	36	165	72

Description	Calories	Pro (g)	Carb (g)	Fat (g)
Regular Ranch	730	18	82	36
Large Cajun	1440	37	165	71
Regular Cajun	720	18	83	35
Flavorbaked Chicken	110	19	0	3
Flavorbaked Chicken Sandwich	290	24	27	10
Popcorn Chicken	250	15	17	14
Batter-Dipped Chicken (1 Piece)	120	8	11	6

Shrimp

Description	Calories	Pro (g)	Carb (g)	Fat (g)
Popcorn Shrimp	280	11	27	15
Large South of the Border	1380	32	169	64
Regular South of the Border	690	16	84	32
Large Classic	1460	32	172	72
Regular Classic	730	16	86	36
Large Ceasar	1460	32	169	73
Regular Ceasar	730	16	84	37
Large Ranch	1460	32	171	72
Regular Ranch	720	16	86	35
Large Cajun	1450	32	172	71
Regular Cajun	720	16	86	35
Batter-Dipped Shrimp (1 Piece)	35	1	2	2.5

Side Items

Description	Calories	Pro (g)	Carb (g)	Fat (g)
Fries	250	3	28	15
Cheese Sticks	160	6	12	9
Hushpuppy (1 Piece)	60	1	9	2.5
Corn Cobbette	140	3	19	8
Corn Cobbette (w/out Butter)	80	3	19	.5
Green Beans	30	2	5	.5
Rice Pilaf	140	3	26	3
Coleslaw	140	1	20	6
Baked Potato	210	4	49	0
Side Salad	25	1	4	0

McDonald's

Sandwiches, Fries & Chicken

Description	Calories	Pro (g)	Carb (g)	Fat (g)
Hamburger	270	12	34	10
Cheeseburger	320	15	35	14
Quarter Pounder	430	23	37	21
Quarter Pounder w/ Cheese	530	28	38	30
Big Mac	530	25	47	28
Arch Deluxe	570	29	43	31
Arch Deluxe w/ Bacon	610	33	43	34
Crispy Chicken Deluxe	530	27	47	26
Fish Fillet Deluxe	510	24	59	50
Grilled Chicken Deluxe	330	27	42	6
Small French Fries	210	3	26	10
Large French Fries	450	6	57	22
Super Size French Fries	540	8	68	26
Chicken McNuggets (4 Piece)	190	12	10	11
Chicken McNuggets (6 Piece)	290	18	15	17
Chicken McNuggets (9 Piece)	430	27	23	26

Breakfast & Salad

Description	Calories	Pro (g)	Carb (g)	Fat (g)
Egg McMuffin	290	17	27	12
Sausage McMuffin	360	13	26	23
Sausage McMuffin w/ Egg	440	19	27	28
English Muffin	140	4	25	2

Description	Calories	Pro (g)	Carb (g)	Fat (g)
Sausage Biscuit	430	10	32	29
Sausage Biscuit w/ Egg	510	16	33	35
Bacon, Egg & Cheese Biscuit	440	17	33	26
Biscuit	260	4	32	13
Sausage	170	6	0	16
Scrambled Eggs (2)	160	13	1	11
Hash Browns	130	1	14	8
Hotcakes (plain)	310	9	53	7
Hotcakes (Marg. 2 pats & Syrup)	580	9	100	16
Breakfast Burrito	320	13	23	20
Low-fat Apple Bran Muffin	300	6	61	3
Apple Danish	360	5	51	16
Cheese Danish	410	7	47	22
Cinnamon Roll	400	7	47	20
Garden Salad	35	2	7	0
Grilled Chicken Salad Deluxe	110	21	5	1
Desserts/Shakes				
Vanilla Low-fat Ice Cream Cone	120	4	23	.5
Strawberry Low-fat Ice Cream Sundae	240	6	5	11
Hot Caramel Low-fat Ice Cream Sundae	300	7	62	3
Hot Fudge Sundae	290	8	53	5
Nuts (Sundae)	40	2	2	3.5
Baked Apple Pie	260	3	34	13
Chocolate Chip Cookie	170	2	22	10
McDonaldland Cookies	180	3	32	5
Low-fat Vanilla Shake (small)	340	12	60	5
Low-fat Chocolate Shake (small)	340	12	62	5
Low-fat Strawberry Shake (small)	340	12	61	5

Pizza Hut

Data is based on 1 slice of Medium Pizza.

Description	Calories	Pro (g)	Carb (g)	Fat (g)
Cheese				
Thin 'N Crispy Crust	205	11	21	8
Hand Tossed Crust	235	13	29	7
Pan Crust	261	12	28	11
Beef				
Thin 'N Crispy Crust	229	13	21	11
Hand Tossed Crust	260	15	29	9
Pan Crust	286	14	28	13
Ham				
Thin 'N Crispy Crust	184	10	21	7
Hand Tossed Crust	213	12	29	5
Pan Crust	239	11	28	9
Pepperoni				
Thin 'N Crispy Crust	215	11	21	10
Hand Tossed Crust	238	12	29	8
Pan Crust	265	11	28	12
Italian Sausage				
Thin 'N Crispy Crust	236	11	21	12
Hand Tossed Crust	267	13	29	11
Pan Crust	293	12	27	15
Pork Topping				
Thin 'N Crispy Crust	237	12	21	12
Hand Tossed Crust	268	14	29	10

Description	Calories	Pro (g)	Carb (g)	Fat (g)
Pan Crust	294	13	28	14
Meat Lover's				
Thin 'N Crispy Crust	288	15	21	13
Hand Tossed Crust	314	17	29	11
Pan Crust	340	16	28	18
Veggie Lover's				
Thin 'N Crispy Crust	186	9	22	7
Hand Tossed Crust	216	11	30	6
Pan Crust	243	10	29	10
Pepperoni Lover's				
Thin 'N Crispy Crust	289	15	22	16
Hand Tossed Crust	306	16	30	14
Pan Crust	332	15	28	17
Supreme				
Thin 'N Crispy Crust	257	14	21	13
Hand Tossed Crust	284	16	30	12
Pan Crust	311	15	28	15
Super Supreme				
Thin 'N Crispy Crust	270	14	22	14
Hand Tossed Crust	296	16	30	13
Pan Crust	323	15	28	17
Bigfoot Pizza is based on 1 slice of Bigfoot Pizza				
Cheese Bigfoot	186	10	25	6
Pepperoni Bigfoot	205	10	25	7
Pepperoni, Mushroom & Italian Sausage Bigfoot	214	11	25	8
Personal Pan Pizza (whole Pizza) Pepperoni	637	27	69	28
Supreme	722	33	70	34

Roy Rogers

Hamburgers & Chicken

Description	Calories	Pro (g)	Carb (g)	Fat (g)
Bacon Cheeseburger	581	32	25	39
Cheeseburger	563	30	28	37
Hamburger	456	24	27	28
RR Bar Burger	611	36	28	39
Roast Beef Sandwich	317	27	29	10
Chicken Breast	412	33	17	24
Chicken Leg	140	12	6	8
Chicken Thigh	296	18	12	20
Chicken Wing	192	11	9	13
Side Orders				
Biscuit	231	4	27	12
Cole Slaw	110	1	11	7
Regular French Fries	268	4	32	14
Potato w/ Bacon & Cheese	397	17	33	22
Potato w/ Broccoli & Cheese	397	14	40	18
Potato w/ Sour Cream & Chives	408	7	48	21
Potato Salad	107	2	11	6
Breakfasts				
Apple Danish	249	5	32	12
Breakfast Crescent w/ Bacon	431	15	26	30
Breakfast Crescent (plain)	401	13	25	27
Breakfast Crescent w/ Sausage	449	20	26	30
Egg & Biscuit Platter w/ Bacon	435	20	22	30
Egg & Biscuit Platter (plain)	394	17	22	27
Pancake Platter w/ Sausage	608	14	72	30

Fast Food Guide (*continued*)

Description	Calories	Pro (g)	Carb (g)	Fat (g)
Dessert				
Brownie	264	3	37	11
Hot Fudge Sundae	337	7	53	13
Strawberry Shortcake	447	10	59	19
Chocolate Shake	358	8	61	10
Vanilla Shake	306	8	45	11

Taco Bell

Description	Calories	Pro (g)	Carb (g)	Fat (g)
Tacos				
Taco	170	10	11	10
Soft Taco	210	12	20	10
Taco Supreme	220	11	13	13
Soft Taco Supreme	260	13	22	14
Double Decker Taco	340	16	37	15
Double Decker Taco Supreme	390	16	39	18
Steak Soft Taco	200	14	18	7
BLT Soft Taco	340	11	22	23
Kid's Soft Taco Roll-Up	290	16	20	16
Burritos				
Bean Burrito	380	13	55	12
Burrito Supreme	440	19	50	18
Big Beef Burrito Supreme	520	26	52	23
7-Layer Burrito	540	16	65	24
Chili Cheese Burrito	330	14	37	13
Chicken Club Burrito	540	22	43	31
Bacon Cheeseburger Burrito	560	29	43	30
Specialties				
Tostado	300	11	31	14
Mexican Pizza	570	21	41	36
Big Beef MexiMelt	300	16	21	16
Taco Salad w/ Salsa	840	32	62	52
Taco Salad w/ Salsa w/out Shell	420	26	29	21
Cheese Quesadilla	370	16	32	20
Chicken Quesadilla	420	24	33	22
Border Wraps				
Steak Fajita Wrap	460	20	48	21
Chicken Fajita Wrap	460	18	49	21
Veggie Fajita Wrap	420	11	51	19
Steak Fajita Wrap Supreme	510	21	50	25
Chicken Fajita Wrap Supreme	500	19	51	25
Veggie Fajita Wrap Supreme	460	11	53	23
Border Lights				
Light Chicken Burrito	310	18	41	8
Chicken Burrito	400	19	45	16
Light Chicken Burrito Supreme	430	25	52	13
Chicken Burrito Supreme	550	30	50	26
Light Chicken Soft Taco	180	13	21	5
Chicken Soft Taco	250	15	23	11
Light Kid's Chicken Soft Taco	180	13	20	5
Kid's Chicken Soft Taco	240	15	21	11
Nachos & Sides				
Nachos	310	2	34	18
Big Beef Nachos Supreme	430	12	43	24
Nachos Bell Grande	740	16	83	39

Description	Calories	Pro (g)	Carb (g)	Fat (g)
Pintos 'N Cheese	190	9	18	8
Mexican Rice	190	6	20	10
Cinnamon Twists	140	1	19	6

Wendy's

Description	Calories	Pro (g)	Carb (g)	Fat (g)
Sandwiches				
Plain Single	360	25	31	16
Single w/ Everything	420	26	37	20
Big Bacon Classic	570	34	46	29
Jr. Hamburger	270	15	34	10
Jr. Cheeseburger	320	17	34	13
Jr. Bacon Cheeseburger	380	21	34	19
Jr. Cheeseburger Deluxe	360	18	36	16
Kids' Meal Hamburger	270	15	33	10
Kids' Meal Cheeseburger	320	17	33	13
Grilled Chicken Sandwich	310	27	35	8
Breaded Chicken Sandwich	440	28	44	18
Chicken Club Sandwich	470	31	44	20
Spicy Chicken Sandwich	410	28	43	15
Fresh Salads-To-Go				
Caesar Side Salad	110	8	8	5
Deluxe Garden Salad	110	7	10	6
Grilled Chicken Salad	200	25	10	8
Grilled Chicken Caesar Salad	260	28	17	10
Side Salad	60	4	5	3
Taco Salad	590	29	53	30
Soft Breadstick	130	4	24	3
Desserts & Side Orders				
Chocolate Chip Cookie	270	4	38	11
Frosty Dairy Dessert (small)	340	9	57	10
Frosty Dairy Dessert (medium)	460	12	76	13
Frosty Dairy Dessert (large)	570	15	95	17
French Fries (small)	260	3	33	13
French Fries (medium)	380	5	47	19
French Fries (biggie)	460	6	58	23
Plain Baked Potato	310	7	71	0
Bacon & Cheese Baked Potato	540	17	78	18
Broccoli & Cheese Baked Potato	470	9	80	14
Cheese Baked Potato	570	14	78	23
Chili & Cheese Baked Potato	620	20	83	24
Sour Cream & Chives Baked Potato	380	8	74	6
Small Chili	210	15	21	7
Large Chili	310	23	32	10

The Calorie Guide

This calorie guide is designed to help you understand the dietary content of the foods you eat. It is not intended to be an all inclusive guide. Other, more complete calorie guides are available in most book stores. The foods listed here should help you as you go through The LEARN Program.

Calories are listed for average serving sizes whenever possible. You may wish to convert some measurements to others to simplify matters. For example, some beverages are listed in fluid ounces while others are listed in cups. Several measurement equivalents are shown below to help with this task.

The protein, carbohydrate, and fat content of all the foods listed in the Calorie Guide are presented in grams (g). Unfortunately, the nutrient content for all food items was not availabel at press time, therefore, some of this information may be missing.

Helpful Measures		
3t = 1T	= ½ fl oz	
16T = 1 cup	= 8 fl oz	= ½ pint
2 cups = 1 pint	= ½ quart	= ⅛ gallon
1 quart = 2 pints	= ¼ gallon	= .946 liter
1 gallon = 4 quarts	= 3.785 liter	1 liter = 1.057 quarts
1 oz = 28.35 g	1 lb = 16 oz	= 453.59 g

Description	Cal	Pro (g)	Carb (g)	Fat (g)
Alcohol (see Beverages)				
Almonds				
dried (1 oz) *24 nuts*	167	5.7	5.8	14.8
dry roasted (1 oz)	167	4.6	6.9	14.7
oil roasted (1 oz) *22 nuts*	176	5.8	4.5	16.4
Anchovy, raw (3 oz)	111	17.3	.0	4.1
Apples				
raw, w/skin (1 med)	81	.3	21.1	.5
raw, w/o skin (1 med)	72	.2	19.0	.4
boiled, w/o skin (1 cup)	91	.5	23.3	.6
Apple juice, canned (1 cup)	116	.2	29.0	.3
Apple sauce				
canned, unsweetened (½ cup)	53	.2	13.8	.1
canned, sweetened (½ cup)	97	.2	25.5	.2
Apricots				
raw (3 med)	51	1.5	11.8	.4
canned in water (4 halves)	20	.6	4.9	.0
canned in heavy syrup (4 halves)	75	.5	19.3	.1
dried, uncooked (10 halves)	83	1.3	21.6	.2
Apricott nectar, canned (1 cup)	141	.9	36.1	.2
Artichoke, boiled (1 med)	53	2.8	12.4	.2
Artichoke hearts, boiled (½ cup)	37	1.9	8.7	.1
Asparagus				
boiled (½ cup - 6 spears)	22	2.3	4.0	.3
canned (½ cup)	24	2.6	3.0	.8
frozen, boiled (4 spears)	17	1.8	2.9	.3
Avocado (1 med)	306	3.6	12.0	30.0
Bacon				
broiled, pan fried (3 med pieces)	109	5.8	.1	9.4
Canadian, grilled (2 slices)	86	11.3	.6	.4
Bagel (1 med)	163	6.0	30.9	1.4
Baking powder (1 t)	3.	.0	.7	.0
Bamboo shoots, raw (½ cup)	21	2.0	4.0	.2
Banana (1 med)	105	1.2	26.7	.6
Barbecue sauce (1 T)	12	.3	2.0	.3
Bass				
baked (3 oz)	215	17.7	2.3	14.6
stuffed, baked (3 oz)	222	13.9	9.8	13.5
Beans				
green, fresh, boiled (½ cup)	22	1.2	4.9	.2
green, canned (½ cup)	13	.8	3.1	.1
green, frozen, boiled (½ cup)	18	.9	4.2	.1
kidney, boiled (½ cup)	113	7.7	20.2	.4
kidney, canned (½ cup)	104	6.6	19.0	.4
lima, boiled (½ cup)	121	7.3	19.6	.6
lima, canned (½ cup)	96	5.9	17.9	.2
navy, boiled (½ cup)	130	7.9	23.9	.5
navy, canned (½ cup)	148	9.8	26.8	.6
northern, great, boiled (½ cup)	105	7.4	18.6	.4
northern, great, canned (½ cup)	150	9.6	27.6	.5
pinto, canned (½ cup)	93	5.5	17.5	.4
refried, canned (½ cup)	135	7.9	23.4	1.4
white, boiled (½ cup)	125	8.7	22.4	.3
white, canned (½ cup)	153	9.5	28.7	.4
yellow, boiled (½ cup)	127	8.1	22.3	1.0
yellow, canned (½ cup)	180	9.0	30.0	3.0
Bean sprouts, raw (½ cup)	16	1.6	3.1	.1
Beef, cooked (3.5 oz)				
brisket, lean	241	29.4	.0	12.8
chipped, dried	165	29.0	1.4	3.9

Description	Cal	Pro (g)	Carb (g)	Fat (g)
chuck pot roast, lean	231	33.0	.0	10.0
chuck blade roast, lean	270	31.1	.0	15.3
corned beef brisket, cured	251	18.2	.5	19.0
flank steak, lean	244	28.0	.0	13.8
ground, extra lean	250	24.5	.0	16.1
ground, lean	268	23.9	.0	18.3
ground, regular	287	23.0	.0	20.9
porterhouse steak, lean	218	28.2	.0	10.8
rib eye, lean	225	28.0	.0	11.6
round steak, lean	184	28.5	.0	7.0
sirloin steak, lean	208	30.4	.0	8.7
T-bone steak, lean	214	28.1	.0	10.4
Beef stew				
w/ vegetables (1 cup)	218	15.7	15.2	10.5
w/o vegetables, creamed (1 cup)	377	20.1	17.4	25.2
Beer (see Beverages)				
Beets				
boiled (½ cup slices)	26	.9	5.7	.0
canned (½ cup slices)	27	.8	6.1	.1
Beverages (nonalcoholic)				
cider, apple (6 oz)	90	.0	21.0	.0
choc milk, 1% fat (1 cup)	158	8.1	26.1	2.5
choc milk, 2% fat (1 cup)	179	8.0	26.0	5.0
choc milk, whole (1 cup)	208	7.9	25.9	8.5
coffee, black (1 cup)	5	.1	1.1	.0
coffee w/ sugar (1 cup)	35	.1	9.1	.0
coffee w/ sugar & cream (1 cup)	109	.9	10.1	7.6
lemonade, frozen conc (8 oz)	133	.1	34.7	.1
lemonade, from powder (8 oz)	102	.0	26.9	.0
milk, skim (8 oz)	86	8.4	11.9	.4
milk, 1% fat (8 oz)	102	8.0	11.7	2.6
milk, 2% fat (8 oz)	121	8.1	11.7	4.7
milk, whole (8 oz)	150	8.0	11.0	8.0
milk shake, thick vanilla (8 oz)	350	12.1	55.6	9.5
milk shake, thick choc (8 oz)	356	9.2	63.5	8.1
soft drinks (12 oz)				
cola	151	.1	38.5	.1
cola, diet	2	.2	.3	.0
cream soda	191	.0	49.3	.0
eggnog	513	14.6	51.6	28.5
fruit punch	200	.0	49.9	.0
ginger ale	124	.1	31.9	.0
grape soda	161	.0	41.7	.0
orange soda	177	.0	45.8	.0
orange soda, diet	2	.0	.6	.0
root beer	152	.1	39.2	.0
tea, black (1 cup)	3	.0	.5	.0
tea, w/ sugar (1 cup)	33	.1	8.5	.0
tea, w/ sugar & cream (1 cup)	107	.9	9.5	7.6
Beverages (alcoholic)				
beer and ale (12 oz)				
ale	150	1.7	10.0	.0
beer, regular	150	1.1	11.1	.0
beer, light	100	.7	4.8	.0
distilled spirits				
brandy (1 oz)	70	.0	.0	.0
cognac (1 oz)	70	.0	.0	.0
gin, 100 proof (1.5 oz jigger)	124	.0	.0	.0
rum, 100 proof (1.5 oz jigger)	124	.0	.0	.0
vodka, 100 proof (1.5 oz jigger)	124	.0	.0	.0
whiskey, 100 proof (1.5 oz jigger)	124	.0	.0	.0

Description	Cal	Pro (g)	Carb (g)	Fat (g)
liqueurs and cordials (1 oz)				
absinthe	84	.0	.0	.0
anisette	111	.0	.0	.0
Benedictine	112	.0	.0	.0
brandy, fruit	86	.0	.0	.0
Cherry Herring	80	.0	.0	.0
creme de menthe	125	.0	.0	0.1
Drambuie	110	.0	.0	.0
Southern Comfort	120	.0	.0	.0
triple sec	83	.0	.0	.0
mixed drinks				
daiquiri (3.5 oz)	194	.0	7.2	.0
highball, 4 oz	83	.0	.0	.0
Manhattan (3.5 oz cocktail)	224	.0	3.2	.0
martini (3.5 oz cocktail)	218	.0	.3	.0
old fashioned (4 oz)	180	.0	.0	.0
pina colada (6.8 oz can)	525	1.3	61.3	16.9
screwdriver (7 oz)	174	1.2	18.4	.1
tequilla sunrise (5.5 oz)	189	.6	14.7	.2
tom collins (7.5 oz)	121	.1	3.0	.0
whiskey sour (3.5 oz)	144	.2	5.8	.1
wines & wine beverages (3.5 oz)				
sparkling coolers	63	.2	8.8	.2
dessert, dry	130	.2	4.2	.0
dessert, sweet	158	.2	12.3	.0
table, red	74	.2	1.8	.0
table, rose	73	.2	1.5	.0
table, white	70	.1	.8	.0
Biscuits, 1 medium (homemade)	102	2.1	12.8	4.8
Blackberries				
raw (½ cup)	37	.5	9.2	.3
canned, heavy syrup (½ cup)	118	1.7	29.6	.2
frozen, unsweetened (1 cup)	97	1.8	23.7	.7
Blackeyed peas (cowpeas)				
boiled (½ cup)	99	6.6	17.8	4.5
canned (½ cup)	92	5.7	16.4	.7
Blueberries				
raw (½ cup)	41	.5	10.2	.6
canned, heavy syrup (½ cup)	112	.8	28.2	.4
frozen, sweetened (1 cup)	187	.9	50.5	.3
Bluefish, raw (3 oz)	124	14.7	.0	6.8
Bologna (see sausage)				
Bouillon, beef broth (1 cube)	6	.6	.6	.1
Bouillon, chicken broth (1 cube)	9	.7	1.1	.2
Brains, simmered beef (3.5 oz)	160	11.1	.0	12.5
Bran flakes (1 oz)	100	4.0	20.0	1.0
Braunschweiger (see sausage)				
Breads (1 slice or piece)				
bread sticks (2 sticks)	77	2.4	15.1	.6
cinnamon raisin	80	2.0	15.0	1.0
corn	178	3.8	27.5	5.8
cracked wheat	66	2.3	12.5	.9
french	81	2.7	14.8	1.1
hoagie or submarine roll	400	13.0	73.0	7.0
italian	78	2.8	14.9	.6
mixed grain	64	2.5	11.7	.9
oatmeal	71	2.4	13.0	1.2
pita pocket (1 pocket)	106	4.0	20.6	.6
pumpernickel	82	2.9	15.4	.8
raisin	70	2.1	13.2	1.0

Description	Cal	Pro (g)	Carb (g)	Fat (g)
rye	66	2.1	12.0	.9
white	64	2.0	11.7	.9
whole wheat	61	2.3	11.3	1.0
Breadcrumbs (1 cup)	392	12.6	73.4	4.6
Bread pudding (1 cup)	496	14.8	75.3	16.2
Bread stuffing (1 cup)	416	8.8	39.4	25.6
Broccoli				
raw (½ cup chopped)	12	1.3	2.3	.2
boiled (½ cup)	23	2.3	4.3	.2
Brussels sprouts, boiled (½ cup)	30	2.0	6.8	.4
Buns				
cinnamon (1 bun)	179	4.5	36.7	1.9
hot cross	111	2.0	18.0	3.0
Butter (1 T)				
regular	108	.1	.0	12.2
whipped	81	.1	.0	9.2
Cabbage, green				
raw (½ cup shredded)	8	.4	1.9	.1
boiled (½ cup shredded)	16	.7	3.6	.1
Cakes (1/12 of cake)				
angel food, homemade	161	4.8	35.7	0.1
angel food, from mix	126	3.2	28.6	.2
Boston cream pie	207	3.5	34.2	6.5
carrot, from mix	187	1.6	36.1	4.0
cheesecake	257	4.6	24.3	16.3
chocolate chip, from mix	189	1.8	35.6	4.4
coffee cake, from mix	116	2.2	18.9	3.5
cupcake (1 cupcake)	172	2.2	28.4	6.0
cottage pudding	93	1.8	14.7	3.0
devils food, homemade	227	3.4	30.4	11.3
devils food, from mix	312	4.0	53.6	11.3
fruit cake, homemade	163	2.1	25.7	6.6
german chocolate, from mix	250	3.0	36.0	11.0
gingerbread, homemade	267	3.0	35.0	12.9
honey spice, from mix	363	4.2	62.7	11.1
pineapple upside-down	236	2.5	37.4	9.1
pound	142	1.7	14.1	8.9
sponge	188	4.8	35.7	3.1
white	285	4.6	40.9	11.6
yellow	283	4.3	38.9	12.4
Cake icing (½ cup)				
chocolate	518	4.4	92.8	19.2
chocolate fudge	586	3.4	103.8	22.2
white	600	.8	130.2	10.4
Candy				
almond joy (1 oz)	136	1.5	16.4	2.3
baby ruth (2 oz bar)	260	4.0	36.0	12.0
butterfinger (2 oz bar)	260	4.0	38.0	12.0
butterscotch (1 oz)	113	.0	26.9	1.0
candy corn (¼ cup)	182	.1	44.8	1.0
caramels (1 oz)	113	1.1	21.7	2.9
chocolate				
almonds, coated (1 oz)	161	3.5	11.2	12.4
bar (1.65 oz bar)	254	3.8	27.1	14.5
chips (1 oz)	148	1.6	17.8	7.8
cherries, coated (2 pieces)	175	1.0	32.0	4.5
kisses (1.5 oz –9 pieces)	222	3.4	23.7	12.5
milk (1 oz)	147	2.2	16.1	9.2
peanuts, coated (1 oz)	159	4.6	11.1	11.7
semi-sweet (1 oz)	144	1.2	16.2	10.1
sweet (1 oz)	150	1.2	16.4	10.0

Description	Cal	Pro (g)	Carb (g)	Fat (g)
fudge (1 oz)	113	.8	21.3	3.5
gum drops (1 oz)	98	.0	24.8	0.2
hard (1 oz)	109	.0	27.6	.3
jelly beans (1 oz)	104	.0	26.4	.1
life savers, all flavors (1 piece)	9.1	.0	3.0	.0
marshmallow (1 large)	19	.1	4.8	.0
mints (3 cup)	100	.0	24.7	.6
peanut brittle (1 oz)	119	1.6	23.0	2.9
peanut butter chips (1.5 oz)	228	8.9	19.3	12.8
peanut butter cups (1.8 oz)	281	6.4	25.9	16.7
Cantaloupe, raw (1 cup)	57	1.4	13.4	.4
Carrots				
raw (1 med)	31	.7	7.3	.1
boiled (½ cup slices)	35	.9	8.2	.1
canned (½ cup slices)	17	.5	4.0	.1
Carrot juice, canned (1 cup)	97	2.3	22.8	.4
Casaba melon, raw (1 cup)	45	1.5	10.5	.2
Cashew nuts				
dry roasted (1 oz)	163	4.4	9.3	13.2
oil roasted (1 oz)	163	4.6	8.1	13.7
Catfish				
channel, raw (3 oz)	99	15.5	.0	3.6
breaded & fried (3 oz)	194	15.4	6.8	11.3
Catsup *(see ketchup)*				
Cauliflower				
raw (½ cup slices)	12	1.0	2.5	.1
boiled (½ cup slices)	15	1.2	2.9	.1
Caviar, black & red (1 T)	42	3.9	.6	2.9
Celery				
raw, 1 stalk (7.5" long)	6	.3	1.5	.1
boiled (½ cup diced)	11	.4	2.6	.1
Cereals (1 oz)				
all-bran (⅓ cup)	71	4.0	21.1	.5
almond delight (¾ cup)	110	2.1	23.0	1.6
alpha bits (1 cup)	110	2.3	24.1	.7
booberry (1 cup)	110	1.0	24.0	1.0
bran, 100% (½ cup)	76	3.5	20.7	1.4
bran chex (⅔ cup)	90	2.9	23.0	.7
bran flakes (¾ cup)	93	3.6	22.2	.5
cap'n crunch (¾ cup)	121	1.4	22.9	2.6
cheerios (⅓ cup)	111	4.3	19.6	1.8
cinnamon toast crunch (¾ cup)	120	1.0	23.0	3.0
cocoa krispies (¾ cup)	110	1.5	25.2	.4
coco puffs (1 cup)	110	1.0	25.0	.1
corn chex (1 cup)	110	2.0	25.0	.2
corn flakes (1 cup)	110	2.0	25.0	.1
cream of rice, cooked (¾ cup)	95	1.6	21.1	.1
cream of wheat, cooked (¾ cup)	100	2.9	20.8	.4
farina, cooked (¾ cup)	87	2.5	18.5	.1
froot loops (1 cup)	111	1.7	25.0	.5
frosted mini-wheats (4 biscuits)	102	2.9	23.4	.3
golden grahams (¾ cup)	109	1.6	24.1	1.1
granola (3 cup)	138	3.5	15.6	7.7
grape-nuts (⅞ cup)	104	2.8	22.7	.8
honey comb (1⅓ cups)	110	1.4	25.4	.3
honey nut cheerios (¾ cup)	107	3.1	22.8	.7
kix (1½ cups)	110	2.5	23.4	.7
life (⅔ cup)	111	5.2	18.6	1.8
lucky charms (1 cup)	110	2.6	23.2	1.1
malt-o-meal, cooked (¾ cup)	92	2.6	19.4	.2

Description	Cal	Pro (g)	Carb (g)	Fat (g)
maypo, cooked (¾ cup)	128	4.4	23.9	1.8
oatmeal, cooked (¾ cup)	109	4.6	18.4	1.9
product 19 (¾ cup)	108	2.8	23.5	.2
puffed rice (2 cups)	114	1.8	25.6	.2
puffed wheat (2 cups)	104	4.2	22.6	.4
rice chex (1⅛ cups)	110	1.7	25.0	.3
rice krispies (1 cup)	112	1.9	24.8	.2
shredded wheat (4 biscuits)	102	3.1	22.6	.6
special K (1⅓ cups)	111	5.6	21.3	.1
sugar frosted flakes (¾ cups)	108	1.4	25.7	.1
sugar smacks (¾ cup)	106	2.0	24.7	.5
super sugar crisp (7/8 cup)	106	1.8	25.6	.3
total (1 cup)	100	2.8	22.3	.6
trix (1 cup)	109	1.5	25.2	.4
wheat chex (⅔ cup)	100	2.9	23.0	.7
wheaties (1 cup)	99	2.7	22.6	.5
Cheese (1 oz)				
american, processed	106	6.3	.5	8.9
blue	100	6.1	.7	8.2
brick	105	6.6	.8	8.4
camembert, domestic	85	5.6	.1	6.9
cheddar	114	7.1	.4	9.4
colby	112	6.7	.7	9.1
cottage, creamed	30	3.5	.8	1.3
cream cheese (2 T)	99	2.1	.8	9.9
edam	101	7.1	.4	7.9
fontina	110	7.3	.4	8.8
gouda	101	7.1	.6	7.8
gruyere	117	8.5	.1	9.2
limburger	93	5.7	.1	7.7
monterey	106	6.9	.2	8.6
mozzarella	80	5.5	.6	6.1
muenster	104	6.6	.3	8.5
neufchatel	74	2.8	.8	6.6
parmesan, grated (1 T)	23	2.1	.2	1.5
parmesan, hard	111	10.1	.9	7.3
pimento, processed	106	6.3	.5	8.8
provolone	100	7.3	.6	7.6
ricotta, part skim (½ cup)	171	14.1	6.4	9.8
romano	110	9.0	1.0	7.6
roquefort	105	6.1	.6	8.7
swiss	107	8.1	1.0	7.8
velveeta	84	5.2	2.2	6.1
Cherries				
raw (10 cherries)	49	.8	11.3	.7
sour, canned in syrup (½ cup)	116	.9	29.8	.1
sour, canned in water (½ cup)	43	.9	10.9	.1
sweet, canned in syrup (½ cup)	107	.8	27.4	.2
sweet, canned in water (½ cup)	57	1.0	14.6	.2
Chewing gum (1 piece)	10	.0	2.0	.0
Chicken, (3.5 oz)				
dark, fried w/ skin	285	27.2	4.1	16.9
dark, fried w/o skin	239	29.0	2.6	11.6
dark, roasted w/ skin	253	26.0	0.0	15.8
dark, roasted w/o skin	205	27.4	.0	9.7
light, fried w/ skin	246	30.5	1.8	12.1
light, fried w/o skin	192	32.8	.4	5.5
light, roasted w/ skin	222	29.0	.0	10.9
light, roasted w/o skin	173	30.9	.0	4.5

Description	Cal	Pro (g)	Carb (g)	Fat (g)
parts, w/ skin				
breast, fried (½ breast)	218	31.2	1.6	8.7
breast, roasted (½ breast)	193	29.2	.0	7.6
drumstick, fried (1 drumstick)	120	13.2	.8	6.7
drumstick, roasted (1 drumstick)	112	14.1	.0	5.8
thigh, fried (1 thigh)	162	16.6	2.0	9.3
thigh, roasted (1 thigh)	153	15.5	.0	9.6
wing, fried (1 wing)	103	8.4	.8	7.1
wing, roasted (1 wing)	99	9.1	.0	6.6
Chicken a la king, homemade (1 c)	468	27.4	12.3	34.3
Chicken fricassee, homemade (1 c)	386	36.7	7.4	22.3
Chicken pot pie, homemade (1 slice)	545	23.4	42.5	31.3
Chickpeas (garbanzo beans)				
boiled (½ cup)	135	7.2	22.5	2.2
canned (½ cup)	143	5.9	27.2	1.4
Chili/chili con carne				
with beans (1 cup)	286	14.6	30.4	14.0
without beans (1 cup)	412	15.4	12.1	33.5
Chili powder (1 t)	8	.3	1.4	.4
Chocolate (see candy)				
Chocolate syrup (2 T)	82	.7	22.1	.3
Chop suey (1 cup)	300	26.0	12.8	17.0
Chow mein, chicken (1 cup)	255	31.0	10.0	10.0
Cider (see beverages)				
Clams				
raw (3 oz)	63	10.9	2.2	.8
steamers (3 oz)	126	21.7	4.4	1.7
breaded & fried (3 oz)	171	12.1	8.8	9.5
Clam sauce (4 oz)				
red sauce	81	3.6	9.3	3.2
white sauce	121	4.5	4.2	9.6
Cocoa (see beverages)				
Coconut, dried (1 oz)	187	2.0	6.7	18.3
Codfish				
raw (3 oz)	70	15.1	.0	.6
broiled (3 oz)	89	19.4	.0	.7
frozen & breaded (3 oz)	174	12.0	6.0	12.0
Coffee (see beverages)				
Cola (see beverages)				
Cold cuts (see sausage)				
Coleslaw (½ cup)	42	.8	7.5	1.6
Collards, boiled (1 cup chopped)	27	2.1	5.0	.3
Cookies				
animal crackers (10 pieces)	112	1.7	20.8	2.4
apple newtons (2 cookies)	147	1.3	28.0	2.7
applesauce raisin (2 cookies)	140	2.0	17.0	8.0
brownies w/ nuts (2" square)	97	1.3	10.2	6.3
butter (10 cookies)	229	3.1	35.5	8.5
cherry newtons (2 cookies)	147	1.3	26.7	2.7
chocolate chip (1 cookie)	46	.5	6.4	2.7
choc fudge sandwich (3 cookies)	150	2.0	19.0	7.0
choc coated grahams (2 cookies)	124	1.4	17.6	6.2
choc & cream sandwich (1 cookie)	49	.5	7.1	2.1
fig bar (1 bar)	53	.5	10.6	1.0
fig newtons (2 cookies)	100	1.0	20.0	2.0
gingersnaps (1 cookie)	34	.3	4.7	1.6
ladyfingers (2 ladyfingers)	79	1.7	14.2	1.7
macaroon (2 cookies)	181	2.0	25.1	8.8
marshmallow sandwich (4)	120	1.0	22.0	3.0
molasses (1 cookie)	137	2.0	24.7	3.4

Description	Cal	Pro (g)	Carb (g)	Fat (g)
nilla wafers (7 cookies)	130	1.1	21.0	4.0
nutter butter peanut butter (2)	140	3.0	18.0	6.0
oatmeal (1 cookie)	62	.8	8.9	2.6
oatmeal raisin (4 cookies)	235	3.2	38.2	8.0
oreo (3 cookies)	140	1.0	20.0	6.0
peanut butter (1 cookie)	50	.8	5.9	2.6
shortbread (1 cookie)	42	.5	4.9	2.3
sugar (2 cookies)	71	1.0	10.9	2.7
sugar wafers (2 cookies)	92	.9	13.9	3.7
vanilla wafers (5 cookies)	92	1.1	14.9	3.2
Cooking oil (see oils)				
Corn, grits				
dry (1 cup)	579	13.7	124.2	1.8
cooked (1 cup)	146	3.5	31.4	.5
Corn, yellow				
boiled (½ cup)	89	2.7	20.6	1.1
canned, cream style (½ cup)	93	2.2	23.2	.5
canned, vacuum pack (½ cup)	83	2.5	20.4	.5
Cornbread (see breads)				
Corn muffins (see muffins)				
Corn oil (see oil)				
Cornstarch (1 T)	30	.0	7.2	.0
Cornsyrup (see syrup)				
Cottage cheese (see cheese)				
Crab				
raw (3 oz)	71	15.6	.0	.5
canned (3 oz)	84	17.4	.0	1.0
steamed (3 oz)	87	17.2	.0	1.5
Crackers				
cheese (5 crackers)	81	1.4	7.8	4.9
graham (2 squares)	60	1.0	10.8	1.5
oyster (10 crackers)	33	.7	5.3	1.0
ritz (4 crackers)	70	1.0	9.0	4.0
ry-krisp (3 large square)	40	1.5	13.0	.2
saltines (2 crackers)	26	.6	4.4	.6
soda (10 crackers)	125	2.6	20.1	3.7
triscuit (3 crackers)	60	1.0	10.0	2.0
wheat thins (8 crackers)	70	1.0	9.0	3.0
zwieback (1 piece)	30	.7	5.2	.6
Cranberries, raw (1 cup)	46	.4	12.1	.2
Cranberry juice, canned (1 cup)	147	.1	37.7	.1
Cranberry sauce, jelled (½ cup)	209	.3	53.7	.2
Crayfish				
raw (3 oz)	76	15.9	.0	.9
steamed (3 oz)	97	20.3	.0	1.2
Cream & cream substitutes				
creamer, non-dairy liquid (½ oz)	22	.0	2.1	1.6
creamer, non-dairy powder (1 t)	11	.1	1.1	.7
half & half (1 T)	20	.4	.6	1.7
heavy whipping (1 T)	52	.3	.4	5.6
light (1 T)	29	.4	.6	2.9
light whipping (1 T)	44	.3	.4	4.6
medium, 25% fat (1 T)	37	.4	.5	3.8
sour, cultured (1 oz)	52	.8	1.0	5.0
sour, half & half cultured (1 oz)	40	.8	1.2	3.6
sour, imitation (1 oz)	59	.7	1.9	5.5
Cream puff w/ filling (1 cream puff)	303	8.5	26.7	18.1
Cucumber (½ cup slices)	7	.3	1.5	.1
Custard, baked (1 cup)	305	14.3	29.4	14.6
Dates, pitted (10 dates)	228	1.6	61.0	.4

Description	Cal	Pro (g)	Carb (g)	Fat (g)
Dips (1 oz)				
bacon	71	1.0	2.0	6.0
blue cheese	100	6.1	.7	8.2
clam	67	1.0	3.0	5.0
onion	70	1.0	2.0	6.0
Doughnuts (1 doughnut)				
cake	105	1.3	12.2	5.8
chocolate coated	130	1.0	14.0	8.0
glazed old fashioned	310	3.0	34.0	18.0
powdered sugar	110	1.0	15.0	5.0
raised / yeast	176	2.7	16.0	11.3
Duck, roasted (3.5 oz)				
w/ skin	337	19.0	.0	28.4
w/o skin	201	23.5	.0	11.2
Eggs				
boiled, hard/soft (1 large)	79	6.1	.6	5.6
fried (1 large)	83	5.4	.5	6.4
omelette, plain (1 large)	95	6.0	1.4	7.1
poached (1 large)	79	6.0	.6	5.6
scrambled w/ milk & fat (1 large)	95	6.0	1.4	7.1
white, fresh/frozen (1 large)	16	3.4	.4	.0
whole, fresh/frozen (1 large)	79	6.1	.6	5.6
yolk, fresh (1 large)	63	2.8	.0	5.6
Eggnog (see beverages)				
Eggplant				
raw (½ cup pieces)	11	.5	2.6	.0
boiled (½ cup)	13	.4	3.2	.1
Farina (see cereals)				
Figs				
raw (1 med)	37	.4	9.6	.2
dried (10 figs)	477	5.7	122.2	2.2
Fish (see individual kinds)				
Fish fillets, frozen				
batter-dipped (3 oz)	180	10.0	15.0	10.0
Fish sticks, frozen				
1 stick (about 1 oz)	76	4.4	6.7	3.4
batter-dipped (3 oz)	165	7.5	11.2	11.2
Flounder / sole				
raw (3.5 oz)	68	14.9	.0	.5
baked (3.5 oz)	202	30.0	.0	8.2
frozen, breaded (3.5 oz)	210	10.5	10.5	14.0
Flour				
enriched, 1 cup	455	12.9	95.4	1.2
wheat, 1 cup sifted	400	15.0	80.0	2.0
Frankfurters (see sausage)				
French toast, 1 slice	150	5.0	11.0	9.0
Frog legs, 3.5 oz	73	16.1	.0	0.3
Frostings (see cake icing)				
Frozen custard (see ice cream)				
Fruit (see individual listing)				
Fruit cocktail				
canned, water pack (½ cup)	40	.5	10.4	.1
canned, heavy syrup (½ cup)	93	.5	24.2	.1
canned, juice pack (½ cup)	56	.6	14.7	.0
Garbanzo beans (see chickpeas)				
Garlic, raw (3 cloves)	13	.6	3.0	.1
Gelatin				
plain, 1 pkt	25	6.0	.0	.0
fruit flavors, ½ cup	80	2.0	19.0	.0
diet, ½ cup	8	2.0	.0	.0

Description	Cal	Pro (g)	Carb (g)	Fat (g)
Gin (see beverages)				
Ginger ale (see beverages)				
Gingerbread (see cakes)				
Ginger root, raw (¼ cup)	17	.4	3.6	.2
Granola Bar, (.8 oz bar)	109	2.0	16.0	4.0
Grape juice, canned (1 cup)	155	1.0	37.0	.2
Grapefruit				
raw, pink & red (½ cup)	43	.6	11.1	.1
raw, white (½ cup)	42	1.0	10.5	.1
canned, juice pack (½ cup)	44	.7	11.2	.1
Grapefruit juice, canned (1 cup)	96	1.2	22.7	.2
Grapes (1 cup)	57	.5	14.2	.5
Gravy (½ cup)				
beef	62	44	5.6	1.4
chicken	94	2.2	6.4	6.8
mushroom	60	1.6	6.6	3.2
Grits (see corn grits)				
Gum (see chewing gum)				
Haddock				
raw (3 oz)	74	16.1	.0	.6
broiled (3 oz)	95	20.6	.0	.8
smoked (3 oz)	99	21.4	.0	.8
Halibut				
raw (3 oz)	93	17.7	.0	2.0
broiled (3 oz)	119	22.7	.0	2.5
frozen, batter--dipped (3 oz)	195	7.5	11.2	11.2
Ham (see pork)				
Hamburger (see beef, ground)				
Hash, corned beef (see beef)				
Herbs	0	.0	.0	.0
Herring, atlantic				
raw (3 oz)	135	15.3	.0	7.8
baked, broiled (4 oz)	230	26.1	.0	13.1
pickled (4 oz)	297	16.1	10.9	20.4
Hollandaise sauce, ½ cup	119	2.4	6.9	9.9
Hominy, canned				
white (½ cup)	69	1.0	15.0	.4
yellow (½ cup)	64	1.3	13.9	.3
Honey, 1 T	60	.0	16.0	.0
Honeydew melon, raw (½ cup)	66	1.6	15.4	.6
Horseradish, 1 T	10	.0	1.0	.0
Ice cream (½ cup)				
chocolate	280	5.0	35.0	14.0
strawberry	230	4.0	20.0	15.0
vanilla	270	5.0	26.0	17.0
French, vanilla	189	3.5	19.1	11.3
sherbet, orange	135	1.1	29.4	1.9
Ice cream bar, vanilla w/choc (3 fl oz)	320	1.0	34.0	20.0
Ice cream cone, plain	60	1.0	11.0	1.0
Ice cream sandwich (2.7 fl oz)	204	2.2	30.1	8.3
Ice milk, vanilla (½ cup)	92	2.6	14.5	2.8
Ice milk bar	140	3.0	22.0	5.0
Icings (see cake icings)				
Jams, 1 T	53	.0	13.5	.0
Jellies, 1 T	53	.0	13.5	.0
Jello	81	2.0	19.0	.0
sugar free	80	2.0	19.0	.0
Juice (see types)				
Kale, boiled (½ cup chopped)	21	1.2	3.7	.3
Ketchup, 1 T	16	.2	4.1	.1

Description	Cal	Pro (g)	Carb (g)	Fat (g)
Kiwifruit, raw (1 med)	46	.8	11.3	.3
Knockwurst (see sausage)				
Kumquats, raw (1 med)	12	.2	3.1	.0
Lamb (3 oz)				
leg, roasted, lean	163	24.0	.0	6.6
loin chops, broiled, lean	269	21.4	.0	19.7
Lard, 1 T	115	.0	.0	12.8
Leeks				
raw (½ cup chopped)	32	.8	7.4	.2
boiled (½ cup chopped)	16	.4	4.0	.1
Lemon, raw (1 med)	22	1.3	11.6	.3
Lemonade, 8 oz	80	.0	20.0	.0
Lemon juice				
fresh (1 T)	4	.1	1.3	.0
fresh (1 cup)	60	.9	21.1	.0
Lentils, boiled (1 cup)	231	17.9	39.9	.7
Lettuce (fresh)				
iceberg, raw (3 leaves)	9	.6	1.2	.0
looseleaf, raw (1 cup)	15	1.2	3.0	.3
romaine, raw (1 cup)	8	1.0	1.4	.2
Lima beans (see beans)				
Lime, raw (1 med)	20	.5	7.1	.1
Liver (cooked)				
beef, 4 oz	183	27.6	3.9	5.5
chicken, 4 oz	178	27.6	1.0	6.2
Liverwurst, (see sausage)				
Lobster, steamed (4 oz)	111	23.2	1.5	.7
Lobster Newberg, 1 cup	468	17.2	11.	39.4
Lox (see salmon)				
Luncheon meats (see sausage)				
Macadamia nuts, dried (1 oz)	199	2.43	.9	20.9
Macaroni (cooked)				
shells, small, 1 cup	162	5.5	32.6	.8
spirals, 1 cup	189	6.4	38.0	.9
Macaroni & cheese (1 cup)	420	20.0	50.0	16.0
Mackerel, broiled (3 oz)	223	20.3	.0	15.1
Mandarin oranges, canned				
juice packed (½ cup)	46	.8	11.9	.0
light syrup (½ cup)	76	.6	20.4	.1
Mango, raw (1 med)	135	1.1	35.2	.6
Margarine (1 T)	100	.0	.0	11.0
Marshmallow (see candy)				
Mayonnaise (see salad dressing)				
Meatloaf (see sausage)				
Meats (see beef, lamb, pork)				
Melba toast, 1 slice	25	1.0	6.1	.5
Melons (see types)				
Milk, cow (1 cup)				
whole (3.7% fat)	157	8.0	11.4	8.9
skim	86	8.4	11.9	.4
low fat (2% fat)	121	8.1	11.7	4.7
dry, whole, regular	635	33.7	49.2	34.2
dry, nonfat, regular	435	43.4	62.4	.9
dry, nonfat, instant	326	31.9	47.5	.7
Milk shake (see beverages)				
Molasses, 1 T	60	.0	14.0	.0
Muffins				
blueberry (1.5 oz)	130	2.0	18.0	5.0
bran, raisin (2.5 oz)	190	3.0	30.0	7.0

Description	Cal	Pro (g)	Carb (g)	Fat (g)
corn (2.5 oz)	220	4.0	33.0	8.0
English	130	4.3	25.4	1.3
oat bran (2.75 oz)	180	5.0	27.0	7.0
wheat bran	140	2.0	24.0	4.0
Mushrooms				
raw (½ cup pieces)	9	.7	1.6	.2
boiled (½ cup pieces)	21	1.7	4.0	.4
canned (½ cup pieces)	19	1.5	3.9	.2
Mussels				
raw (3 oz)	73	10.1	3.1	1.9
steamed (3 oz)	147	20.2	6.3	3.8
Mustard, 1 T	14	1.0	1.0	1.0
Mutton (see lamb)				
Nectarine, raw (1 med)	67	1.3	16.0	.6
Noodles, 1 cup				
egg, cooked	212	7.6	39.7	2.4
chow mein, canned	237	3.8	25.9	13.8
Nuts (see individual kinds)				
Nuts, mixed, 1 oz	170	8.0	3.0	14.0
Oat bran				
raw (1 cup)	231	16.3	62.2	6.6
cooked (1 cup)	87	7.0	25.1	1.9
Oatmeal (see cereal)				
Ocean perch				
raw (3 oz)	80	15.8	.0	1.4
broiled (3 oz)	103	20.3	.0	1.8
Oils, all vegetable, 1T	120	.0	.0	14.0
Okra, boiled (½ cup slices)	34	1.9	7.5	.3
Olives, pitted (1 oz)	33	.2	1.8	3.0
Omelette (see eggs)				
Onion				
raw (½ cup)	27	.9	5.9	.2
boiled (½ cup)	29	1.0	6.6	.2
canned (½ cup)	21	1.0	4.5	.1
Onion rings, frozen (7 rings)	285	3.7	26.7	18.7
Oranges				
navel, raw (1 med)	65	1.4	16.6	.1
valencia, raw (1 med)	59	1.3	14.4	.4
Orange juice, fresh (1 cup)	111	1.7	25.8	.5
Oysters				
raw (3 oz) about 6 med	58	5.9	3.3	2.1
steamed (3 oz) about 12 med	117	12.0	6.7	4.2
canned (3 oz)	58	6.0	3.3	2.1
breaded & fried (3 oz)	167	7.5	9.9	10.7
Pancakes, plain (3.6 oz)	183	5.7	36.5	2.4
Papaya, raw (1 med)	117	1.9	29.8	.4
Parsley (¼ cup chopped)	10	.7	2.1	.1
Parsnips, boiled (½ cup)	63	1.0	15.2	.2
Pastries				
cream puff with custard filling	303	8.5	26.7	18.1
Danish, 1 small	161	2.6	18.8	8.8
Peach				
raw (1 med)	37	.6	9.7	.1
canned, heavy syrup (1 cup)	190	1.2	51.0	.3
canned, light syrup (1 cup)	136	1.1	36.5	.1
canned, juice pack (1 cup)	109	1.6	28.7	.1
canned, water pack (1 cup)	58	1.1	14.9	.1
Peach nectar, canned (1 cup)	134	.7	34.7	.1

Description	Cal	Pro (g)	Carb (g)	Fat (g)
Peanuts				
boiled (½ cup)	102	4.3	6.8	7.0
dry roasted (1 oz)	164	6.6	6.0	13.9
oil roasted (1 oz)	165	7.6	5.3	14.0
Peanut butter				
creamy/smooth (1 T)	95	4.6	2.5	8.2
chunk style/crunchy (1 T)	94	3.9	3.5	8.0
Pear				
raw, (1 med)	98	.7	25.1	.7
canned, heavy pack (1 cup)	188	.5	48.9	.3
canned, juice pack (1 cup)	123	.9	32.1	.2
canned, light syrup (1 cup)	144	.5	38.1	.1
canned, water pack (1 cup)	71	.5	19.1	.1
Peas, green				
raw (½ cup)	63	4.2	11.3	.3
boiled (½ cup)	67	4.3	12.5	.2
canned (½ cup)	59	3.8	10.7	.3
frozen (½ cup)	63	4.1	11.4	.2
Pecans				
dried (1 oz)	190	2.2	5.2	19.2
dry roasted (1 oz)	187	2.3	6.3	18.4
oil roasted (1 oz)	195	2.0	4.6	20.2
Peppers, sweet				
raw, chopped (½ cup)	13	.4	3.2	.1
boiled, chopped (½ cup)	19	.6	4.6	.1
canned (½ cup)	13	.6	2.7	.2
Perch (see ocean perch)				
Pickles				
Bread and butter (1 oz)	30	.0	7.0	.0
dill, 1 medium	12	.4	2.7	.1
sweet, 1 large	41	.1	11.1	.1
sweet relish (1 T)	21	.1	5.1	.1
Pies (1/6 pie)				
apple	250	2.0	37.0	11.0
banana cream	180	2.0	21.0	10.0
blueberry	270	3.0	40.0	11.0
Boston cream (see cakes)				
cherry	250	3.0	36.0	11.0
chocolate cream	190	2.0	24.0	10.0
coconut creme	190	2.0	22.0	11.0
custard	200	5.0	28.0	8.0
lemon meringue (1/8 of pie)	210	2.0	38.0	5.0
mince	280	2.0	48.0	9.0
peach	245	3.0	35.0	11.0
pecan (1/8 of pie)	330	3.0	51.0	13.0
pumpkin	200	3.0	29.0	8.0
strawberry cream	170	2.0	20.0	9.0
sweet potato	150	2.0	21.0	7.0
Pie crust, 1/6 of pie shell (1 oz)	130	1.0	12.0	8.0
Pike, northern, broiled (4 oz)	128	28.0	.0	1.0
Pineapple				
raw, (1 cup)	77	.6	19.2	.7
canned, heavy syrup (1 cup)	199	.9	51.5	.3
canned, juice pack (1 cup)	150	1.0	39.2	.2
Pineapple juice (1 cup)	139	.8	34.4	.2
Pistachios, shelled (1 oz)	172	4.2	7.8	15.0
Pizza				
cheese (½ of pie)	270	10.0	28.0	14.0
sausage & cheese (¼ pie)	350	22.0	34.0	14.0

Description	Cal	Pro (g)	Carb (g)	Fat (g)
Plum				
raw (1 med)	36	.5	8.6	.4
canned, heavy syrup (3 plums)	119	.5	30.9	.1
canned, juice pack (3 plums)	55	.5	14.4	.0
Pomegranate, raw (1 med)	104	1.5	26.4	.5
Popcorn				
popped, plain, air popped (1 cup)	30	1.0	6.0	.4
popped in oil, plain (1 oz)	220	3.0	20.0	15.0
microwave (3 cups)	140	2.0	14.0	9.0
Popovers, 1 medium	90	3.5	10.3	3.7
Pork (4 oz)				
bacon (see bacon)				
ham, canned	266	23.8	.4	18.2
ham, cured, roasted	276	24.5	.0	19.0
ham, fresh, roasted	333	28.4	.0	23.5
ham luncheon meat (1 oz)	31	4.7	1.1	.9
ham, spread, deviled (1 T)	35	2.0	.0	3.0
loin, braised	310	37.4	.0	16.6
loin, chops	291	31.7	.0	17.4
spareribs, braised (6.3 oz)	703	51.4	.0	53.6
Pork and beans (½ cup)	133	6.5	25.2	2.0
Potato salad (½ cup)	179	3.4	14.0	10.3
Potatoes				
au gratin, fresh (½ cup)	160	6.2	13.7	9.3
raw, w/o skin (1 med)	88	2.3	20.1	.1
baked, w/ skin (1 med)	220	4.7	51.0	.2
baked, w/o skin (1 med)	145	3.1	33.6	.2
canned, w/o skin (½ cup)	54	1.3	12.3	.2
french fried, (10 pieces)	158	2.0	20.0	8.3
hash brown, fresh (½ cup)	163	1.9	16.6	10.9
mashed, flakes (½ cup)	118	2.0	15.8	5.9
mashed, fresh (½ cup)	111	2.0	17.5	4.4
scalloped, fresh (½ cup)	105	3.5	13.2	4.5
sweet, baked (1 med)	118	2.0	27.7	.1
sweet, boiled (½ cup mashed)	172	2.7	39.8	.5
sweet, candied (1 med)	144	.9	29.3	3.4
sweet, canned (1 cup pieces)	183	3.3	42.3	.4
Potato chips (1 oz)	148	1.8	14.7	10.1
Potato salad (½ cup)	179	3.4	14.0	10.3
Pretzels				
Dutch style (1 oz)	110	3.0	24.0	.0
sticks (1 oz)	110	3.0	22.0	1.0
Prunes				
canned, heavy syrup (5 prunes)	90	.8	23.9	.2
dried (10 prunes)	201	2.2	52.7	.4
dried, cooked (½ cup)	113	1.2	29.8	.2
Prune juice (1 cup)	181	1.6	44.7	.1
Puddings (½ cup)				
banana	150	2.0	24.0	5.0
butterscotch	170	2.0	26.0	7.0
chocolate	170	3.0	28.0	6.0
chocolate-vanilla	170	3.0	28.0	6.0
rice	120	3.0	20.0	3.0
tapioca, vanilla	170	3.0	27.0	4.0
vanilla	180	3.0	28.0	6.0
Pumpkin				
boiled (½ cup mashed)	24	.9	6.0	.1
canned (½ cup mashed)	41	1.3	9.9	.3
Pumpkin seeds, salted (1 oz)	127	5.3	15.3	5.5

Description	Cal	Pro (g)	Carb (g)	Fat (g)
Quail, breast (1 oz)	35	6.4	.0	.8
Quince (1 med)	53	.4	14.1	.1
Rabbit, roasted (4 oz)	175	25.8	.0	7.2
Radishes, raw (10 med)	7	.3	1.6	.2
Raisins				
seedless (½ cup)	227	2.6	59.6	.4
seeded (½ cup)	222	1.9	58.9	.4
Raspberries				
raw (1 cup)	61	1.1	14.2	.7
canned, heavy syrup (½ cup)	117	1.1	29.9	.2
Relish (see pickles)				
Rice				
brown, cooked (1 cup)	232	4.9	49.7	1.2
white, cooked (1 cup)	223	4.1	49.6	.2
wild, raw (1 cup)	565	22.6	120.5	1.1
Rice mixes (commercial)				
beef (½ cup)	152	3.0	25.2	4.1
chicken (½ cup)	153	3.1	25.1	4.2
fried (½ cup)	159	3.2	25.2	4.8
Rockfish, broiled (3 oz)	103	20.4	.0	1.7
Rolls and buns (1 med)				
brown & serve, club	100	3.0	19.0	1.0
dinner, plain	60	2.0	11.0	1.0
French	108	4.2	21.3	1.5
hoagie or submarine	400	13.0	73.0	7.0
hamburger bun	115	4.3	22.0	2.2
hot dog	108	3.7	20.9	2.0
kaiser	184	7.0	35.4	2.9
sweet roll	133	1.8	17.5	6.6
Root beer (see beverages)				
Roughy, orange, raw (3 oz)	107	12.5	.0	6.0
Rum (see beverages)				
Safflower oil (see oil)				
Salad dressings (1 T)				
bleu cheese	77	.7	1.1	8.0
bleu cheese, diet	30	.0	2.0	2.0
Caesar	70	1.0	2.0	7.0
French	67	.1	2.7	6.4
French, diet	18	.0	3.0	1.0
Italian	69	.1	1.5	7.1
Italian, diet	6	.0	1.0	.0
mayonnaise	57	.1	3.5	4.9
Ranch	78	.1	1.1	8.3
Ranch, reduced calorie	16	.0	4.0	.0
Thousand Island	59	.1	2.4	5.6
Thousand Island, reduced calorie	20	.0	3.0	1.0
vinegar and oil	67	.5	2.3	6.5
Salad oil (see oils)				
Salads				
coleslaw (see coleslaw)				
chicken & celery (1 oz)	64	3.0	3.0	5.0
fruit, mixed, canned in water (4 oz)	34	.4	8.9	.1
fruit, mixed, cnd, light syrup (4 oz)	66	.4	17.2	.1
fruit, mxd, cnd, heavy syrup (4 oz)	83	.4	21.7	.1
garden (½ cup)	80	1.5	18.1	.3
gelatin (see gelatin)				
macaroni (½ cup)	200	40	21.0	10.0
potato (see potato salad)				
tuna (4 oz)	212	18.2	10.7	10.5

Description	Cal	Pro (g)	Carb (g)	Fat (g)
Salami (see sausage)				
Salmon, chinook				
raw (3 oz)	153	17.1	.0	8.9
smoked (3 oz)	99	15.5	.0	3.7
Salt	0	.0	.0	.0
Sardines				
canned in soybean oil (2 sardines)	50	5.9	.0	2.8
canned in tomato sauce (1 sardine)	68	6.2	.0	4.6
Sauces and Toppings (1 T)				
barbecue	12	.3	2.0	.3
butterscotch	60	.0	13.0	1.0
cheese (4 oz)	240	5.0	11.0	20.0
chili	24	.9	4.1	1.3
chocolate	50	1.0	11.0	.0
cream, half & half	20	.4	.6	1.7
soy	9	.9	1.5	.0
tartar	70	.0	2.0	7.0
tomato, canned (½ cup)	37	1.6	8.8	.2
Worcestershire	10	.0	2.0	.0
Sauerkraut, canned (½ cup)	22	1.1	5.1.	2
Sausage, cold cuts				
beef (1 link)	75	3.8	.0	6.1
bologna (1-oz slice)	80	4.0	1.0	7.0
Braunschweiger (1 oz)	80	4.0	.0	7.0
brown & serve sausage (1 link)	60	3.5	1.0	4.1
frankfurter (1 link)	160	5.0	2.0	14.0
knockwurst (2 oz)	180	7.0	1.0	16.0
liverwurst (1 oz)	97	4.0	1.0	9.0
meatloaf (4 oz)	200	10.0	8.0	14.0
minced ham (1 oz)	68	4.6	.1	5.3
mortadella (1 oz)	88	4.6	.9	7.2
Polish sausage (1 oz)	92	4.0	.5	8.1
pork sausage, cooked (1 oz)	105	5.6	.3	8.8
salami (1 oz)	119	6.5	.7	9.7
scrapple (1 slice)	65	2.7	4.2	3.7
Scallions (see onions)				
Scallops, raw (3 oz)	75	14.3	2.0	.6
Scrapple (see sausage)				
Sesame seeds, dried kernels (1 T)	47	2.1	.8	4.4
Shad, baked (1 oz)	56	4.8	.0	3.9
Sherbet (see ice cream)				
Shortbread (see cookies)				
Shortcake, strawberry (3 oz)	170	2.0	30.0	5.0
Shortening (1 T)	113	.0	.0	12.8
Shrimp				
raw (3 oz)	90	17.3	.8	1.5
breaded & fried (3 oz)	206	18.2	9.8	10.4
cocktail (4 oz)	113	7.0	19.0	1.0
canned (3 oz)	102	19.6	.9	1.7
steamed (3 oz)	84	17.8	.0	.9
Soft drinks (see beverages)				
Sole (see flounder)				
Soup (commercial, 1 cup)				
asparagus, cream	87	2.3	10.7	4.1
bean	190	9.0	30.9	3.4
bean, black	116	5.6	19.8	.05
beef broth	18	2.0	1.0	.0
beef noodle	84	4.8	9.0	3.1
celery, cream	90	1.7	8.8	5.6
chicken broth	39	4.9	.9	1.4

Description	Cal	Pro (g)	Carb (g)	Fat (g)
chicken, cream	116	3.4	9.3	7.4
chicken, gumbo	56	2.6	8.4	1.4
chicken, noodle	75	4.0	9.4	2.5
chicken with rice	60	3.5	7.2	1.9
chicken vegetable	74	3.6	8.6	2.8
clam chowder, Manhattan	78	4.2	12.2	2.3
clam chowder, New England	95	4.8	12.4	2.9
green pea	164	8.6	26.5	2.9
minestrone	83	4.3	11.2	2.5
mushroom, cream	129	2.3	9.3	9.0
onion	57	3.8	8.2	1.7
split pea with ham	189	10.3	28.0	4.4
tomato	86	2.1	16.6	1.9
turkey noodle	69	3.9	8.6	2.0
vegetable, vegetarian	72	2.1	12.0	1.9
vegetable beef	79	5.6	10.2	1.9
Soybean nuts				
dry roasted (½ cup)	387	34.0	28.1	18.6
roasted (½ cup)	405	30.3	28.9	21.8
roasted & toasted (1 oz)	129	10.5	8.7	6.8
Soybean tofu, raw (½ cup)	183	19.9	5.4	11.0
Soybean oil (see oils)				
Soybeans				
green, boiled (½ cup)	127	11.1	10.0	5.8
mature, boiled (½ cup)	149	14.3	8.5	7.7
Soy sauce (see sauces)				
Spaghetti				
cooked, with egg (4 oz)	149	5.8	28.3	1.2
with meatballs (4 oz)	116	4.4	17.6	4.0
with meat sauce (4 oz)	134	3.9	18.6	5.2
Spanish rice, cooked (1 cup)	90	2.0	20.0	.0
Spices	0	.0	.0	.0
Spinach				
raw (½ cup chopped)	6	.8	1.0	.1
boiled (½ cup)	21	2.7	3.4	.2
canned (½ cup)	25	3.0	3.6	.5
Squash				
acorn, baked (½ cup)	57	1.1	14.9	.1
acorn, boiled (½ cup)	41	.8	10.7	.1
crookneck, boiled (½ cup)	18	.8	3.9	.3
hubbard, boiled (½ cup)	35	1.8	7.6	.4
scallop, boiled (½ cup)	14	.9	3.0	.2
zucchini, raw (½ cup)	9	.8	1.9	.1
zucchini, boiled (½ cup)	14	.6	3.5	.1
Stew (see beef & vegetable stew)				
Strawberries				
raw (1 cup)	61	1.1	14.2	0.7
canned, heavy syrup (½ cup)	117	1.1	29.9	.2
Stuffing, cornbread (1 oz)	110	3.0	22.0	1.0
Sturgeon, cooked (4 oz)	153	23.5	.0	5.9
Succotash				
boiled (½ cup)	111	4.9	23.4	.8
canned (½ cup)	81	3.31	7.9	.6
Sugar (beet or cane)				
brown, packed (1 cup)	821	.0	212.1	.0
granulated (1 cup)	770	.0	199.0	.0
granulated (1 T)	46	.0	11.9	.0
granulated, 1 lump (2 cubes)	19	.0	5.0	.0
granulated, 1 packet (.2 oz)	23	.0	6.0	.0

Description	Cal	Pro (g)	Carb (g)	Fat (g)
powdered (1 cup unsifted)	462	.0	119.4	.0
powdered (1 T unsifted)	31	.0	8.0	.0
Sunflower seeds, hulled				
dried (1 oz)	162	6.5	5.3	14.1
dry roasted (1 oz)	165	5.5	6.8	14.1
oil roasted (1 oz)	175	6.1	4.2	16.3
Sweetpotatoes (see potato)				
Swordfish				
raw (3 oz)	103	16.8	.0	3.4
baked (3 oz)	132	21.6	.0	4.4
Syrups (1 T)				
Chocolate	46	.3	12.4	.2
Corn, light or dark	60	.0	15.0	.0
Maple	50	.0	12.8	.0
Molasses	60	.0	14.0	.2
Sorghum	53	.0	14.0	.0
Tangerine, raw (1 med)	37	.5	9.4	.2
Tapioca (see puddings)				
Tartar sauce (see sauces)				
Tea (see beverages)				
Tomatoes				
green, raw (1 med)	30	1.5	6.3	.3
red, raw (1 med)	24	1.1	5.3	.3
red, boiled (½ cup)	30	1.3	6.8	.3
red, canned (½ cup)	35	1.0	6.0	1.0
red, paste, canned (½ cup)	110	5.0	24.7	1.2
red, stewed (½ cup)	34	1.2	8.3	.2
puree, (½ cup)	51	2.1	12.5	.2
Tomato juice (1 cup)	43	1.9	10.2	.1
Tomato juice, cocktail (1 cup)	51	1.7	12.2	.2
Tomato ketchup (see ketchup)				
Toppings (see candy & sauces)				
Tortilla, flour (7 in. diam.)	80	2.0	14.0	2.0
Trout				
mixed species, raw (3 oz)	126	17.7	.0	5.6
rainbow, raw (3 oz)	100	17.5	.0	2.9
rainbow, baked (3 oz)	129	22.4	.0	3.7
Tuna				
canned in oil, light (3 oz)	169	24.8	.0	7.0
canned in oil, white (3 oz)	158	22.6	.0	6.9
canned in water, light (3 oz)	111	25.1	.0	.4
canned in water, white (3 oz)	116	22.7	.0	2.1
Tuna Salad (see salads)				
Turkey, roasted (4 oz)				
dark, with skin	251	31.2	.0	13.1
dark, without skin	212	32.4	.0	8.2
white, with skin	223	32.4	.0	9.4
white, without skin	178	33.9	.0	3.7
Turnip, boiled (4 oz)	26	1.7	4.9	.3
Turnip greens				
raw (½ cup)	7	.4	1.6	.1
boiled (½ cup)	15	.8	3.1	.2
canned (½ cup)	17	1.6	2.8	.4
Veal, roasted (4 oz)				
ground	195	27.6	.0	8.6
loin	246	28.1	.0	14.0
rib	259	27.2	.0	15.8
Vegetable juice (1 cup)	45	1.4	11.0	.3
Vegetables (see types)				
Vegetables, mixed (½ cup)	39	2.1	7.6	.2

Description	Cal	Pro (g)	Carb (g)	Fat (g)
Vegetable stew (8 oz)	170	5.0	20.0	8.0
Venison, roasted (4 oz)	179	34.3	.0	3.6
Vinegar, white (1 cup)	30	.4	12.0	.4
Vodka (see beverages)				
Waffles (2 pieces)	280	6.0	51.0	6.0
Walnuts, dried (1 oz)	172	6.9	3.4	16.1
Water chestnuts, raw (½ cup)	66	.9	14.8	.1
Watermelon (1 cup)	50	1.0	11.5	.7
Wheat (see cereals, flours)				
Wheat germ, crude (1 cup)	414	26.6	59.6	11.2
Whiskey (see beverages)				
Whitefish				
raw (3 oz)	114	16.2	.0	5.0
baked, stuffed (3.5 oz)	215	15.2	5.8	14.0
smoked (3 oz)	92	19.9	.0	.8
Wine (see beverages)				
Yeast, baker's, dry (.6 oz)	15	2.0	2.0	.0
Yogurt (1 cup)				
plain, skim milk	127	13.0	17.4	.4
plain, whole milk	139	7.9	10.6	7.4
coffee, low-fat	194	11.2	31.3	2.8
strawberry, low-fat	250	9.0	48.0	2.0
vanilla, low-fat	194	11.2	31.3	2.8

This manual and the other materials distributed through The LEARN Education Center are not available in bookstores. You may write, call, or visit us on the Internet to obtain current pricing and shipping charges. Discounts are available for bulk orders. Below are listed other materials and services available.

The LEARN Education Center

The LEARN Education Center was established to respond to the increasing demand for scientifically sound, state-of-the-art publications, training courses and services. The Center is dedicated to the development of health and wellness materials, including audio tapes, newsletters, professional training guides, leadership training programs, and professional counseling services.

For your ordering convenience, a toll free number is available and may be called 24 hours a day. In addition, you can order via our Internet address at www.LearnEducation.com. Payments can be made with a major credit card, check, or money order.

All orders are shipped with 24 hours of receipt, and next day and second day delivery service is available. As you use our publications, we sincerely welcome any comments you may have to improve these materials, and we encourage you to tell us how we are doing.

For ordering or general information, please write or call us at:

The LEARN Education Center
P.O. Box 37328, Dept. 70
Dallas, Texas 75235-0328

Toll free telephone	1-800-736-7323
In Dallas telephone	817-545-4500
Fax	817-545-2211

E-mail address	LearnCtr@aol.com
Internet address:	
	www.LearnEducation.com

The LEARN Institute for LifeStyle Management

The LEARN Institute was established to provide state-of-the-art training programs to health professionals working with overweight clients. The LEARN Institute is the first to offer specific training and certification in the field of weight control. The **LifeStyle Counselor Certification Program** has been developed to provide a comprehensive cross-disciplinary training program to health professionals working in the field of weight and stress management.

Two certifications are currently offered and training is provided in various cities throughout the United States. Certifications currently being offered include:

Certification in Weight Control
Certification in Stress Management

For more detailed information on The LifeStyle Counselor Certification Program or a free brochure call or write to:

The LEARN Institute for
LifeStyle Management
P.O. Box 35328, Dept. 50
Dallas, Texas 75235-0328

Toll free telephone	1-800-736-7323
In Dallas telephone	817-545-4500
Fax	817-545-2211

E-mail address	LearnCtr@aol.com
Internet address	
	www.LearnEducation.com

The American Association of LifeStyle Counselors

The American Association of LifeStyle Counselors is a nonprofit corporation dedicated to providing its members and the general public with the most current, safe, and sound lifestyle-management programs and services. Individuals who complete the LifeStyle Counselor Certification Program become eligible for membership into the American Association of LifeStyle Counselors (AALC). Only members of the AALC can use the distinguished title of **Certified LifeStyle Counselor**. If you would like to locate a Certified LifeStyle Counselor in your area you may write, call, or visit the AALC's Internet site as follows:

**The American Association
of LifeStyle Counselors
P.O. Box 35328, Dept. 55
Dallas, Texas 75235-0328**

In Dallas telephone	**817–545–3220**
Fax	**817–545–2211**
E-mail address	LearnCtr@aol.com
Internet address	**www.AALC.com**

Other Materials

Publications currently available from The LEARN Education Center are as follows:

Weight Management

The LEARN Program for Weight Control—7th Edition by Kelly D. Brownell, Ph.D.

The LEARN Program for Weight Control—Medication Edition by Kelly D. Brownell, Ph.D. and Thomas A. Wadden, Ph.D.

The LEARN Program Monitoring Forms

The LEARN Program Cassettes by Kelly D. Brownell, Ph.D.

The LEARN Weight Maintenance and Stabilization Guide, by Kelly D. Brownell—Available January, 1998.

The Health & Fitness Club Leader's Guide—Administering A Weight Management Program by Ross Andersen, Ph.D., Kelly D. Brownell, Ph.D., and William L. Haskell, Ph.D.

The LifeStyle Counselor's Guide for Weight Control, by Brenda L. Wolfe, Ph.D., et al., eds.

The Weight Control Digest—annual subscription.

Weight Sex & Marriage by Richard B. Stuart, Ph.D. and Barbara Jacobson

Eating Disorders

Binge Eating by Christopher G. Fairburn, M.D. and G. Terence Wilson, Ph.D.

Overcoming Binge Eating by Christopher Fairburn, M.D.

Eating Disorders and Obesity, Kelly D. Brownell, Ph.D. and Christopher G. Fairburn, M.D., eds.

Physical Activity and Exercise

Living with Exercise—by Steven N. Blair, P.E.D.

Stress Management

The LifeStyle Counselor's Guide for Stress Management, by Leslie A. Telfer, Ph.D., et al.

Mastering Stress—A LifeStyle Approach by David H. Barlow, Ph.D. and Ronald M. Rapee, Ph.D.

Mind Over Mood by Dennis Greenberger, Ph.D. and Christine A. Padesky, Ph.D.

Other Materials:

The Balancing Act by Georgia Kostas, M.P.H., R.D.

Body Images—Development, Deviance, and Change by Thomas F. Cash, Ph.D. and Thomas Pruzinsky, Ph.D.

Body Image Therapy—A Program for Self-Directed Change by Thomas F. Cash, Ph.D.

More of What's Cooking by Veronica C. Coronado with Patty Kirk, R.D., L.D.

Motivational Interviewing by William R. Miller and Stephen Rollnick.

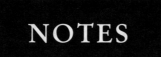

NOTES

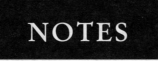

NOTES

NOTES

NOTES

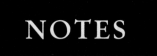

NOTES

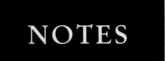

NOTES

Kelly D. Brownell, Ph.D. is an internationally known expert on weight control. He received training at Purdue University, Rutgers University, and Brown University. After serving on the faculty of the University of Pennsylvania School of Medicine for 13 years, he joined the faculty at Yale University, where he is Professor of Psychology, Professor of Epidemiology and Public Health, Director of the Yale Center for Eating and Weight Disorders, and Master of Silliman College. He has written 12 books and more than 200 research papers and book chapters, and holds appointments on 10 editorial boards.

Dr. Brownell has received awards from the American Psychological Association and the New York Academy of Sciences, and has been awarded research grants from the National Institutes of Health, the MacArthur Foundation, and the National Institute of Mental Health. He has been the President of the Society of Behavioral Medicine, the Division of Health Psychology of the American Psychological Association, and the Association for the Advancement of Behavior Therapy. He has been an advisor to the U.S. Navy, American Airlines, Johnson & Johnson and other organizations.

He has appeared on the *Today Show*, *Good Morning America*, *Nova* and *20/20*, and his work has been featured in the *New York Times*, *Washington Post*, *Glamour*, *Redbook*, *Family Circle*, *Vogue*, and other publications.

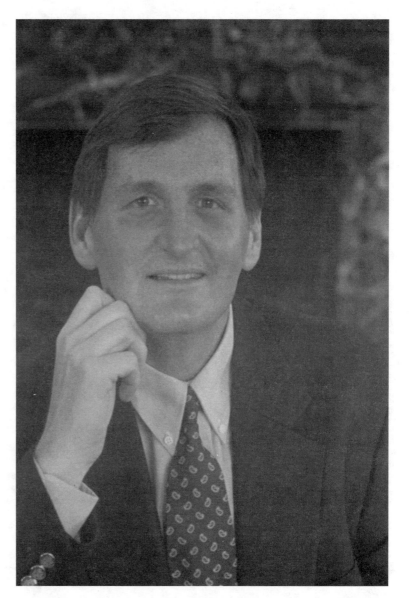